Cranial Osteomyelitis

Ali Akhaddar

Cranial Osteomyelitis

Diagnosis and Treatment

Springer

Ali Akhaddar
Department of Neurosurgery
Avicenne Military Hospital of Marrakech
University of Mohammed V in Rabat
Marrakech, Morocco

ISBN 978-3-319-30266-9 ISBN 978-3-319-30268-3 (eBook)
DOI 10.1007/978-3-319-30268-3

Library of Congress Control Number: 2016934694

Printed on acid-free paper

This Springer imprint is published by Springer Nature
The registered company is Springer International Publishing AG Switzerland

To His Majesty Mohammed VI, King of Morocco

To my parents, my wife, and my children with love
To my teachers with gratitude
To my patients, my inspiration

Foreword I

Cranial osteomyelitis is an uncommon but important entity that has not been systematically addressed. This unique book, edited and authored by Pr Ali Akhaddar, is therefore very welcome and achieves its goals in a comprehensive and effective fashion. Cranial osteomyelitis can be difficult to treat. The differential diagnosis, imaging aspects, bacteriology, and options for treatment are thoroughly discussed. Important sections on the prognosis and prevention of this illness are included. This is a most welcome reference source that is well crafted and up to date.

Edward R. Laws, MD, FACS
Professor of Neurosurgery
Brigham & Women's Hospital
Harvard Medical School
Boston, Massachusetts, USA
elaws@partners.org

Foreword II

Cranial Osteomyelitis: Diagnosis and Treatment written by Professor Ali Akhaddar is a welcome addition to the world of neurosurgical infectious disease. This 16 chapter contribution represents a comprehensive reference book that describes the most important aspects of cranial osteomyelitis which are important for numerous clinicians involved in diagnosing and managing this disease process. These medical specialists include but are not limited to Neurosurgeons, Otolaryngologists, Radiologists, Neurologists, and Infectious Disease Consultants that are either in training or practicing physicians. Due to the controversial management of this infection, the author strives to determine a rational approach for directing those involved in the treatment of patients harboring this complicated multifaceted problem.

The work is organized into six well-conceived parts containing from one to four individual chapters that each address a critical component of the condition. Beginning with a definition of the infection and the historical aspects of the disease, the author then provides the essential basic components of the infection namely the epidemiology, risk factors, causative pathogens, histopathological findings, and pathophysiology of dissemination. Making an accurate diagnosis based on the clinical presentation while excluding others diagnostic possibilities relies on the laboratory results and the appearance of the imaging studies is covered in the next part. Clearly an essential section for the book that is of major clinical interest is the management of the infection with respect to surgical and medical therapy. Antimicrobial agents are the mainstay of medical treatment but the use of hyperbaric oxygen is reviewed in its own chapter. The overall prognosis and the resulting outcomes are considered together. As with many medical disorders, there can be unforeseen clinical situations that arise and unusual pathogenic organisms that are causative, both of which are discussed in individual chapters. The last and final part of the text is perhaps one of the most important for clinicians to reflect on and that is how to prevent the development of such an infection.

The bibliography of each chapter is current and the work is richly illustrated to provide visual examples for the clinicians to appreciate. The ultimate goal of this thoroughly researched reference text is for the reader to choose the most appropriate way to manage those patients that are unfortunate enough to fall victim to this uncommon infection that is significantly important to numerous physicians in multiple medical specialties. The author should be applauded for the succinct compilation of such an authoritative compendium on a disease entity that has been virtually overlooked in the infectious disease realm. This unique work will serve as the definitive source for the surgical and medical management of cranial osteomyelitis for years to come.

Walter A. Hall, MD, MBA
Professor of Neurosurgery
State University of New York (SUNY)
Upstate Medical University
Syracuse, New York, USA
hallw@upstate.edu

Acknowledgements

The author wishes to thank the following colleagues for providing this book with some illustrations and pictures:

- **Pr. Mohamed Boucetta**, M.D. Mentor and Former Chairman. Department of Neurosurgery. Mohammed V Military Teaching Hospital. Rabat, Morocco
- Pr. Mostafa El Ouennass, M.D. Department of Microbiology. Mohammed V Military Teaching Hospital. Rabat, Morocco
- Pr. Mohamed Zalagh, M.D. Department of Otorhinolaryngology. Moulay Ismail Military Hospital. Meknes, Morocco
- Pr. Mohamed Lakouichmi, M.D. Department of Maxillofacial Surgery. Avicenne Military Hospital. Marrakech, Morocco
- Dr. Youssef Zoubeir, M.D. Department of Histopathology. Avicenne Military Hospital. Marrakech, Morocco
- Pr. Mohamed Benzagmoute, M.D. Department of Neurosurgery. University Hospital Hassan II. Fez. Morocco
- Pr. Joseph Peterson, Ph.D. Department of Geology, University of Wisconsin, Oshkosh, Wisconsin, United States of America
- Dr. Johannes Trück, M.D. Clinical Lecturer. Paediatric Infectious Diseases and Immunology, University Department of Paediatrics, Oxford, United Kingdom
- Dr. Nisa Lluís, M.D., Ph.D. Department of Clinical Research, University of Bern/Inselspita, Switzerland
- Mr. Saïd Mahfoud. English teacher. Marrakech, Morocco
- Team of Springer (New York) for anatomical illustrations

Contents

Part I
General Introduction

Chapter 1
Introduction, Definitions and Historical Aspects

"One must study to know, know to understand, understand to judge."

Narada (*Ancient Hindu philosopher*)

"Life is short, and Art is long; the opportunity fleeting, experience perilous, and decision difficult."

Hippocrates (*Greek physician*) *460 BC–377 BC*

Contents

Introduction

Osteomyelitis of the skull (more particularly the neurocranium) is an uncommon true bony infection with numerous variations that can lead to intracranial complications, systemic illness, bone loss, aesthetic concerns, and significant neurological morbidity and mortality. These make cranial osteomyelitis more challenging to manage especially with changing traits of this disease in the past two decades. In developed countries, cranial osteomyelitis presents most frequently as a postoperative complication and especially in some immunocompromised patients. On the other hand, in developing nations, the original profile of otorhinogenic dominated cranial bone infections; in this condition cranial osteomyelitis should be considered the transitional point between a primary extracranial infection and its secondary intracranial extension. Although still uncommon in day-to-day practice, it is increasingly important to be aware of osteomyelitis of the skull and to consider them in the differential diagnosis of appropriate cases as the early diagnosis and treatment have a significant impact on improved outcome.

A. Akhaddar, *Cranial Osteomyelitis*, DOI 10.1007/978-3-319-30268-3_1

Different terminologies and classifications are used for cranial osteomyelitis based on a variety of features such as clinical course, pathological/anatomical or imaging features, etiology, and pathogenesis. Acute osteomyelitis develops into "secondary chronic" osteomyelitis after a mean duration of 4 weeks [1–4]. Acute osteomyelitis and chronic ones are therefore regarded to be the same disease at different stages. Anyway, both acute and chronic osteomyelitis are considered true bone infections that are accompanied with more or less extensive suppuration.

Until now, medical and surgical specialists continue to manage osteomyelitis of various types with the recognition that cranial osteomyelitis differs significantly from osteomyelitis of the long bones and at other skeletal sites of the body. Neuro-cranial bones are unique and the danger of their infection stems from their closeness to the meninges and brain and the possibility of spreading disease. Today, most osteomyelitis in the skull region are encountered preferably as a consequence of otorhinologic infections or cranial surgeries, but also following a post-traumatic lesion, spontaneous scalp infection or, more infrequently, as hematogenic metastasis. But, in some rare cases, no causes can be identified (cryptogenic forms). Depending on the intensity of the infection, its localization, and the host bone response, the clinical presentation and course may vary considerably which ranges from asymptomatic to critical illness. Although the diagnosis is somewhat quickly made clinically, an imaging study can be used for early detection and confirmation when the diagnosis is uncertain or to help measure the severity of infection and the degree of involvement. However, in spite of all the advances in imaging techniques, biological/infectious investigations and therapeutic methods, its optimal management is still controversial owing to the limited individual experience and the variable clinical course of the condition. Classically, the goals of treatment are drainage of purulent collections, surgical cranial bone debridement, control of infection, and protection of vital intracranial structures. In addition, it is important for the treating physician to consider host compromise and treat any compromising condition, when feasible, concomitantly with the cranial infection.

To the best of our knowledge, there is no comprehensive universally accepted guideline on the management of patients with skull osteomyelitis to date: some believe that immediate neurosurgical intervention is necessary, whilst others insist that a more conservative approach with or without neurosurgical intervention carries similar results. Despite these divergences, the majority of authors adheres to the fact that the cornerstone to an appropriate therapy is a precise diagnosis and a close collaboration between neurosurgical, otorhinolaryngologic, microbiologic and infectious disease specialists. Overall, the prognosis of this complex loco-regional infectious disease is related to the severity of infection, its localization and extension (especially intracranial complication), the delay in diagnosis, and the underlying medical condition of the host.

Personal interest in this topic was stimulated by the difficulty to manage many patients with skull osteomyelitis since the beginning of my neurosurgical training, 20 years ago. In addition, there was minimal to no neurosurgical research devoted to this topic as demonstrated by the few publications on this subject, most often in the form of isolated case reports. But, in recent years, the literature in this field has increased in complexity and quantity probably because of change in our societies and advances in modern medicine (see Chap. 2). Indeed, cranial infections have an undoubted potential to return with a vengeance [5]. For all these reasons a need has become evident for a timely and concise book that provides a comprehensive and updated review to better elucidate biological aspects, clinical characteristics, neuroradiological findings and treatment strategies for skull osteomyelitis. This richly illustrated book is designed to bring further light to this complex infectious disease and to serve as a succinct appropriate resource for medical students, residents, neurosurgeons, otorhinolaryngologists, neuroradiologists, microbiologists, and infectious disease specialists with an interest in cranial infections. Cases of facial osteomyelitis including mandibular (jaw), malar and maxillary bones are completely separated from the present subject matter.

Definitions

Various terms have been used by different authors to denote inflammation/infection of bones: osteitis, periosteitis, myelitis, osteoperiosteitis, periosteomyelitis and osteomyelitis [6]. Osteomyelitis is the term more universally employed nowadays. The word "**osteomyelitis**" describes an inflammatory condition of bone (osteitis) and bone marrow (myelitis) caused by pus-producing bacteria. Although other etiological factors, such as traumatic injuries, tumors, radiation and chemical substances, among others may also produce inflammation of bone and bone marrow space, the term "osteomyelitis" is mostly used in medical literature to describe a true infection by pyogenic microorganisms [1, 7]. However, for many authors, this definition may be extended to cover all other no-pyogenic microorganisms including specific and no-specific bacteria, fungi and parasites.

Additionally, osteitis can occur independently of marrow infection or, more commonly, as a phenomenon related to it [8]. For that reason, common medical literature also extends the definition of "osteomyelitis" to an inflammation process of the entire bone including the cortical bone and periosteum (periosteitis). Classically, it can be considered as an inflammatory condition of the bone, beginning in the medullar cavity (marrow space) and Haversian systems and extending to involve the subperiosteal space or the periosteum of the affected area. The infection becomes established in calcified portion of the bone when pus and edema in the medullary cavity and beneath the periosteum compromises or obstructs the local blood supply. Following ischemia, the infected bone becomes necrotic and leads to *sequester formation*, which is considered a classical sign of osteomyelitis [9–11]. Radiographic and pathologic differentiation of osteomyelitis and osteitis can be extremely difficult. Some authors affirm that *osteitis* and *osteomyelitis* are synonyms and the two terms are often used interchangeably [12–14], this is particularly true in the skull where the thickness of the marrow space and diploic venous system vary greatly from one cranial bone to another (see Chap. 5), between individuals and with age [15, 16]. In the German literature, osteitis and

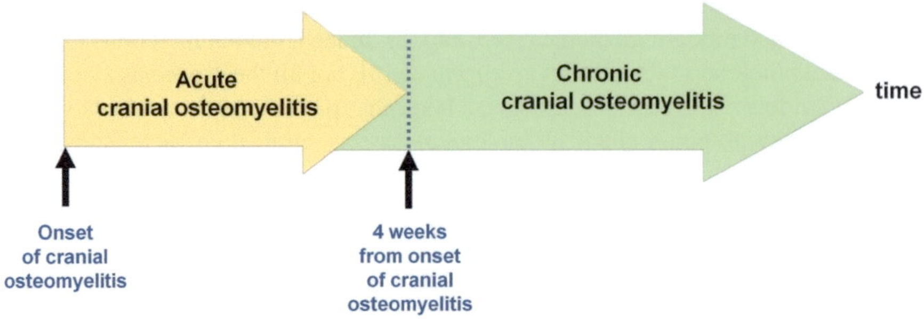

Fig. 1.1 Process of evolution of the two main types of Cranial osteomyelitis

osteomyelitis are two clearly distinct pathological entities. Osteitis is caused by direct contact of the tissue with bacteria during trauma or surgery. Whereas, osteomyelitis is caused by bacterial seeding from the blood (hematogenous spread) [8]. According to Tiemann and Hofmann, the main difference between osteitis and osteomyelitis is the way that the infection affects the bone: centripetal for osteitis or centrifugal for osteomyelitis. However, they assume that the clinical and investigative findings of osteitis and osteomyelitis may be very similar particularly in their later stages where it might be quite difficult to differentiate between the two [13].

Various microorganisms (non-specific and specific bacteria, fungi and parasites) may be encountered in cranial osteomyelitis but *Staphylococcus aureus* remains the most frequent. Pathogens may reach the skull bone using various conceivable portals of entry and mechanisms of spread in order to establish infection. The most usual possibilities are secondary to direct inoculation (by surgical manipulation or trauma), following contiguous source of adjacent infection mainly paranasal sinusitis or otomastoiditis or rarely via hematogenous bloodborne route.

Depending on the literature, mainly two different types of osteomyelitis are distinguished: *acute* (illness duration less than 1 month) and *chronic* osteomyelitis (more than 1 month) (Fig. 1.1), although some authors add a sub-acute category (between 2 weeks and 3 months) [1, 8, 17, 18]. However, the "sub-acute" subgroup is rarely distinguished in cranial osteomyelitis and therefore rarely used in otorhinolaryngology and neurosurgical practices. For many authors, acute and chronic forms of cranial osteomyelitis are primarily the same disease, depending on the length of time the infection or symptoms persist. As we shall see further, the limit between acute and chronic osteomyelitis can only be arbitrary defined with a clear-cut time interval after beginning of the deep bone infection [2–4]. Both acute and chronic forms represent a true microbiologic infection of the skull where suppuration, fistula formation, and sequestration are distinctive features.

The term "refractory osteomyelitis" is applied to chronic osteomyelitis that persists or recurs after appropriate interventions have been performed or where acute osteomyelitis has not responded to accepted management techniques [19]. This form develops generally, where there is some reason why the bone is not able to heal itself correctly. Refractory osteomyelitis may persist for a life-time with severe consequences.

On another side, osteomyelitis includes a large spectrum of different diseases. This is due to many-sided presentation of bone infection. Different classifications are used based on a variety of features such as duration of disease, imaging features, route of infection, presence of implant, underlying etiology, pathogenesis, physiological host response and age of onset. Traditionally, most of these classifications were established by orthopedic surgeons and infectious disease specialists [3, 11, 20–26]. This is principally due to the fact that osteomyelitis mainly involves long bones and foreign devices are widely used. However, it is well recognized that the topic of cranial osteomyelitis differs significantly from osteomyelitis of the tubular bones and at other skeletal sites [7].

In this book and to simplify the management of cranial osteomyelitis, the seven following parameters were considered: age of onset (children, adults), duration of infection (acute or chronic), pathogenesis (spread from an otorhinogenic disease, contiguous source following cranial surgeries or head injuries, and hematogenous spread), anatomic location (cranial vault, skull base), extension of infection (extra-cranial, cranial and intracranial structures), comorbidities (immunosuppressive diseases and other underlying medical conditions) and causative microorganisms (specific and unspecific bacteria, fungi, and parasites).

The skull base is an uncommon location of osteomyelitis which is often described as a complication of malignant (necrotizing) otitis externa. However, the expression "malignant external otitis" was improperly used by many otorhino-laryngologists to describe skull base osteomyelitis [7, 27, 28]. This term is confusing and must be used to describe features limited to lateral temporal osteomyelitis which is a less serious condition than medial or central temporal osteomyelitis. From this perspective, the concept of central skull base osteomyelitis "CSBO" has been recently defined as an osteomyelitis of the temporal bone and the skull base including the bony labyrinth, the media part of petrous bone, the sphenoidal, the occipital and the clivus, even reaching the infratemporal fossa [29–31]. According to some authors, central skull base osteomyelitis must be unrelated to otogenic source etiology [29, 31]. In the present monograph, the focus will be predominately on the medial temporal bone osteomyelitis and the central form of skull base osteomyelitis.

Historical Aspects

Evidence of osteomyelitis in the skull has been encountered at such an early period of history of the earth, long before the advent of man. Paleopathologists (specialists in ancient disease and injury) recognized the disease in many species of dinosaurs specially *Pachycephalosaurus wyomingensis* who had an important thickened cranial roof [32, 33]. The high frequency of cranial bone osteomyelitis (20 %) seen in pachycephalosaurids is, therefore, consistent with the hypothesis that the cranial dome was employed in intraspecific combat (head injuries) [32] (Fig. 1.2).

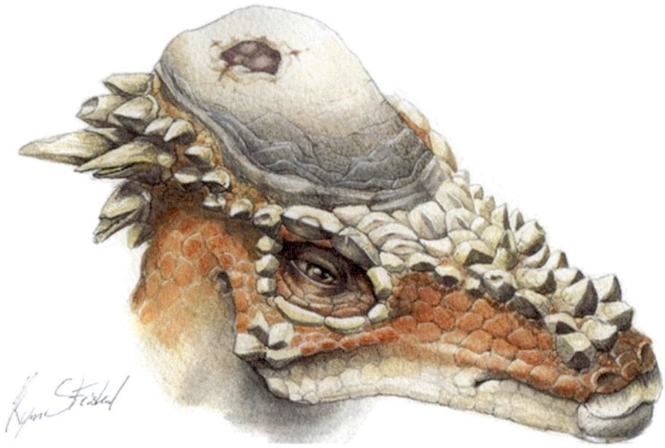

Fig. 1.2 Schematic reconstruction of *Pachycephalosaurus wyomingensis* with cranial vault osteomyelitis lesion (Reproduced with permission from Peterson JE, Dischler C, Longrich NR. Distributions of cranial pathologies provide evidence for head-butting in dome-headed dinosaurs (Pachycephalosauridae). PLoS One. 2013 Jul 16;8(7):e68620. doi: 10.1371/journal.pone.0068620) [32]

Ancient Civilizations

In human, skull trepanation or trephination performed with primitive tools and techniques, is one of the most intriguing surgical practices in our history used since antiquity to treat a range of medical conditions (correction of head injuries, epilepsy, treatment of headaches…) or for mystical reasons (issues of religion, ritual, release of demons…) [34–40]. This neurosurgical operation involves the removal of one or more pieces of bone without causing any damage to the blood vessels, the meninges that cover the brain, or the brain itself; it is a procedure that requires both skill and care from the part of the surgeon. Many prehistoric skulls show evidence of healing, suggesting that these early patients survived the surgery for more or less long time [40–44] (Fig. 1.3). Infections rate were unexpectedly low after trepanation (only 15 %) as represented by surrounded bony inflammatory reactions. One report described a pre-Columbian South American mummy with a severe cranial periostitis after this type of primitive surgery [45]. Progressively, survival rates increased for patients over time. About 80 % of patients survived the operation in those times, provided that the dura mater was not damaged either by the traumatic incident or during operation [46].

In the prehistoric world, some skulls also showed evidence of cranial osteomyelitis after traumatic calvarial injuries [47]. In one case, a man had survived an arrow injury to his forehead. However, he subsequently developed severe periorbital osteomyelitis, probably resulting in a generalized fatal infection [45].

On the other hand, several diseases are present in the archaeological records. Sequelae of mastoid osteomyelitis in the skeletons of ancient Egyptians mummies were frequently met [48]. Cranial syphilis is by far the most common. The

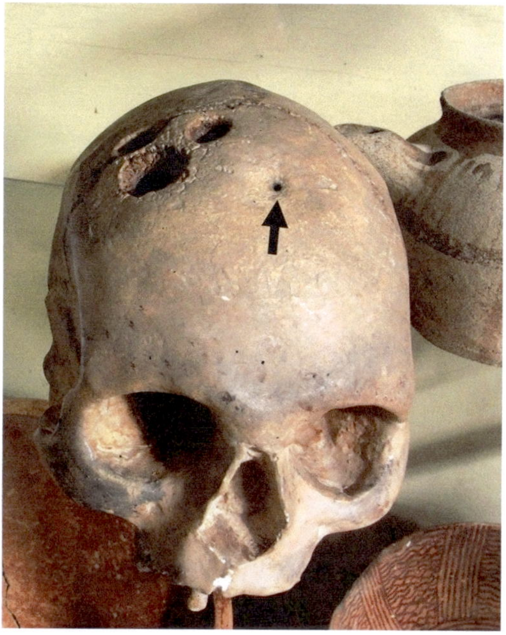

Fig 1.3 Bronze Age skull (2200–2000 BCE) from Jericho, exhibited in the Jordan Archaeological Museum (modern cast of human skull). This skull shows evidence of four separate holes made by the ancient surgical process of trepanation. This individual survived the first one, as indicated by the almost complete healing of one hole near the front center of the skull (*arrow*). The later three operations were apparently less successful and he dead shortly afterward

pathognomonic lesion of syphilis is that of tertiary gummatous osteoperiosteal lesion that was defined as "caries sicca" (Fig. 1.4) by Virchow who subdivided the condition into three categories: (1) Caries and necrosis of bone subsequent to ulcers eroding local soft tissues. (2) Peripheral caries and necrosis related to suppurative periostitis or deeper sero-sanguinous ulceration. (3) Internal caries and necrosis developing from a gummatous or suppurative osteomyelitis [9, 49, 50]. In tuberculosis, cranial erosion begins in the inner table with very little new bone formation. Therefore, hypertrophic osseous expansion is rarely found. Klaus reported a Muchik child from north coast Peru (AD 900–1750) with two distinct tuberculous lesions of the posterior cranium: theses irregular destructive foci perforated the inner and outer tables and were surrounded by jagged margins lacking evidence of inflammation. Radiographic and CT-scan studies reveal lesions originating in the diploë [51]. Classically, pyogenic osteomyelitis produces sequestrum and cloacae formation, lesions that are rarely observed in syphilis. In addition, pyogenic osteomyelitis does not involve as many bones as does syphilis [49].

More than 2500 years ago, Hippocrates the Greek physician and philosopher described in his "*Corpus Hippocraticum, Diseases II*" the clinical signs and course of craniocerebral infections. He points out that he involvement of bone indicates a direct surgical approach: [If a sphacelus (of the skull) occurs. . .the patient swells up and becomes livid. . .When this happens, you must incise wherever the swelling is, and clean and scrape the bone until you arrive at the diploe. Then treat as you would in the case of a fracture (Chapter 23)] [52]. In the first century AD, Celcius described scraping away or debridement of the dead bone until it bleeds. But most patients

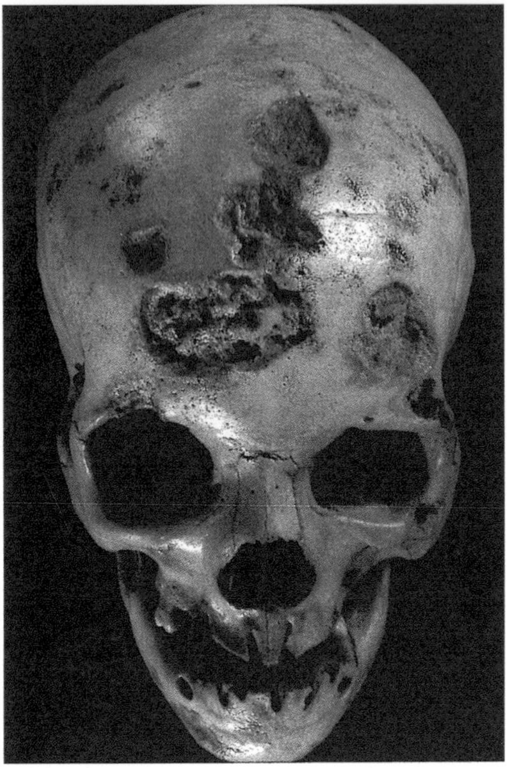

Fig 1.4 Syphilitic skull "*Caries sicca.*" The frontal bone is extensively destroyed by gummas with only a modest periosteal response in the lesions' periphery (Reproduced with permission from the Cambridge University Press. Aufderheide A.C., & Rodriguez-Martin C. Cambridge Encyclopaedia of Paleopathology 1998, page 161, ISBN 978-0-521-55203-5) [49]

with open fractures subsequently died before elucidation of the germ theory or understanding of the principles of infection [53].

Modern Times

Osteomyelitis was first described by Chassaignac in 1852. However, a century earlier (1764), Hunter described pockets of dead cortical bone with abscess, which he termed "sequestra." He also described "involucrum" or new bone formed in response to the sequestra [53]. In the skull, the most interesting description was reported in 1760 by Percival Pott (Fig. 1.5), a surgeon at St Bartholomew's Hospital (London), in "*Observations on the nature and consequences of those injuries to which the head is liable from external violence.*" published in 1768. He defined the "Pott's puffy tumor" as one or more superiosteal abscesses of the frontal bone associated with underlying osteomyelitis [54, 55]. This condition was related to earlier forehead trauma (bone contusion). Pott assumed that every severe head contusion detachment of the dura mater is caused by an extradural hematoma which irritates the dura, and this irritation increases and causes suppurative

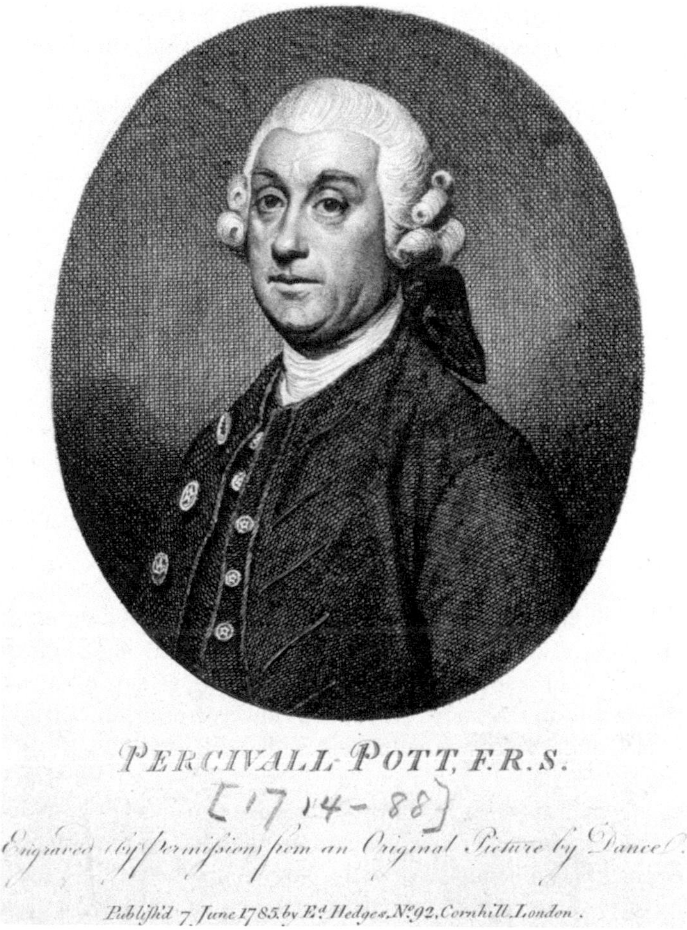

Fig. 1.5 Sir Percivall Pott (1714–1788). This work is in the public domain in the United States because it was published (or registered with the U.S. Copyright Office) before January 1st, 1923

inflammation [54–56]. In 1775, Pott reported another case as a result from sinusitis. Surgical exploration revealed a subperiosteal abscess and osteomyelitis in the presence of frontal sinus infection [56]. Lannelongue proved in 1879 that cranial paraosseous abscesses were due to disease of the underlying bone itself, although the relationship was suspected by Chassaignac in 1859 [57, 58]. Fischer in 1882, wrote of apparently spontaneous inflammation of the skull that it was probably caused by progressive suppuration in the neighboring tissues [59, 60]. Cases of cranial osteomyelitis having an origin in the paranasal sinuses were also reported by Luc and Tilley in 1889 [61, 62].

An otologic origin of cranial osteomyelitis was reported few years later. Lastly, Von Bergmann recognized a metastatic/hematogenous origin (secondary to a primary septic focus elsewhere in the body) of cranial osteomyelitis in 1900 in his "Handbook of Practical Surgery" [60]. However, in 1904, Schilling points out that metastatic osteomyelitis of the skull are rare compared with those located in long bones [63]. This is true particularly since Rodet produced the first experimental acute hematogenous osteomyelitis in 1884: *Staphylococcus aureus* "un micrococcus qui possède une couleur jaune orange" was injected to rabbits and resulted in the occurrence of multiple bone abscesses [64]. Behind cranial vault osteomyelitis, skull base localization was described in the 1920s mainly in postmortem examination [65]. Interestingly, in 1904, Gradenigo presented some cases of paralysis of the abducens nerve of post-otitic origin. These cases formed the basis for the description of a syndrome currently known as *Gradenigo's syndrome* which consists of homolateral trigeminal neuralgia and paresis or paralysis of the homolateral abducens nerve in the context of chronic or acute suppuration of the ear after involvement of the apex of the petrous part of the temporal bone known as petrous apicitis or apical petrositis [66, 67]. For some authors, this syndrome is related to a form of skull base osteomyelitis [68, 69]. Toulmouche was the first physician to have described a case of progressive osteomyelitis of temporal bone in 1938 [70]. Later in 1959, Meltzer and Keleman reported a patient with Pyocyaneous chondritis, osteomyelitis of the external auditory canal and temporal bone [71]. Because of the high mortality rate in early series, this condition is often referred to as "malignant otitis externa" [72]. Since then, the term "skull base osteomyelitis" was also improperly used to describe osteomyelitis in the temporal bone, osteomyelitis of the mastoid and middle ear cleft, osteitis of the base of the skull and necrotizing otitis externa [7, 71, 72]. However, as mentioned above, there is a certain lack of clarity in presenting this condition.

The prevalence, clinical course, and management of cranial osteomyelitis have changed greatly in the twentieth century. This is due to using antisepsis and aseptic techniques into the operating room by Lister and introduction of antibiotic therapy, especially penicillin by Fleming. Currently, new antimicrobials allow the treatment of almost every pathogen with reasonable risk of toxicity. Further factors have additionally led to improvement in the management of skull bone osteomyelitis as the advances made in neurosurgical techniques, anesthesia, modern diagnostic imaging, biologic investigation and hyperbaric oxygen therapy. But, despite the introduction of modern surgical and pharmacological therapy, cranial bone infection still continues to be difficult to treat. They still have undoubted potential for permanent nervous system damage or fatal consequences and continue to pose a significant challenge to the contemporary neurosurgeon worldwide.

References

1. Marx RE. Chronic osteomyelitis of the jaws. Oral Maxillofac Surg Clin North Am. 1991;3 (2):367–81.
2. Meier DE, Tarpley JL, OlaOlorun DA, Howard CR, Price CT. *Haematogenous osteomyelitis* in the developing world: a practical approach to classification and treatment with limited resources. Contemp Orthop. 1993;26:495–502.

3. Solagberu BA. A new classification of osteomyelitis for developing countries. East Afr Med J. 2003;80(7):373–8.
4. Bonakdar-pour A, Gaines VD. The radiology of osteomyelitis. Orthop Clin North Am. 1983;14(1):21–37.
5. Nathoo N, Narotam PK, Nadvi S, van Dellen JR. Taming an old enemy: a profile of intracranial suppuration. World Neurosurg. 2012;77(3–4):484–90. doi:10.1016/j.wneu.2011.04.023.
6. Eid EM. Osteomyelitis: historical overview. Pan Arab J Orth Trauma. 2003;7(2):95–109.
7. Prasad KC, Prasad SC, Mouli N, Agarwal S. Osteomyelitis in the head and neck. Acta Otolaryngol. 2007;127(2):194–205.
8. Kemmer A, Stein T, Hierholzer C. Persistent osteomyelitis. In: Mathieu D, editor. Handbook on hyperbaric medicine. Netherlands: Springer; 2006.
9. Turk JL. Syphilitic caries of the skull. The changing face of medicine. J R Soc Med. 1995;88 (3):146–8.
10. Strumas N, Antonyshyn O, Caldwell CB, Mainprize J. Multimodality imaging for precise localization of craniofacial osteomyelitis. J Craniofac Surg. 2003;14(2):215–9.
11. Waldvogel FA, Medoff G, Swartz MN. Osteomyelitis: a review of clinical features, therapeutic considerations and unusual aspects. N Engl J Med. 1970;282(4):198–206.
12. Horn KL, Erasmus MD, Akiya FI. Suppurative petrous apicitis: osteitis or osteomyelitis? An imaging case report. Am J Otolaryngol. 1996;17(1):54–7.
13. Tiemann AH, Hofmann GO. Principles of the therapy of bone infections in adult extremities : are there any new developments? Strategies Trauma Limb Reconstr. 2009;4(2):57–64.
14. McConnell G. A manual of pathology. Philadelphia: W.B. Saunders Company; 1906.
15. Herrmann BW, Chung JC, Eisenbeis JF, Forsen Jr JW. Intracranial complications of pediatric frontal rhinosinusitis. Am J Rhinol. 2006;20(3):320–4.
16. Kombogiorgas D, Seth R, Athwal R, Modha J, Singh J. Suppurative intracranial complications of sinusitis in adolescence. Single institute experience and review of literature. Br J Neurosurg. 2007;21(6):603–9.
17. Riise ØR, Kirkhus E, Handeland KS, Flatø B, Reiseter T, Cvancarova M, Nakstad B, Wathne KO. Childhood osteomyelitis-incidence and differentiation from other acute onset musculoskeletal features in a population-based study. BMC Pediatr. 2008;8:45. doi:10.1186/1471-2431-8-45.
18. Dartnell J, Ramachandran M, Katchburian M. Haematogenous acute and subacute paediatric osteomyelitis: a systematic review of the literature. J Bone Joint Surg Br. 2012;94(5):584–95. doi:10.1302/0301-620X.94B5.28523.
19. Strauss MB. Refractory osteomyelitis. J Hyperbaric Med. 1987;2:147–59.
20. Cierny G, Mader JT. Adult chronic osteomyelitis. Orthopedics. 1984;7(10):1557–64. doi:10.3928/0147-7447-19841001-07.
21. Lew DP, Waldvogel FA. Osteomyelitis. Lancet. 2004;364(9431):369–79.
22. Kelly PJ. Infected nonunion of the femur and tibia. Orthop Clin North Am. 1984;15 (3):481–90.
23. McPherson EJ, Woodson C, Holtom P, Roidis N, Shufelt C, Patzakis M. Periprosthetic total hip infection: outcomes using a staging system. Clin Orthop Relat Res. 2002;403:8–15.
24. Bowen TR, Widmaier JC. Host classification predicts infection after open fracture. Clin Orthop Relat Res. 2005;433:205–11.
25. Romanò CL, Romanò D, Logoluso N, Drago L. Bone and joint infections in adults: a comprehensive classification proposal. Eur Orthop Traumatol. 2011;1(6):207–17.
26. Schmidt HG, Diefenbeck M, Krenn V, Abitzsch D, Militz M, Tiemann AH, Haustedt N, Gückel P, Bühler M, Gerlach UJ. Classification of haematogenous and post-traumatic osteomyelitis. Z Orthop Unfall. 2014;152(4):334–42. doi:10.1055/s-0034-1368620.German.
27. Rothholtz VS, Lee AD, Shamloo B, Bazargan M, Pan D, Djalilian HR. Skull base osteomyelitis: the effect of comorbid disease on hospitalization. Laryngoscope. 2008;118 (11):1917–24. doi:10.1097/MLG.0b013e31817fae0d.

28. Chen JC, Yeh CF, Shiao AS, Tu TY. Temporal bone osteomyelitis: the relationship with malignant otitis externa, the diagnostic dilemma, and changing trends. ScientificWorldJournal. 2014;2014:591714. doi:10.1155/2014/591714.
29. Cavel O, Fliss DM, Segev Y, Zik D, Khafif A, Landsberg R. The role of the otorhinolaryngologist in the management of central skull base osteomyelitis. Am J Rhinol. 2007;21 (3):281–5.
30. Ridder GJ, Breunig C, Kaminsky J, Pfeiffer J. Central skull base osteomyelitis: new insights and implications for diagnosis and treatment. Eur Arch Otorhinolaryngol. 2015;272 (5):1269–76. doi:10.1007/s00405-014-3390-y.
31. Johnson AK, Batra PS. Central skull base osteomyelitis: an emerging clinical entity. Laryngoscope. 2014;124(5):1083–7. doi:10.1002/lary.24440.
32. Peterson JE, Dischler C, Longrich NR. Distributions of cranial pathologies provide evidence for head-butting in dome-headed dinosaurs (Pachycephalosauridae). PLoS One. 2013;8(7): e68620. doi:10.1371/journal.pone.0068620.
33. Whinney LA, Rothschild BM, Carpenter K. Posttraumatic chronic osteomyelitis in *Stegosaurus* dermal spikes. In: Carpenter K, editor. The armored dinosaurs. Bloomington: Indiana University Press; 2001.
34. Goodrich JT. Landmarks in the history of neurosurgery. In: Rengachary SS, Ellenbogen RG, editors. Principles of neurosurgery. 2nd ed. Philadelphia: Elsevier Mosby; 2005.
35. Horsley V. Brain surgery in the Stone Age. Br Med J. 1887;1:582–7.
36. Rifkinson-Mann S. Cranial surgery in ancient Peru. Neurosurgery. 1988;23(4):411–6.
37. Daland J. Depressed fracture and trephining of the skull by the Incas of Peru. Ann Med Hist. 1935;7:550–8.
38. Ferembach DI. Anthropologie. In: Ferembach D, Dastugue J, Poitrat Targowla MJ, editors. La Nécropole Épipaléolithique de Taforalt (Maroc oriental). Paris: Éditions du CNRS; 1962.
39. El Ouarzazi A. Was skull surgery born in Morocco? In: El Khamlichi A, editor. Proceedings of the 13th World Congress of Neurological Surgery; 2005 June 19–24; Marrakesh, Morocco. Bologna: Medimond; 2005. p. 517–22.
40. Holliday DY. Occipital lesions: a possible cost of cradleboards. Am J Phys Anthropol. 1993;90 (3):283–90.
41. MacCurdy GC. Human skeletal remains from the highlands of Peru. Am J Phys Anthropol. 1923;6:217–67.
42. Cushing H. Surgery of the head. In: Keen WW, editor. Surgery, its principles and practice. Philadelphia: WB Saunders; 1908.
43. Petrone P, Niola M, Di Lorenzo P, Paternoster M, Graziano V, Quaremba G, Buccelli C. Early medical skull surgery for treatment of post-traumatic osteomyelitis 5,000 years ago. PLoS One. 2015;10(5):e0124790. doi:10.1371/journal.pone.0124790.
44. Weber J, Wahl J. Neurosurgical aspects of trepanations from Neolithic Times. Int J Osteoarchaeol. 2006;16:536–45.
45. Gerszten PC, Gerszten E, Allison MJ. Diseases of the skull in pre-Columbian South American mummies. Neurosurgery. 1998;42(5):1145–51.
46. Heidecker KM. Trepanation of the skull in classical antiquity. Wurzbg Medizinhist Mitt. 2006;25:113–31.
47. Manzon VS, Hohenstein UT, Gualdi-Russo E. Injuries on a skull from the Ancient Bronze Age (Ballabio, Lecco, Italy): a natural or an anthropic origin? J Archaeol Sci. 2012;39 (11):3428–35.
48. Smith GE, Dawson WR, editors. Egyptian Mummies. London: George Allen and Unwin Ltd; 1924.
49. Aufderheide AC, Rodriguez-Martin C, editors. The Cambridge Encyclopedia of human paleopathology. Cambridge, UK: Cambridge University Press; 1998.
50. Virchow R. Ueber die Natur der constitutionell syphilitischen Affectionen. Arch Pathol Anat. 1858;15:217–336.

51. Klaus HD, Wilbur AK, Temple DH, Buikstra JE, Stone AC, Fernandez M, Wester C, Tam ME. Tuberculosis on the north coast of Peru: skeletal and molecular paleopathology of late pre-Hispanic and postcontact mycobacterial disease. J Archaeol Sci. 2010;37(10):2587–97.
52. Viale GL, Deseri S, Gennaro S, Sehrbundt E. A craniocerebral infectious disease: case report on the traces of Hippocrates. Neurosurgery. 2002;50(6):1376–8.
53. Babu RP, Todor R, Kasoff SS. Pott's puffy tumor: the forgotten entity. Case report. J Neurosurg. 1996;84(1):110–2.
54. Pott P. Observations on the nature and consequences of those injuries to which the head is liable from external violence. London: L Hawes, W Clarke, R Collins; 1768.
55. Flamm ES. Percivall Pott: an 18th century neurosurgeon. J Neurosurg. 1992;76(2):319–26.
56. Ravitch MM. Surgery in 1776. Ann Surg. 1977;186(3):291–300.
57. Lannelongue OM. De l'ostéomyélite aigue pendant la croissance. Paris: Asselin & Cie; 1879.
58. Chassaignac E. Traité pratique de la suppuration et du drainage chirurgical. Paris: Masson; 1859.
59. Fischer H. Die Osteomyelitis Traumatica Purulenta Cranii. Deut Zeit Chir. 1900;56:449–72.
60. Wilensky AO. Osteomyelitis of the skull. Arch Surg. 1933;27(1):83–158.
61. Luc H. La méthode de Killian pour la cure radicale de l'empyème frontal chronique. Annales des maladies de l'oreille, du larynx, du nez et du pharynx. Décembre 1902, p 497
62. Tilley H. Remarks on the operative treatment of a case of double frontal sinus empyema, complicated by double antral suppuration. Br Med J. 1897;1(1882):197–9.
63. Schilling R. Ueber die Osteomyelitis der Flachen Schadelknochen im Anschlusse an Entzundungen der Stirnhohle und des Mittelohres. Zeit f Ohrenheilk. 1904;48:52.
64. Rodet A. Etude expérimentale sur l'ostéomyélite infectieuse. Comptes Rendus de l'Académie des Sciences. 1884;99:569–71.
65. Kramer R. Intracranial complications following sphenoid infection. Laryngoscope. 1929;39 (9):573–88.
66. Gradenigo G. On circumscribed leptomeningitis and on abducens paralysis of post-otitic origin—Sulla leptomeningite circoscritta e sulla paralisi dell' abducente di origine otitica. G Accad Med Torino. 1904;10:59–64. Italian.
67. Matis GK, de A Silva DO, Chrysou OI, Karanikas MA, Birbilis TA. Giuseppe Gradenigo: much more than a syndrome! Historical vignette. Surg Neurol Int. 2012;3:122. doi:10.4103/2152-7806.102343.
68. Niho S, Niho M, Yoshio K, Iwatake T, Takahata N. Petrositis and osteomyelitis temporalis. Yokohama Med Bull. 1954;5(2):125–38.
69. Hehl K, Tisch M, Lampl L, Draf W, Stussak G, Frey G. Bilateral Gradenigo syndrome—on the value of an integrated therapy concept including hyperbaric oxygenation and chronic destructive inflammation of the skull base. HNO. 1992;40(8):318–21. German.
70. Toulmouche MA. Observations d'*otorrhée* cérébrale suivis des réflexions. Gaz Med Paris. 1938;6:422–6.
71. Meltzer PE, Keleman G. Pyocyaneous osteomyelitis of the temporal bone, mandible and zygoma. Laryngoscope. 1959;69:1300–6.
72. Chandler JR. Malignant external otitis. Laryngoscope. 1968;78(8):1257–94.

Part II
Basic Information for Cranial Osteomyelitis

Chapter 2
Epidemiology and Risk Factors

Contents

Abbreviations

CNS Central nervous system
ENT Ear, nose, and throat
SSI Surgical site infection

Epidemiology

Osteomyelitis may affect any bone, with a predilection for the tubular bones of the arms and legs [1]. Osteomyelitis is primarily a disease of young children presumably because of the rich vascular supply of their rapidly growing bones [2]. The skull (neurocranium) was recognized as a rare anatomic site, but potentially serious. However, cranial osteomyelitis is regularly seen in countries with lesser sanitary capacities. Migratory flows, the ease of travelling, and number of trips have led to the possibility of the discovery and development of infectious diseases that are usually uncommon in developed countries. We must keep in mind the changing traits of cranial osteomyelitis. The presumed rarity of osteomyelitis of the skull, led us to conduct a simple search study with MEDLINE as the mean search engine. To obtain the highest number of skull osteomyelitis, the following Boolean operator combinations were used: ((“skull” and “osteomyelitis”) OR (“cranial” and “osteomyelitis”)) in English-language literature from 1955 to 2014. The search yielded

A. Akhaddar, *Cranial Osteomyelitis*, DOI 10.1007/978-3-319-30268-3_2

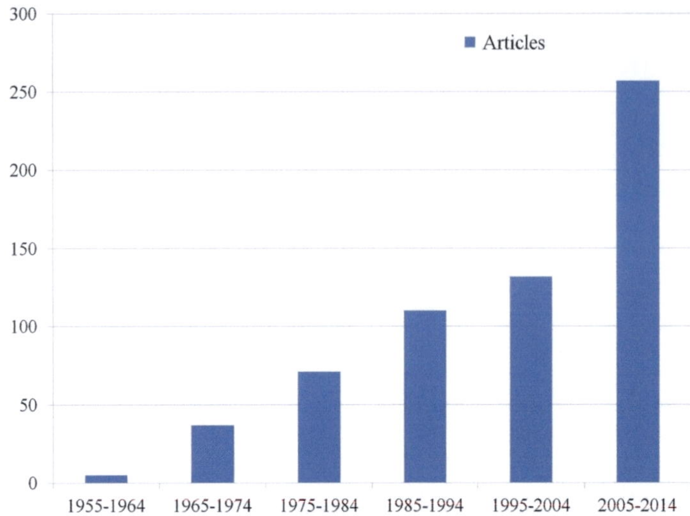

Fig. 2.1 Bar graph showing progression of number of English language articles about *cranial osteomyelitis* found in MEDLINE database over time (from 1955 to 2014)

612 articles and we can see a significant increase in the number of articles published recently in peer-reviewed literature particularly in the first decade of the new millennium (Fig. 2.1). For many authors, this high article number seen recently suggests that this complication is far more common than supposed [3–13]. The exact reason is most likely due to either of the following:

- Firstly, a more adequate access to radiological imaging has allowed more accurate modality for the diagnosis of complications of dental, paranasal sinus and ear infections.
- Secondly, an increased awareness of physicians for cranial infections.
- Finally, a rise in the frequency and complexity of cranial neurosurgical procedures currently performed.

Many sources of osteomyelitis are described in the skull (Fig. 2.2). In developing countries, paranasal sinusitis and scalp infections remain the most common causes of cranial osteomyelitis, while in industrialized nations, postsurgical craniotomy infections have become the predominant source [8, 11, 14, 15]. However, in many developed countries, otorhinolaryngologic infections have increased the relative incidence of contiguous cranial osteomyelitis that nowadays equals that of post-operative osteomyelitis [4, 6, 12, 13, 16].

In the world literature, there are no valid data about the exact incidence of skull osteomyelitis in general. So, its prevalence was difficult to estimate from previous case series as a result from small patient numbers, the frequent inclusion of patients with acute/chronic osteomyelitis without confirmed diagnosis and variation in the diagnostic methods used. In developed countries, cranial osteomyelitis account for about 0.3–1.5 % of all skeletal localizations [1, 17, 18]. While the incidence of

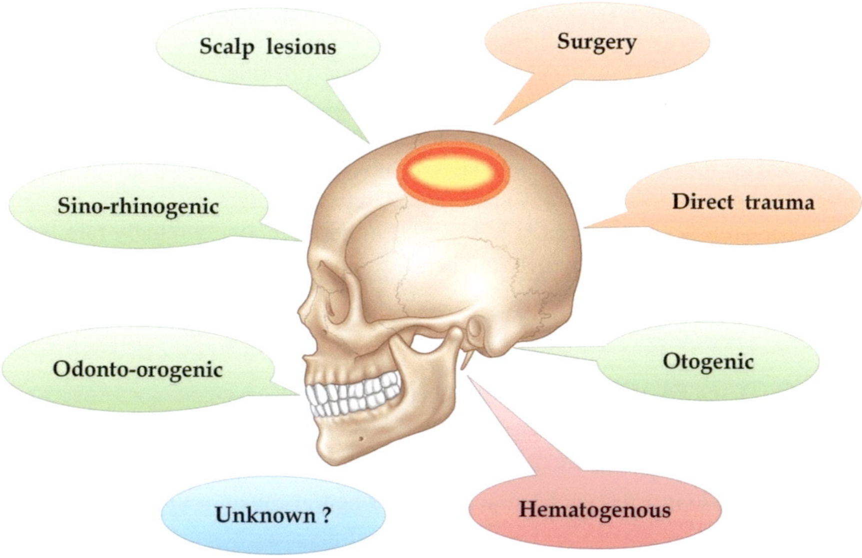

Fig. 2.2 Schematic drawing of sources of osteomyelitis formation in the skull bones

cranial vault tuberculosis is estimated to be between 0.2 and 1.3 % of all cases of skeletal tuberculosis [19]. Epidemiologic evaluation of some institutes would suggest that between one to four cases of cranial osteomyelitis would be seen per year in general neurosurgical practice. In our experience, during a 13-year-study period from 2000 to 2012, 29 cases of osteomyelitis of the skull were treated in the department of neurosurgery of Mohammed V Military teaching hospital, Rabat, Morocco, under the direction of professor Boucetta (mean of 2.4 cases per year). Nineteen patients were male (65.5 %) and the mean age at diagnosis was 41.9 years (range from 11 to 76 years). The cranial vault was involved in 25 patients (86.2 %) and 4 cases (13.8 %) had a skull base osteomyelitis. Contiguous spread of infection from paranasal sinusitis or odonto/otogenic infections was found in 13 patients (44.8 %). Also, post-craniotomy osteomyelitis was seen in 13 cases (44.8 %). One patient (3.4 %) had a penetrating head injury and a hematogenous spread infection was suspected in two patients (6.9 %). Some concurrent illnesses were found with skull osteomyelitis such as diabetes (3 cases), malignancy (3 cases), previous radiation therapy (3 cases) and renal failure (2 cases).

On the other hand, the overall incidence of skull osteomyelitis seems higher in other developing countries particularly in sub-Saharan regions of Africa, where access to health care and advanced diagnostic testing is limited [18]. Recently, 8 cases (12.7 %) of cranial osteomyelitis were reported among 63 cases of pediatric osteomyelitis in a tertiary referral centre in Tanzania (East Africa) between 2008 and 2010 [20]. During the period 1983–1997, Nathoo et al. reported 699 patients with cranial subdural empyemas in South Africa. Among them, 47 patients (6.7 %)

presented a skull osteomyelitis which was removed [21]. Infections following open traumatic injuries are less frequent.

Overall in neurosurgical practice, it seems that oro-rhino-otogenic infections account for as many as 40–50 % of cases of skull osteomyelitis. Direct surgical site infections and the use of cranioplasty materials also contribute for about 40–50 % of cases. Other major causes of cranial osteomyelitis include contiguous source following head injuries (5 %) [22] and more rarely hematogenous seeding secondary to bacteremia or fungemia [17, 23–26]. Furthermore, on extremely rare occasions, risk factors or etiology may not be ascertained.

Risk Factors for Skull Osteomyelitis

A multitude of factors have been identified that result in skull osteomyelitis. However, this disease is usually related to the following three main sources (Table 2.1):

Direct Spread from Contiguous Sites

Frontal sinusitis is the most important predisposing factor for osteomyelitis of the skull especially in children, adolescents and young adults than in other age-groups (Fig. 2.3). The predilection for this age-group is explained by the peculiarities of the development of frontal sinuses. Adolescents are likely to have highly vascular diploic bone, which increases valveless bidirectional flow between the frontal sinus mucosa and dural veinous drainage [27]. A cranial osteomyelitis was seen in 0.5–9 % of patients with suppurative intracranial complications of paranasal

Table 2.1 The main sources of infection in cranial osteomyelitis

Sources of infection	Causes
Direct extension from contiguous site of infection	Paranasal sinusitis
	Otitis or otomastoiditis
	Oral or odontogenic infections
	Spontaneous scalp infections
Post-surgical or post-traumatic direct inoculation	Neurosurgical site infections (primary)
	Following cranioplasty (secondary)
	Otologic site infections
	Craniofacial injuries (scalp and/or bone fracture)
	Cephalhematomas
Hematogenous dissemination from remote source of infection	Lung, spine, peripheral arthritis, meningitis
	Cryptogenic

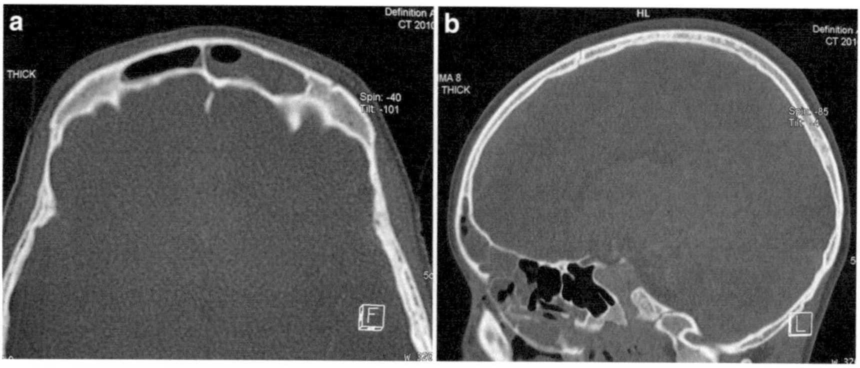

Fig. 2.3 Axial (**a**) and sagittal reconstructions (**b**) cranial CT-scan in bone windows showing left frontal sinusitis

sinusitis in neurosurgical practice [28–31]. In head and neck, incidence of cranial osteomyelitis may be as high as 28 % [8].

As all other forms of cranial osteomyelitis, Pott's puffy tumor is reported as rare in the antibiotic therapy era, although, despite the use of broad-spectrum antibiotics, the number of cases reported has increased since 2000 [32–38]. In 2012, 141 cases of Pott's puffy tumor were reported in the world literature by Nisa et al. [7]. This form of cranial osteomyelitis is more common in male and almost always confined to the second decade of life, more rarely in adults and newborns. The prevalence in young males is attributed to their larger diploic veins, which makes it easier for infections to spread [31, 35].

Besides the frontal sinus, the other paranasal sinuses should be taken into considerations: ethmoidal sinuses (Fig. 2.4), maxillar sinuses (Fig. 2.5) if not all paranasal sinuses (pansinusitis) (Fig. 2.6). Osteomyelitis of the calvaria can also spread from orbital (Fig. 2.7), oral or dental infections [7, 16, 25, 31, 33, 37, 39, 40]. One of our patients developed an occipital osteomyelitis 3 weeks following a dental procedure [41].

The cranial vault is more commonly involved than the skull base. Skull base osteomyelitis is rare, mainly seen in ear, nose, and throat (ENT) practice following ear and mastoid infections (Fig. 2.8) or secondary to sphenoidal sinusitis [42–46] (Fig. 2.9). The patients often are elderly or immunocompromised or have microvascular disease such as diabetes [3, 4]. The invasive form of malignant external otitis, an otitis-associated skull base infection, remains the most frequent appearance [47]. Rothholtz and colleagues (otolaryngologists) from California, have published their experience with skull base osteomyelitis. They found a remarkable higher number of cases than previously reported articles: 820 patients over an 11-year period from 1990 to 2000. The male to female ratio was nearly 1:1. Over 90 % of the patients were over the age of 25 and 38 % of the patients were over the age of 65 years. With respect to race, the white population (69.3 %) was more likely to present with the disease than Native American (13.2 %), African American

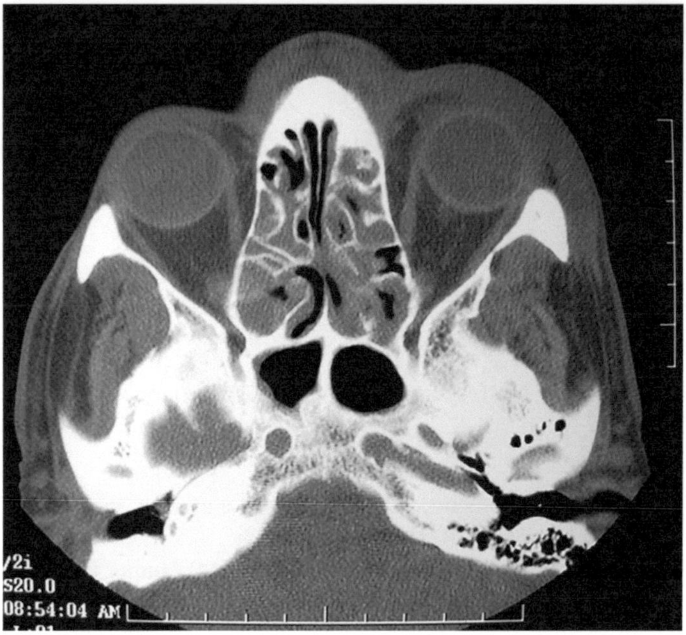

Fig. 2.4 Axial CT-scan in bone windows with bilateral ethmoiditis

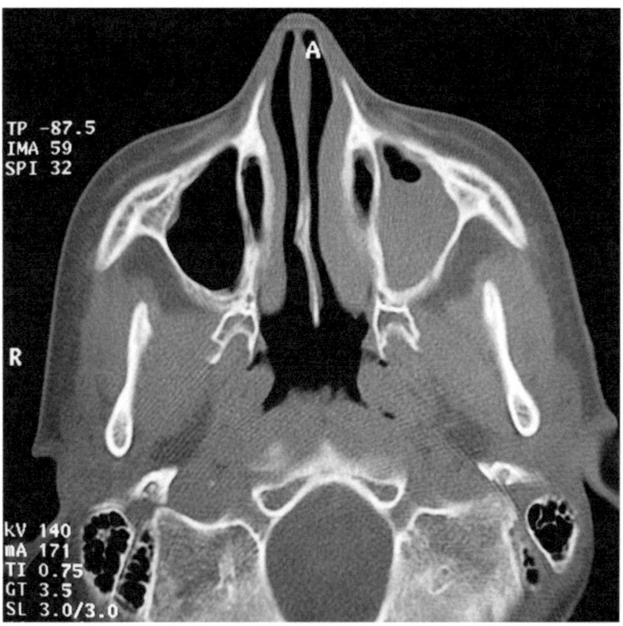

Fig. 2.5 Bone-windows axial CT-scan showing left maxillary sinusitis

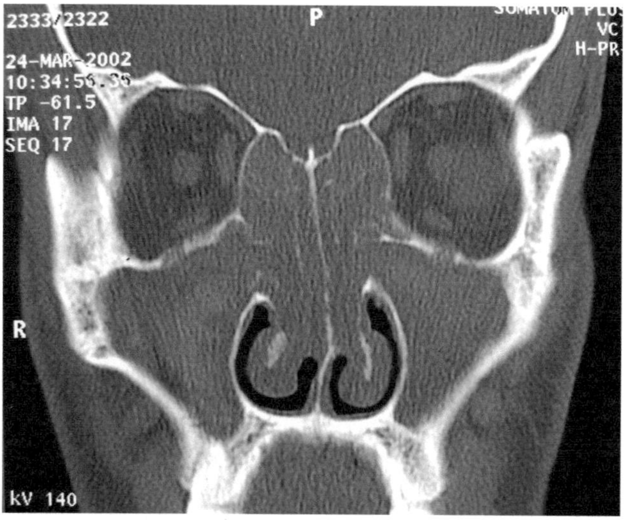

Fig. 2.6 Coronal reconstructions CT-scan in bone windows demonstrating bilateral paranasal pansinusitis

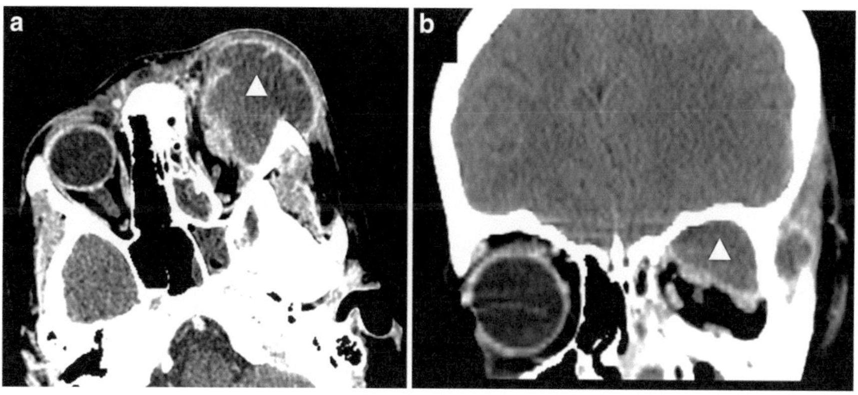

Fig. 2.7 Axial (**a**) and coronal reconstructions (**b**) CT-scan after contrast injection showing a left orbital abscess (*triangle*). Note adjacent sinusitis in the ethmoid cells and sphenoidal sinus

(6.5 %), or Asian (2.9 %) descent [3]. In contrast, only 12 cases were identified in a single department of ENT in New Zealand from 2004 to 2011 [6]. A prospective study in India from 2001 to 2008 found 20 patients with temporal bone osteomyelitis. The most common age-group affected was the 40–60 years (65 % of cases) without sex predilection. Interestingly, there were two sets of identical twin girls of 2 and 3 years of age respectively [5]. A systematic review of case series of central skull base osteomyelitis unrelated to otologic infection from 1946 to 2013 found 42 cases with mean age of 52 years and male female ratio of 2.2 to 1 [4].

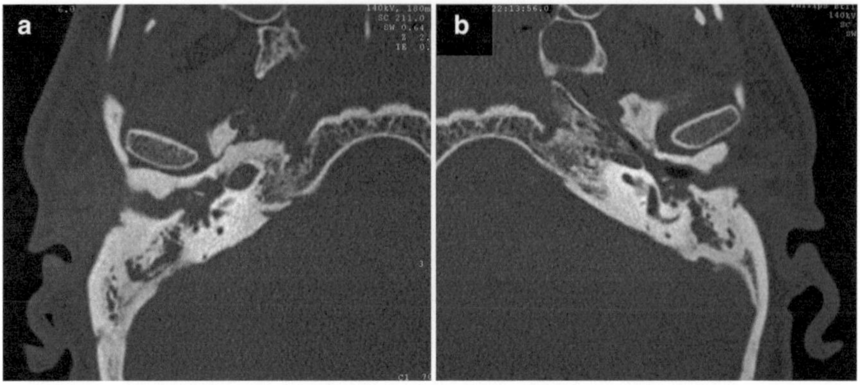

Fig. 2.8 Axial CT-scan in bone windows demonstrating bilateral (**a**, **b**) chronic otomastoiditis

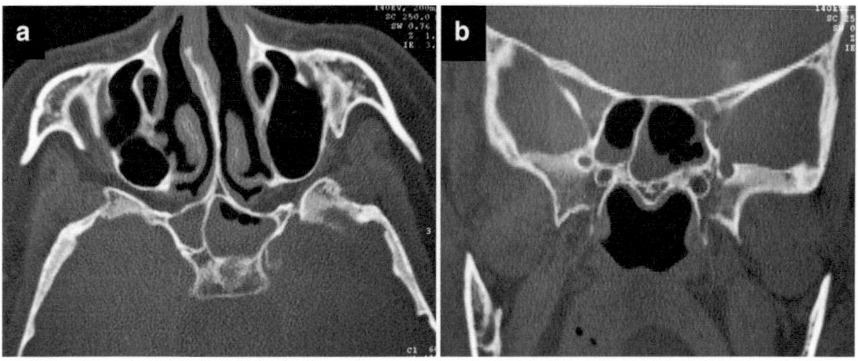

Fig. 2.9 Axial (**a**) and coronal reconstructions (**b**) CT-scan in bone windows showing bilateral sphenoidal sinusitis

As seen above, the epidemiology of temporal bone osteomyelitis, which is classically a part of skull base osteomyelitis, was changed in the last decade. In the past, it was predominantly seen in elderly diabetic and immunocompromised patients with history of episodic otitis externa in the months prior to presentation. In contrast with the typical features, several atypical cases have been reported more recently. Often a source of infection is not found and patients were younger and previously healthy [4, 48]. Paranasal sinuses and hematological spread from distant sites of infection are considered possible sources.

The scalp is a rare site for suppuration. The risk of its infection stems from its proximity to the skull and the possibility of spreading disease. Non healing ulcerations and chronic sinus tracts should be suspected of harboring infection. Previous scalp lesions over the skull can lead to osteomyelitis. Major causes include any spontaneous scalp infections [49, 50] (Fig. 2.10) as well as carbuncle, scalp abscess [51–53] (Fig. 2.11), scalp pressure ulcer [54] (Fig. 2.12), nasal dermal sinus tract

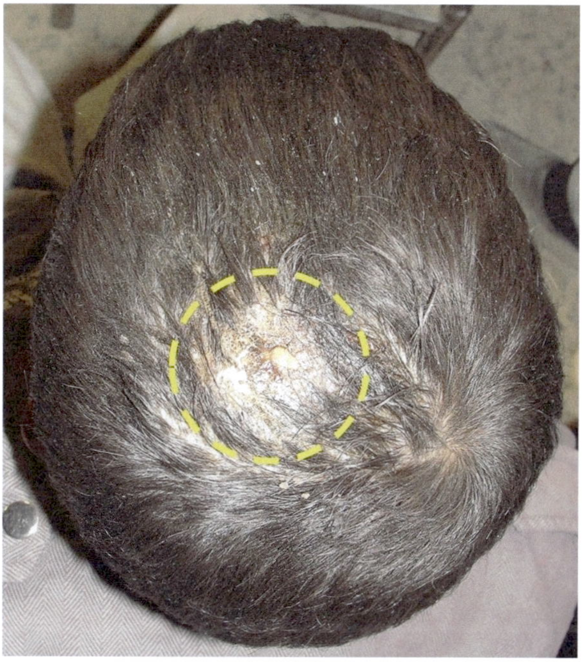

Fig. 2.10 Spontaneous scalp abscess near the vertex

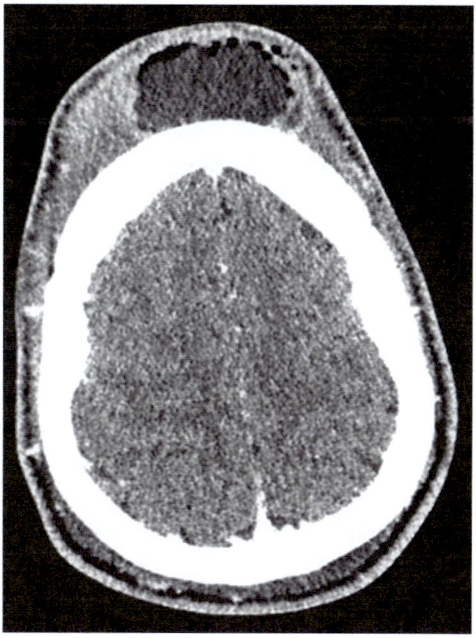

Fig. 2.11 Important subperiosteal frontal extracranial abscess. Air may be seen within the collection

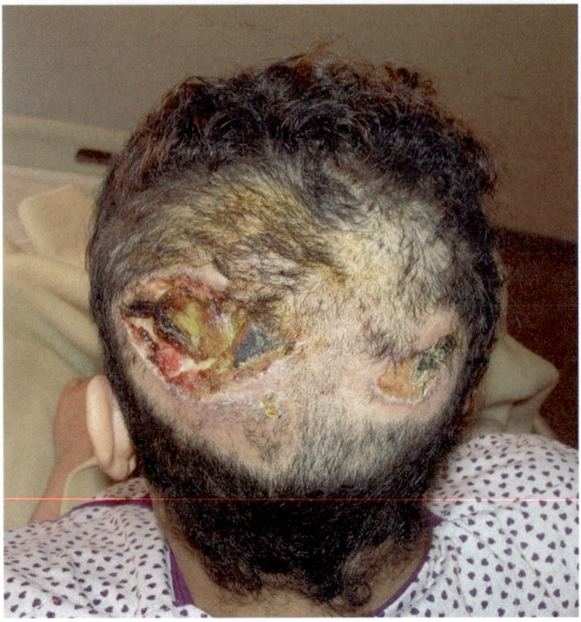

Fig. 2.12 Bilateral chronic parieto-occipital non-healing scalp pressure ulcer

[55], facial cellulitis [56, 57] (Fig. 2.13), scalp necrotizing fasciitis [58] and more rarely epidermal necrolysis of the scalp [59]. Interestingly, a 5-month-old girl was previously reported with 1 cm right parietal bone osteomyelitis under a pox lesion of the scalp related to varicella infection [60].

Postoperative or Secondary to Direct Trauma

According to the criteria of the Centers for Disease Control [61], a surgical site infection (SSI) was considered in the presence of one of the following cases: a purulent discharge from the wound, a serous discharge with positive bacterial culture, a deep or superficial wound abscess with or without positive bacterial culture, wound swelling and erythema with or without pyrexia, or meningitis/ventriculitis with positive bacterial culture or microorganisms seen on the Gram's stain, occurring within 30 days of the surgical procedure. More specifically, a superficial incisional SSI in the scalp was defined as having a purulent discharge or cutaneous dehiscence with positive microbiological testing. A deep incisional SSI, such as osteitis or discitis, was diagnosed on the basis of a positive computed tomographic or magnetic resonance imaging scans associated with or without positive microbiological testing; an organ/space SSI, such as a brain abscess, was determined by both magnetic resonance imaging and computed tomography parenchymal alteration, which was surgically verified and confirmed by histological or microbiological testing. Meningitis was diagnosed by a positive cerebrospinal fluid

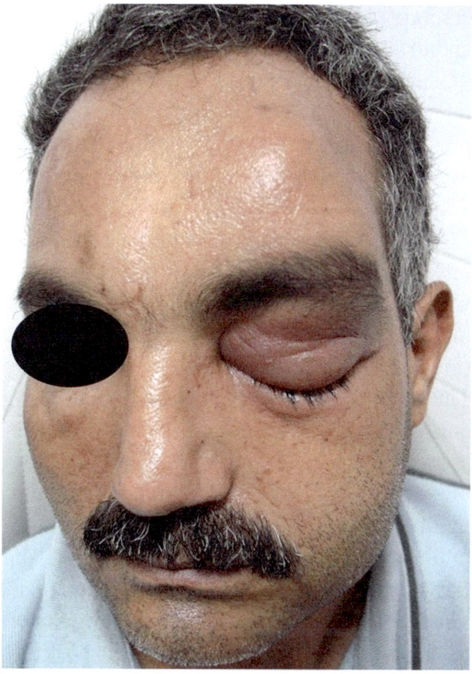

Fig. 2.13 Left frontal swelling with orbito-facial cellulitis on the same side (with the patient's signed permission)

stain or culture or the alteration of cytochemical parameters [62]. In 2008, these criteria were modified in a minor fashion [63].

Despite improvements in prevention, surgical site infections remain a significant clinical problem as they are associated with major source of morbidity and mortality. The primary site of inflammation after a central nervous system (CNS) infection is the choroid plexus, in which about 100,000 bacterial organisms per gram of tissue are needed to produce a postoperative CNS infection [64]. It's well known that postoperative infections represent an important contributor to the cost of care (long hospital stays and costly interventions) and a true frustrating problem for clinicians. The cost for SSI after craniotomy was estimated by O'Keeffe and colleagues to be over £9000 for each case of infection [65]. For Broex et al., healthcare costs for a patient with SSI are, on average, approximately twice the amount of costs for a patient without an SSI [66].

The incidence of SSI in cranial neurosurgery is reported between the range of 0–17.6 % (average rate of around 5 %), depending on the surgical procedure, the surveillance criteria used, and the quality of data collection [10, 62, 65, 67–75]. Interestingly, the infection rates before and after 1940 are nearly the same [75]. Generally, depth of SSI is classified as subgaleal, bone, epidural, subdural, and/or intracerebral. A given layer was considered infected if there was gross purulent material in that layer intraoperatively or if cultures taken from that layer were positive [76]. A variety of risks factors for SSI have been reported and debated in neurosurgery as well as: duration of surgery (longer than 4 h), presence of cerebrospinal fluid leak (which provides a portal of access to deeper wound layers and increase complications from infection), reoperation (especially for glioma), type of surgery (craniofacial, emergency and dirty surgeries carry a greater risk of infection), method of surgery (craniotomy or craniectomy), type of tumor (especially meningioma) method of wound closure (staples or sutures) prior radiation therapy, use of invasive devices and immunosuppression of the patient [10, 14, 62, 69, 70, 75, 77].

The incidence of post-surgical cranial osteomyelitis is often not reported separately from other deep neurosurgical infections and may be considered together with scalp infection, extradural abscess and subdural empyema. Bone flap osteomyelitis after craniotomy is relatively unusual accounting for about a fifth of SSI (mean of 21.2 %) but this incidence can vary greatly from 0 to 60.8 % (Table 2.2). The rarity of this complication demands high case numbers to permit conclusive analysis beyond anecdotal case reports. In this setting, cranial osteomyelitis is more common in adult population than in children. The age of distribution of patients is older than that of sinusitis-related cranial osteomyelitis, reflecting the greater number of older patients requiring cranial surgery. Few recent data have been published. The incidence of postsurgical skull osteomyelitis reported in the literature ranges from 0 to 3.1 % with a mean of 1.2 % (Table 2.2). Surgery with implants like cranioplasty and bone flap fixating material has to be followed up for 12 months in order to rule out infection because of the long latency period for some chronic bone flap infection. One of our patients presented with a suppurative acrylic cranioplasty, exposure of implant, and proximate parietal cranial osteomyelitis 11 years following a craniotomy for an acute subdural hematoma (Fig. 2.14). Another 52-year-old woman was operated 25 years ago for a frontal tuberculoma with cranioplasty (methylmethacrylate). She developed a secondary suppurative denuded cranioplasty with contiguous cranial osteomyelitis (please see chap. 10 for more details about this case report). Blumenkopf et al. reported a 17-year-old man with infected cranioplasty and adjacent skull osteomyelitis revealing by purulent drainage from scalp sinus tract. These complications have occurred 10 years after cranioplasty and ventriculoperitoneal shunt following a brain abscess surgical exploration and post-meningitic hydrocephalus [78]. Even, without implants, bone flap osteomyelitis may occur several years after the first surgery. In 2001, Karabatsou et al. reported a patient with a Pott's puffy tumor manifesting itself 13 years after a hemispherectomy for intractable seizures [79]. Wilson et al. described a case of skull osteomyelitis 24 years after an intracerebral hematoma evacuation secondary to an arteriovenous malformation [80]. Recently, Levitt et al. reported a patient with an asymptomatic postoperative osteomyelitis occurring 23 years after initial craniotomy. The rarity of postoperative cranial osteomyelitis has been attributed to the vascularity of the cranial vault and the preventive efficacy of perioperative antibiotics [81]. However, for some authors, the true efficacy of prophylactic antibiotics remains controversial [62, 67, 69, 73]. Postoperative cranial wound dehiscence may induce bone flap osteomyelitis and several factors may contribute to this complication including a history of prior scalp irradiation, neoadjuvant of postoperative chemotherapy, development of a cerebrospinal fluid

Table 2.2 Incidence of postoperative cranial osteomyelitis in more recently published studies

Authors [reference number]	Year of publication	Country	Time of data collection	Number of patients with CS	Incidence of SSI (number of patients)	Incidence of cranial osteomyelitis relative to patients with CS (number of patients)	Incidence of cranial osteomyelitis relative to patients with SSI
Rasmussen et al. [73]	1990	Denmark	3 years	202	n/a	6.4 % (13)[a]	n/a
Whitby et al. [67]	2000	Australia	2 years	613	2.4 % (15)	0	0
Idali et al. [68]	2004	Morocco	2003	170	17.6 % (30)	1.1 % (2)	6.6 %
Korinek et al. [69]	2005	French	May 1997–2001	4578	6.6 % (303)	1.7 % (77)	25.4 %
McClelland and Hall. [70]	2007	USA	Feb 1991–2005	1587	0.8 % (14)	0	0
Dashti et al. [71]	2008	USA	1997–2007	16,540	0.3 % (50)	0.1 % (22)	44 %
Syrmos et al. [72]	2009	Greece	2006–2008	155	14.8 % (33)	2.5 % (4)	12.1 %
Abu Hamdeh et al. [10]	2014	Sweden	2010	448	4.5 % at 3 months (20) 5.1 % at 12 months (23)	3.1 % (14)	60.8 %

[a]Prophylactic antibiotics were not administered
n/a no data available, *CS* cranial surgery

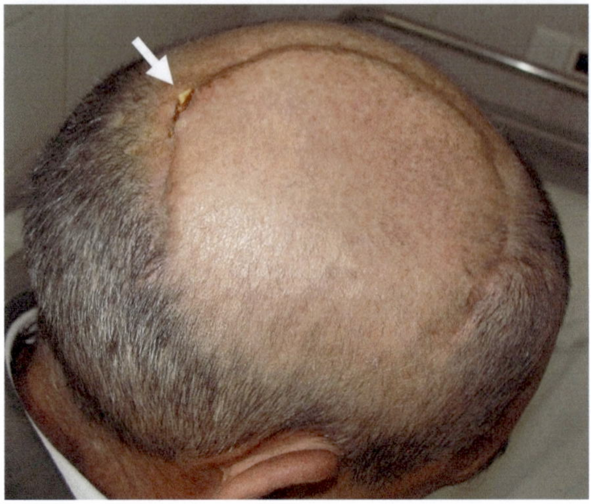

Fig. 2.14 This patient was operated 11 years ago for an acute subdural hematoma with methylmethacrylate cranioplasty. Acrylic plate become exposed over time and infected with contiguous cranial osteomyelitis

leak, and/or an anterior ablative defect. Bone flaps that include part of a sinus wall (particularly the frontal sinus) are especially susceptible to developing bone flap infection [82]. Recently, published reports suggest that the incidence of wound-healing complications was higher in patients who underwent surgery after initiating bevacizumab (Avastin*) treatment compared with those who underwent surgery alone [83, 84]. Gliadel wafers also significantly increased the risk of SSI after procedures to treat tumors [85].

The association between cranial osteomyelitis and other intracranial infections (parameningeal empyemas or brain abscess) is a well known situation [11, 14, 86, 87]. In our series of 13 patients with a postoperative osteomyelitis (4 patients had a primary craniotomy at an outside institution), bone flap osteomyelitis was seen alone (4 cases) or in combination with extradural empyema (6 cases), brain abscess (1 case) or both (2 cases). A wound purulent discharge was seen in 4 patients. Two patients had an osteomyelitis secondary to a polymethylmethacrylate cranioplasty. Interestingly, one of our patients presented with slowly progressive headache, fever, increasing tenderness, warmth and swelling at the initial surgical site 2 months after temporal craniotomy for arterio-venous fistula. Postoperative computed tomography scan and magnetic resonance imaging revealed an aspect of bone flap osteomyelitis with underlying epidural abscess. The infection was likely due to epidural cotton mistakenly left behind during operation [88] (Fig. 2.15). From 1996 to 2000, Larsson et al. treated 31 consecutive patients with postoperative bone flap infections at the Karolinska Hospital of Stockholm (Sweden). Among them, 6 had an acrylic flap [14]. Recently, Abou Hamdeh et al. identified 14 of 448 patients (3.1 %) as having bone flap infection. Postoperative osteomyelitis was seen alone in 6 cases and in conjunction with a brain abscess in 5 additional cases. Bone flap osteomyelitis and subdural empyema were seen together in 2 cases. One patient had bone flap osteomyelitis, brain abscess and meningitis. Osteomyelitis after cranial reconstruction was seen in three patients (synthetic bone substitute in one case and

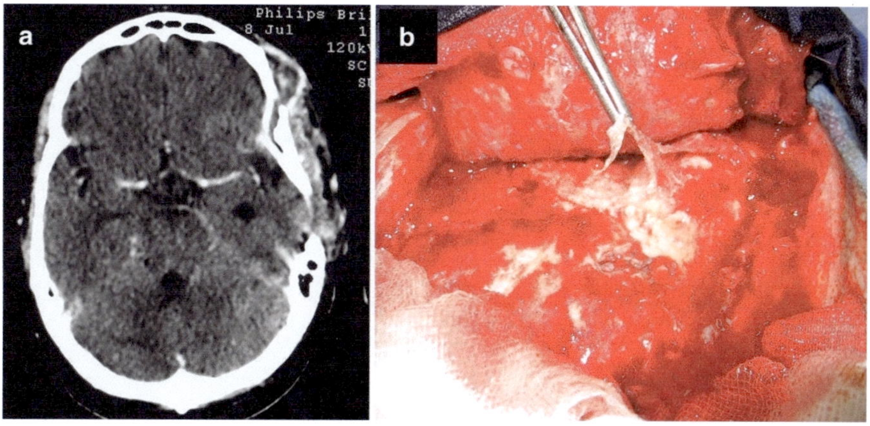

Fig. 2.15 Postoperative computed tomography scan, axial section after contrast injection revealing left epidural abscess with frontal extracranial collection (**a**). Operative view after bone flap removal (**b**). The infection was likely due to epidural cotton left behind during surgical time

on cryo-preserved bone flap in two cases) [10]. In addition, Bhaskar et al. found 5 patients with cranial osteomyelitis among 179 autogenous bone cranioplasties (infection rate of 2.8 %) [89].

True skull base osteomyelitis has been described as occurring after surgical interventions at the site of infection [90, 91]. Ridder et al. described a series of 12 patients including middle ear surgery with mastoidectomy (58 %), operations on the external auditory canal (18 %), cochlear implant (8 %) and an otologic operation of unknown type (8 %). The mean time between the first surgery and diagnosis of skull base osteomyelitis was 44.2 months (ranged from 1 to 456 months, median 2 months) [92]. An interesting case of skull base osteomyelitis that presented 4–8 weeks after a maxillectomy for a plexiform ameloblastoma of the right posterior maxilla was previously reported [93].

Direct injuries are well recorded situations when they occur: in the newborn following infection of a cephalhematoma (particularly after vaccum extraction) [52, 94, 95], secondary to craniofacial injuries with or without fractures [22, 96–98] (Fig. 2.16), penetrating craniocerebral injury [99] (Fig. 2.17), after burns to the scalp or electrical injuries [100–102] (Fig. 2.18), following scalp wound/laceration [103–106] (Fig. 2.19) or traumatic scalp hematoma [107], in patients with sickle cell disease [108, 109], as a complication of halo traction [110–112] and secondary to hear transplantation [113]. War wounds tend to be more extensive and contaminated than civilian wounds [114]. The result from poorer wound healing leads to a propensity for infection. Unfortunately, minor trauma with small scalp wounds are usually ignored, and these may result in serious infections [115]. Many cases of skull osteomyelitis were reported secondary to minor scalp wounds such as human bite [15], scalp laceration [116], insect bite [59], acupuncture [117], needle insertion [118] or self-inflected dermatitis [119]. Onoue et al. presented an interesting case of cranial osteomyelitis after head injury with exaggeration and remission for

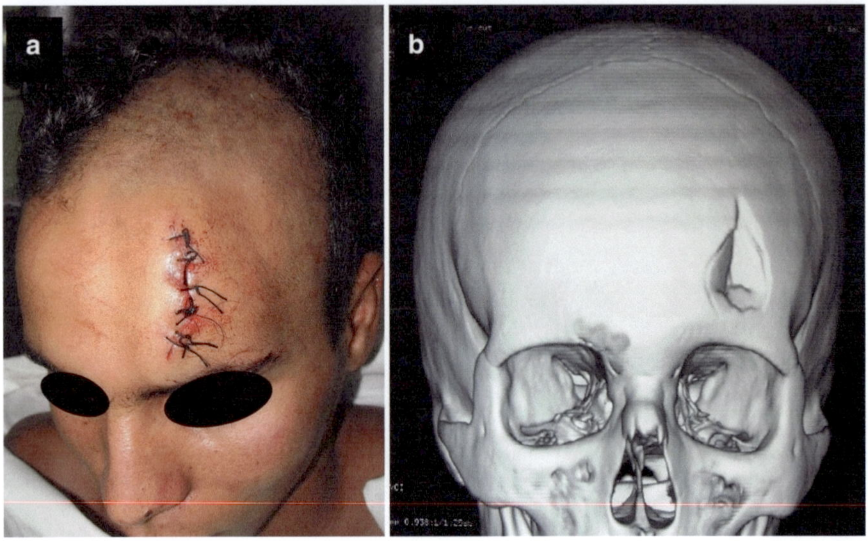

Fig. 2.16 Post-traumatic frontal wound (**a**) with underlying depressed bone fracture on 3-dimensional CT-scan reconstruction (reformatted volume-rendered) (**b**)

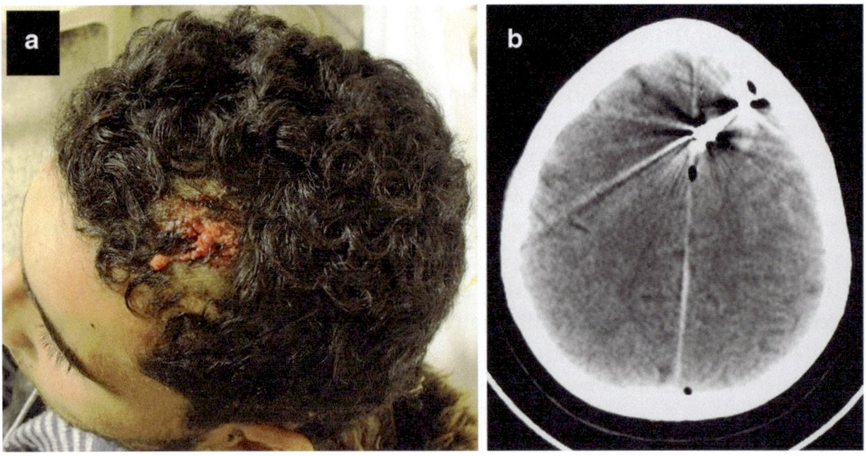

Fig. 2.17 Penetrating craniocerebral injury (open head injury). Note extracranial extrusion of brain matter on the left frontal area (**a**). Axial CT-scan showing multiple intracranial metallic foreign bodies (**b**)

30 years. The mechanism by which osteomyelitis continued over a long course of time was suspected to be the formation of a focus of recurrent inflammation due to the initial head injury [120]. Also, many authors suggest that head injury contributes to the apparent increase in prevalence of Pott's puffy tumor [117, 121–123].

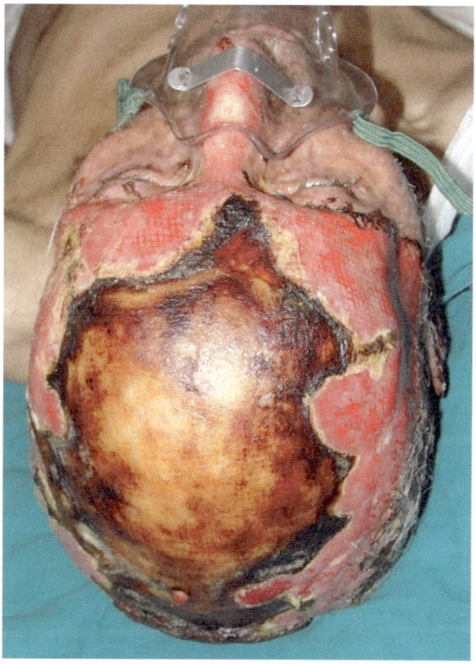

Fig. 2.18 This patient was electrocuted with high tension wire. Picture showing large scalp defect during dressing change. Note frontal and parietal cranial bones exposed with burn eschar

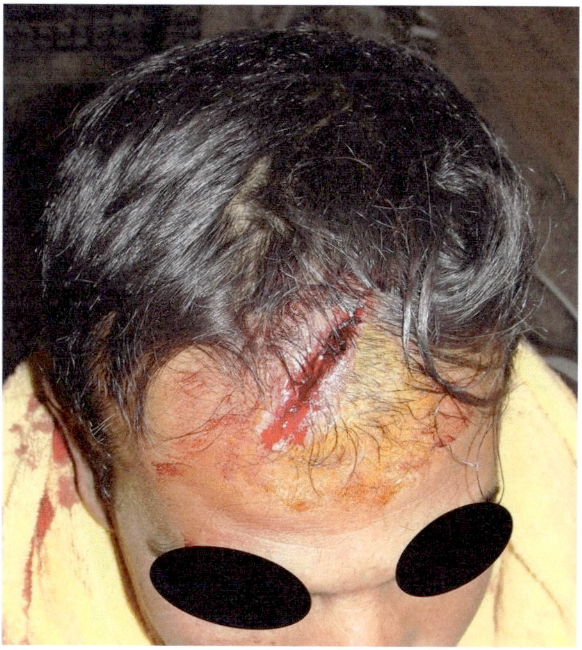

Fig. 2.19 Direct frontal injury with lacerated wound in the forehead

Hematogenous Spread Secondary to Bacteremia or Fungemia

There have been occasional case reports of hematogenous osteomyelitis of the skull [17, 23, 25, 46, 124–126], several large series of osteomyelitis reported by otolaryngologists and neurosurgeons have not mentioned such cases [3, 6, 17, 50]. This most often occurs when the patient has an infection elsewhere in the body that spreads through the blood to the skull bone. Camargo et al. reported a case of *Aspergillus spp.* osteomyelitis of the lumbar spine complicated with right orbital apex syndrome due to orbital and sphenoid wing involvement. They suspected a potential role of the Batson's vascular plexus in disease propagation [23]. Until now, few other anecdotal cases were reported especially with salmonella, secondary syphilis and coccidiodomycosis agents [127–129]. However, the cause of infection may remain cryptogenic in spite of all the investigations [129]. To explain this phenomenon, Prasad et al. suggest that in the first stage an unrecognized infection, or a small focus of infection, heals. By the time, the secondary infection develops and spreads [130]. Interestingly, many cases manifested with septicemia and meningitis especially in children with cephalhematoma were described [95, 131]. In 1991, Yocum and Seligson reported a case of septic arthritis of the knee and osteomyelitis of the skull vault following arthroscopy. The patient had a concomitant cavitary lung lesion caused by Blastomycosis [24]. Recently, Hayashi et al. reported a patient with recurrent meningitis complicated by osteomyelitis of the clivus. They supposed that the septicemia resulted in a secondary septic pulmonary embolism and meningitis and that inflammation had extended to the base of the skull due to the meningitis [25]. In contrast to other hematogenous osteomyelitis of the skeleton, multifocal osteomyelitis is rare in the head.

Comorbidities

In addition to these three principal key sources, some comorbidities or patient-related risk factors should be taken into consideration [3, 49, 59, 70] (Table 2.3). These include vulnerability due to metabolic states (as diabetes mellitus),

Table 2.3 Comorbidities and underlying conditions in skull osteomyelitis

Systemic comorbidity	Local detriment
Obesity and malnutrition Diabetes mellitus Renal or hepatic failure Chronic hypoxia Compromised immune function Malignancy Long period of hospitalization Extremes of age Tobacco abuse	Extensive scarring Radiation fibrosis Small vessel disease Heavy contamination Presence of foreign body Bone necrosis

unbalanced nutritional states (obesity and malnutrition), smoking and tobacco use, specific exposure risks (prolonged preoperative stay, colonization with *Staphylococcus aureus*), compromised immune function (defective immune system, human immunodeficiency virus infection, use of immunosuppressive medications or chronic systemic corticosteroids, irradiation of the head), malignancy, hemodialysis and age (especially newborn and advanced age).

References

1. Peltola H, Pääkkönen M. Acute osteomyelitis in children. N Engl J Med. 2014;370 (4):352–60. doi:10.1056/NEJMra1213956.
2. Waldvogel FA, Medoff G, Swartz MN. Osteomyelitis: a review of clinical features, therapeutic considerations and unusual aspects. N Engl J Med. 1970;282(4):198–206.
3. Rothholtz VS, Lee AD, Shamloo B, Bazargan M, Pan D, Djalilian HR. Skull base osteomyelitis: the effect of comorbid disease on hospitalization. Laryngoscope. 2008;118 (11):1917–24.
4. Johnson AK, Batra PS. Central skull base osteomyelitis: an emerging clinical entity. Laryngoscope. 2014;124(5):1083–7.
5. Prasad SC, Prasad KC, Kumar A, Thada ND, Rao P, Chalasani S. Osteomyelitis of the temporal bone: terminology, diagnosis, and management. J Neurol Surg B Skull Base. 2014;75(5):324–31.
6. Spielmann PM, Yu R, Neeff M. Skull base osteomyelitis: current microbiology and management. J Laryngol Otol. 2013;127 Suppl 1:S8–12.
7. Nisa L, Landis BN, Giger R. Orbital involvement in Pott's puffy tumor: a systematic review of published cases. Am J Rhinol Allergy. 2012;26(2):e63–70. doi:10.2500/ajra.2012.26.3746.
8. Prasad KC, Prasad SC, Mouli N, Agarwal S. Osteomyelitis in the head and neck. Acta Otolaryngol. 2007;127(2):194–205.
9. Szychowski JM, Talbot TR, Daniels T, McGee T. A multidisciplinary intervention to reduce post-craniotomy surgical site infection rates. Am J Infect Control. 2011;39(5):E35–6.
10. Abu Hamdeh S, Lytsy B, Ronne-Engström E. Surgical site infections in standard neurosurgery procedures—a study of incidence, impact and potential risk factors. Br J Neurosurg. 2014;28(2):270–5. doi:10.3109/02688697.2013.835376.
11. Nisbet M, Briggs S, Ellis-Pegler R, Thomas M, Holland D. Propionibacterium acnes: an under-appreciated cause of post-neurosurgical infection. J Antimicrob Chemother. 2007;60 (5):1097–103.
12. Garin A, Thierry B, Leboulanger N, Blauwblomme T, Grevent D, Blanot S, Garabedian N, Couloigner V. Pediatric sinogenic epidural and subdural empyema: the role of endoscopic sinus surgery. Int J Pediatr Otorhinolaryngol. 2015;79(10):1752–60. doi:10.1016/j.ijporl.2015.08.007.
13. Blumfield E, Misra M. Pott's puffy tumor, intracranial, and orbital complications as the initial presentation of sinusitis in healthy adolescents, a case series. Emerg Radiol. 2011;18 (3):203–10. doi:10.1007/s10140-010-0934-3.
14. Larsson A, Engström M, Uusijärvi J, Kihlström L, Lind F, Mathiesen T. Hyperbaric oxygen treatment of postoperative neurosurgical infections. Neurosurgery. 2002;50(2):287–95.
15. Phillips NI, Robertson IJ. Osteomyelitis of the skull vault from a human bite. Br J Neurosurg. 1997;11(2):168–9.
16. Tomovic S, Friedel ME, Liu JK, Eloy JA. Community-acquired methicillin-resistant Staphylococcus aureus skull base osteomyelitis with occipital condylar cerebrospinal fluid leak in an immunocompetent patient. Laryngoscope. 2012;122(5):977–81. doi:10.1002/lary.23253.

17. Wilensky AO. Osteomyelitis of the skull. Arch Surg. 1933;27(1):83–158.
18. Osei-Yeboah C, Neequaye J, Bulley H, Darkwa A. Osteomyelitis of the frontal bone. Ghana Med J. 2007;41(2):88–90.
19. Patankar T, Varma R, Krishnan A, Prasad S, Desai K, Castillo M. Radiographic findings in the tuberculosis of the calvarium. Neuroradiology. 2000;42:518–21.
20. Ali AM, Maya E, Lakhoo K. Challenges in managing paediatric osteomyelitis in the developing world: analysis of cases presenting to a tertiary referral centre in Tanzania. Afr J Paediatr Surg. 2014;11(4):308–11.
21. Nathoo N, Nadvi SS, Gouws E, van Dellen JR. Craniotomy improves outcomes for cranial subdural empyemas: computed tomography-era experience with 699 patients. Neurosurgery. 2001;49(4):872–7.
22. Jung SH, Aniceto GS, Rodríguez IZ, Diaz RG, Recuero II. Posttraumatic frontal bone osteomyelitis. Craniomaxillofac Trauma Reconstr. 2009;2(2):61–6. doi:10.1055/s-0029-1202594.
23. Camargo JF, Seriburi V, Tenner M, El Khoury MY. Aspergillus osteomyelitis of the lumbar spine complicated with orbital apex syndrome: a potential role of the Batson's plexus in disease propagation. Med Mycol Case Rep. 2012;1(1):9–12. doi:10.1016/j.mmcr.2012.02.004.
24. Yocum J, Seligson D. Blastomycosis of the knee and skull after arthroscopy. Am J Sports Med. 1991;19(6):670–2.
25. Hayashi T, Uchiumi H, Yanagisawa K, Ogawa Y, Handa H, Tsukamoto N, Nojima Y. Recurrent Gemella haemolysans meningitis in a patient with osteomyelitis of the clivus. Intern Med. 2013;52(18):2145–7.
26. DeVries S. Metastatic epidural bacterial abscess in a 4-year-old boy. JAMA Neurol. 2013;70 (5):648–9. doi:10.1001/jamaneurol.2013.1942.
27. Kaplan R. Neurologic complications of infections of the head and neck. Otolaryngol Clin North Am. 1976;9:729–49.
28. Gallagher RM, Gross CW, Phillips CD. Suppurative intracranial complications of sinusitis. Laryngoscope. 1998;108(11 Pt 1):1635–42.
29. Oxford LE, McClay J. Complications of acute sinusitis in children. Otolaryngol Head Neck Surg. 2005;133(1):32–7.
30. Ali A, Kurien M, Mathews SS, Mathew J. Complications of acute infective rhinosinusitis: experience from a developing country. Singapore Med J. 2005;46(10):540–4.
31. Clayman GL, Adams GL, Paugh DR, Koopmann Jr CF. Intracranial complications of paranasal sinusitis: a combined institutional review. Laryngoscope. 1991;101(3):234–9.
32. Kombogiorgas D, Solanki GA. The Pott puffy tumor revisited: neurosurgical implications of this unforgotten entity. Case report and review of the literature. J Neurosurg. 2006;105 (2 Suppl):143–9.
33. Shama SA. Osteomyelitis of the central skull base: otogenic and odontogenic sources. Multidetector CT study. Egypt J Radiol Nuc Med. 2012;43:519–26.
34. Ketenci I, Unlü Y, Tucer B, Vural A. The Pott's puffy tumor: a dangerous sign for intracranial complications. Eur Arch Otorhinolaryngol. 2011;268(12):1755–63. doi:10.1007/s00405-011-1660-5.
35. Bambakidis NC, Cohen AR. Intracranial complications of frontal sinusitis in children: Pott's puffy tumor revisited. Pediatr Neurosurg. 2001;35(2):82–9.
36. Salomão JF, Cervante TP, Bellas AR, Boechat MC, Pone SM, Pone MV, de A Pereira B. Neurosurgical implications of Pott's puffy tumor in children and adolescents. Childs Nerv Syst. 2014;30(9):1527–34. doi:10.1007/s00381-014-2480-x.
37. Adams JR, Bryant DG. Cranial osteomyelitis: a late complication of a dental infection. Br J Oral Maxillofac Surg. 2008;46(8):673–4. doi:10.1016/j.bjoms.2008.03.025.
38. Suwan PT, Mogal S, Chaudhary S. Pott's puffy tumor: an uncommon clinical entity. Case Rep Pediatr. 2012;2012:386104. doi:10.1155/2012/386104.
39. Chandy B, Todd J, Stucker FJ, Nathan CO. Pott's puffy tumor and epidural abscess arising from dental sepsis: a case report. Laryngoscope. 2001;111(10):1732–4.

40. Calayatud-Perez V, Trull Gimbernat JM, González LJ. Parietal osteomyelitis of dental origin: a case report. J Craniomaxillofac Surg. 1993;21(3):127–9.
41. Akhaddar A, El Mostarchid B, Gazzaz M, Boucetta M. Cerebellar abscess due to Lactococcus lactis. A new pathogen. Acta Neurochir (Wien). 2002;144(3):305–6.
42. Niv A, Nash M, Slovik Y, Fliss DM, Kaplan D, Leibovitz E, Katz A, Dagan R, Leiberman A. Acute mastoiditis in infancy: the Soroka experience: 1990–2000. Int J Pediatr Otorhinolaryngol. 2004;68(11):1435–9.
43. Laurens MB, Becker RM, Johnson JK, Wolf JS, Kotloff KL. MRSA with progression from otitis media and sphenoid sinusitis to clival osteomyelitis, pachymeningitis and abducens nerve palsy in an immunocompetent 10-year-old patient. Int J Pediatr Otorhinolaryngol. 2008;72(7):945–51. doi:10.1016/j.ijporl.2008.02.025.
44. Hoistad DL, Duvall 3rd AJ. Sinusitis with contiguous abscess involvement of the clivus and petrous apices. Case report. Ann Otol Rhinol Laryngol. 1999;108(5):463–6.
45. Devireddy SK, Kumar RVK, Gali R, Kanubaddy SR, Dasari MR, Akheel M. Mucormycotic skull base osteomyelitis: a case report. J Oral Maxillofac Surg Med Pathol. 2014;26 (3):336–9.
46. Soga Y, Oka K, Sato M, Kabata T, Kawasaki T, Kawano H, Hayano M. Cavernous sinus thrombophlebitis caused by sphenoid sinusitis—report of autopsy case. Clin Neuropathol. 2001;20(3):101–5.
47. Chen JC, Yeh CF, Shiao AS, Tu TY. Temporal bone osteomyelitis: the relationship with malignant otitis externa, the diagnostic dilemma, and changing trends. ScientificWorldJournal. 2014;2014:591714. doi:10.1155/2014/591714.
48. Ganhewa AD, Jafri KJ. A diagnostic dilemma of central skull base osteomyelitis mimicking neoplasia in a diabetic patient. BMJ Case Rep. 2013;2013:bcr2012007183. doi:10.1136/bcr-2012-007183.
49. Rerolle JP, Szelag JC, Diaconita M, Paraf F, Aldigier JC, Le Meur Y. Intracranial granuloma and skull osteolysis: complication of a primary cutaneous cryptococcosis in a kidney transplant recipient. Am J Kidney Dis. 2005;46(6):e113–7.
50. Haines SJ, Chou SN. Infections of the scalp and osteomyelitis of the skull. In: Wilkins RH, Rengachary SS, editors. Neurosurgery. New York: McGraw-Hill; 1985.
51. Nugent NF, Murphy M, Kelly J. Scalp abscess—a cautionary tale. J Plast Reconstr Aesthet Surg. 2010;63(8):e619–21. doi:10.1016/j.bjps.2010.02.011.
52. Chang HY, Cheng KS, Liu YP, Hung HF, Fu HW. Neonatal infected subgaleal hematoma: an unusual complication of early-onset E. coli sepsis. Pediatr Neonatol. 2015;56(2):126–8. doi:10.1016/j.pedneo.2013.03.003.
53. Ramasastry SS, Granick MS, Boyd JB, Futrell JW. Severe perifolliculitis capitis with osteomyelitis. Ann Plast Surg. 1987;18(3):241–4.
54. Holliday DY. Occipital lesions: a possible cost of cradleboards. Am J Phys Anthropol. 1993;90(3):283–90.
55. Rao M, Steele RW, Ward KJ. A "hickey". Epidural brain abscess, osteomyelitis of the frontal bone, and subcutaneous abscess (pott puffy tumor). Clin Pediatr (Phila). 2003;42(7):657–60.
56. Lamoreau KP, Fanciullo LM. Pott's puffy tumour mimicking preseptal cellulitis. Clin Exp Optom. 2008;91(4):400–2. doi:10.1111/j.1444-0938.2007.00234.x.
57. Raja V, Low C, Sastry A, Moriarty B. Pott's puffy tumor following an insect bite. J Postgrad Med. 2007;53(2):114–6.
58. Yuen JC, Puri SK, Feng Z. Scalp necrotizing fasciitis with osteomyelitis of the skull from Aspergillus. J Craniofac Surg. 2002;13(6):762–4.
59. Levitt MR, Benedict WJ, Barton K, Melian E, Gamelli RL, Vandevender D, Rosseau G, Prabhu VC. Management of scalp toxic epidermal necrolysis and cranial osteomyelitis with serratus anterior myocutaneous pedicle flap: a case report. J Burn Care Res. 2007;28 (3):524–9.
60. Gallagher PG. Osteomyelitis of the skull after varicella infection. Clin Pediatr (Phila). 1990;29(1):29.

61. Horan TC, Gaynes RP, Martone WJ, Jarvis WR, Emori TG. CDC definitions of nosocomial surgical site infections, 1992: a modification of CDC definitions of surgical wound infections. Am J Infect Control. 1992;20(5):271–4.
62. Valentini LG, Casali C, Chatenoud L, Chiaffarino F, Uberti-Foppa C, Broggi G. Surgical site infections after elective neurosurgery: a survey of 1747 patients. Neurosurgery. 2008;62 (1):88–95. doi:10.1227/01.NEU.0000311065.95496.C5.
63. Horan TC, Andrus M, Dudeck MA. CDC/NHSN surveillance definition of health care-associated infection and criteria for specific types of infections in the acute care setting. Am J Infect Control. 2008;36(5):309–32. doi:10.1016/j.ajic.2008.03.002.
64. Borges LF. Infections in neurologic surgery: host defenses. Neurosurg Clin N Am. 1992;3 (2):275–8.
65. O'Keeffe AB, Lawrence T, Bojanic S. Oxford craniotomy infections database: a cost analysis of craniotomy infection. Br J Neurosurg. 2012;26(2):265–9. doi:10.3109/02688697.2011.626878.
66. Broex EC, van Asselt AD, Bruggeman CA, van Tiel FH. Surgical site infections: how high are the costs? J Hosp Infect. 2009;72(3):193–201. doi:10.1016/j.jhin.2009.03.020.
67. Whitby M, Johnson BC, Atkinson RL, Stuart G. The comparative efficacy of intravenous cefotaxime and trimethoprim/sulfamethoxazole in preventing infection after neurosurgery: a prospective, randomized study. Brisbane Neurosurgical Infection Group. Br J Neurosurg. 2000;14(1):13–8.
68. Idali B, Lahyat B, Khaleq K, Ibahioin K, El Azhari A, Barrou L. Postoperative infection following craniotomy in adults. Med Mal Infect. 2004;34(5):221–4. French.
69. Korinek AM, Golmard JL, Elcheick A, Bismuth R, van Effenterre R, Coriat P, Puybasset L. Risk factors for neurosurgical site infections after craniotomy: a critical reappraisal of antibiotic prophylaxis on 4,578 patients. Br J Neurosurg. 2005;19(2):155–62.
70. McClelland 3rd S, Hall WA. Postoperative central nervous system infection: incidence and associated factors in 2111 neurosurgical procedures. Clin Infect Dis. 2007;45(1):55–9.
71. Dashti SR, Baharvahdat H, Spetzler RF, Sauvageau E, Chang SW, Stiefel MF, Park MS, Bambakidis NC. Operative intracranial infection following craniotomy. Neurosurg Focus. 2008;24(6):E10. doi:10.3171/FOC/2008/24/6/E10.
72. Syrmos N, Patiakas S, Iliadis C, Grigoriou K, Valadakis V, Chatzinasiou F, Arvanitakis D. Craniotomy infections: the Venizeleio hospital experience. Ann Gen Psychiatry. 2010;9 Suppl 1:S98.
73. Rasmussen S, Ohrström JK, Westergaard L, Kosteljanetz M. Post-operative infections of osteoplastic compared with free bone flaps. Br J Neurosurg. 1990;4(6):493–5.
74. Delgado-López PD, Martín-Velasco V, Castilla-Díez JM, Galacho-Harriero AM, Rodríguez-Salazar A. Preservation of bone flap after craniotomy infection. Neurocirugia (Astur). 2009;20(2):124–31.
75. Lal S, McCutcheon IE. Infections after craniotomy. In: Hall WA, McCutcheon IA, editors. Infections in neurosurgery. Park Ridge, IL: American Association of Neurological Surgeons Publications; 2000.
76. Kshettry VR, Hardy S, Weil RJ, Angelov L, Barnett GH. Immediate titanium cranioplasty after debridement and craniectomy for postcraniotomy surgical site infection. Neurosurgery. 2012;70(1 Suppl Operative):8–14. doi:10.1227/NEU.0b013e31822fef2c.
77. Bruce JN, Bruce SS. Preservation of bone flaps in patients with postcraniotomy infections. J Neurosurg. 2003;98(6):1203–7.
78. Blumenkopf B, Hartshorne MF, Bauman JM, Cawthon MA, Patton JA, Friedman AH. Craniotomy flap osteomyelitis: a diagnostic approach. J Neurosurg. 1987;66(1):96–101.
79. Karabatsou K, Gan YC, Christie M, Sakas D. Pott's puffy tumour: a delayed complication of surgery. Br J Neurosurg. 2001;15(5):441–2.
80. Wilson IF, Candia GJ, Worthington MG, Sullivan JG. Chronic osteomyelitis due to corynebacteria in a postcraniotomy bone flap. Clin Infect Dis. 1999;28(6):1323–4.

81. Levitt MR, Gabikian P, Pottinger PS, Silbergeld DL. Propionibacterium acnes osteomyelitis occurring 23 years after craniotomy: case report and review of literature. Neurosurgery. 2011;69(3):E773–9. doi:10.1227/NEU.0b013e31821964ba.
82. Nibu K, Sasaki T, Kawahara N, Sugasawa M, Nakatsuka T, Yamada A. Complications of craniofacial surgery for tumors involving the anterior cranial base. Neurosurgery. 1998;42 (3):455–61.
83. Editorial Board of Plastic and Reconstructive Surgery. Management of a complex scalp defect. Plast Reconstr Surg. 2008;122(2):623–5. doi:10.1097/PRS.0b013e31817d7f91.
84. Scappaticci FA, Fehrenbacher L, Cartwright T, Hainsworth JD, Heim W, Berlin J, Kabbinavar F, Novotny W, Sarkar S, Hurwitz H. Surgical wound healing complications in metastatic colorectal cancer patients treated with bevacizumab. J Surg Oncol. 2005;91 (3):173–80.
85. Chiang HY, Steelman VM, Pottinger JM, Schlueter AJ, Diekema DJ, Greenlee JD, Howard III MA, Herwaldt LA. Clinical significance of positive cranial bone flap cultures and associated risk of surgical site infection after craniotomies or craniectomies. J Neurosurg. 2011;114(6):1746–54. doi:10.3171/2011.1.JNS10782.
86. Hlavin ML, Kaminski HJ, Fenstermaker RA, White RJ. Intracranial suppuration: a modern decade of postoperative subdural empyema and epidural abscess. Neurosurgery. 1994;34 (6):974–80.
87. Eisenstein VW, Friedman ED, Davison C. Brain abscess of uncommon origin. Relation to osteomyelitis of the skull: a clinicopathologic study. Ann Surg. 1942;115(3):336–55.
88. Akhaddar A, Boulahroud O, Naama O, Al-Bouzidi A, Boucetta M. Paraspinal textiloma after posterior lumbar surgery: a wolf in sheep's clothing. World Neurosurg. 2012;77(2):375–80. doi:10.1016/j.wneu.2011.07.017.
89. Bhaskar IP, Inglis TJ, Lee GY. Clinical, radiological, and microbiological profile of patients with autogenous cranioplasty infections. World Neurosurg. 2014;82(3–4):e531–4. doi:10.1016/j.wneu.2013.01.013.
90. Kim CW, Lee JJ, Kim HS, Won JY. Skull base osteomyelitis following a mastoidectomy. Auris Nasus Larynx. 2013;40(6):584–6. doi:10.1016/j.anl.2012.12.002.
91. Patel SK, McPartlin DW, Philpott JM, Abramovich S. A case of malignant otitis externa following mastoidectomy. J Laryngol Otol. 1999;113:1095–7.
92. Ridder GJ, Breunig C, Kaminsky J, Pfeiffer J. Central skull base osteomyelitis: new insights and implications for diagnosis and treatment. Eur Arch Otorhinolaryngol. 2015;272 (5):1269–76. doi:10.1007/s00405-014-3390-y.
93. Barber AJ, Hanlon R, Rogers SN. Skull base osteomyelitis after maxillectomy: a rare complication. Br J Oral Maxillofac Surg. 2009;47(4):310–2. doi:10.1016/j.bjoms.2009.01.010.
94. Vale B, Morais S, Resende C, Taborda A. Neonatal meningitis associated with osteomyelitis and epidural empyema. BMJ Case Rep. 2013;2013:pii: bcr2013009149. doi:10.1136/bcr-2013-009149.
95. Nakwan N, Nakwan N, Wannaro J, Dissaneevate P, Kritsaneepaiboon S, Chokephaibulkit K. Septicemia, meningitis, and skull osteomyelitis complicating infected cephalhematoma caused by ESBL-producing Escherichia coli. Southeast Asian J Trop Med Public Health. 2011;42(1):148–51.
96. Metzinger SE, Guerra AB, Garcia RE. Frontal sinus fractures: management guidelines. Facial Plast Surg. 2005;21(3):199–206.
97. Parida PK, Surianarayanan G, Ganeshan S, Saxena SK. Pott's puffy tumor in pediatric age group: a retrospective study. Int J Pediatr Otorhinolaryngol. 2012;76(9):1274–7. doi:10.1016/j.ijporl.2012.05.018.
98. Avasthi G, Parti A, Gupta SN, Goel R. Frontal bone osteomyelitis causing recurrent meningitis. J Assoc Physicians India. 1991;39(5):409–10.
99. Domingo Z, Peter JC, de Villiers JC. Low-velocity penetrating craniocerebral injury in childhood. Pediatr Neurosurg. 1994;21(1):45–9.

100. Rockwell WB, Bodily KD. Fate of free muscle transfer covering chronically infected burned skull. J Burn Care Rehabil. 2001;22(4):288–91.
101. Chen J, Yan H, Peng Y, Li X, Hu J, Wu J. Three-dimensional reconstruction of computed tomography scan images for estimating skull damage in electrical burned patients. Int J Low Extrem Wounds. 2012;11(3):157–60.
102. Lu Y, Cen Y, Qing Y, Wang H. Surgical treatment of chronic osteomyelitis of the skull. Zhongguo Xiu Fu Chong Jian Wai Ke Za Zhi. 2011;25(5):558–61. Chinese.
103. Fortún J, Cobo J, Cañal J, Martínez-San MJ. Post-traumatic cranial mucormycosis in an immunocompetent patient. J Oral Maxillofac Surg. 1995;53(9):1099–102.
104. Rodríguez-Hernández MJ, Jiménez-Mejías ME, Montero JM, Regordan C, Ferreras G. Aspergillus fumigatus cranial infection after accidental traumatism. Eur J Clin Microbiol Infect Dis. 2001;20(9):655–6.
105. Kulkarni V, Rajshekhar V. Chronic non-healing ulcers of the scalp after trauma. Postgrad Med J. 2000;76(897):437, 450–1.
106. Valerón-Almazán P, Gómez-Duaso AJ, Rivero P, Vilar J, Dehesa L, Santana N, Carretero G. Extensive, non-healing scalp ulcer associated with trauma-induced chronic osteomyelitis. Ann Dermatol. 2011;23 Suppl 3:S364–7. doi:10.5021/ad.2011.23.S3.S364.
107. Tutela JP, Banta JC, Boyd TG, Kelishadi SS, Chowdhry S, Little JA. Scalp reconstruction: a review of the literature and a unique case of total craniectomy in an adult with osteomyelitis of the skull. Eplasty. 2014;14:e27. eCollection 2014.
108. Saito N, Nadgir RN, Flower EN, Sakai O. Clinical and radiologic manifestations of sickle cell disease in the head and neck. Radiographics. 2010;30(4):1021–34. doi:10.1148/rg.304095171.
109. Emejulu JC, Ekweogwu OC. Complicated Pott's puffy tumour involving both frontal and parietal bones: a case report. J Infect Dis Ther. 2014;2(5):166.
110. Niazi T, Quinoñes-Hinojosa A, Schmidt MH. Management of brain abscesses associated with halo fixation. Neurosurg Focus. 2008;24(6):E14. doi:10.3171/FOC/2008/24/6/E14.
111. Garfin SR, Botte MJ, Triggs KJ, Nickel VL. Subdural abscess associated with halo-pin traction. J Bone Joint Surg Am. 1988;70(9):1338–40.
112. Uppal HS, Issa F, Byren I, Johnson D. A case of pancalvarial osteomyelitis: diagnosis and management. J Plast Reconstr Aesthet Surg. 2010;63(2):e159–60. doi:10.1016/j.bjps.2009.05.015.
113. Jones JW, Ignelzi RJ, Frank DH, Blacklock JB. Osteomyelitis of the skull following scalp reduction and hair plug transplantation. Ann Plast Surg. 1980;5(6):480–2.
114. Margorin EM. Cranium osteomyelitis following gun shot. Voen Med Zh. 1946;(1–2):10–21.
115. Goodman SJ, Cahan L, Chow AW. Subgaleal abscess: a preventable complication of scalp trauma. West J Med. 1977;127:169–72.
116. Pickering SA, Ashpole RD, Wallace ME, Paul SH. Osteomyelitis of calvarium after trivial scalp laceration. J Accid Emerg Med. 1998;15(6):430.
117. Tsai BY, Lin KL, Lin TY, Chiu CH, Lee WJ, Hsia SH, Wu CT, Wang HS. Pott's puffy tumor in children. Childs Nerv Syst. 2010;26(1):53–60. doi:10.1007/s00381-009-0954-z.
118. McGregor JA, McFarren T. Neonatal cranial osteomyelitis: a complication of fetal monitoring. Obstet Gynecol. 1989;73(3 Pt 2):490–2.
119. Riffaud L, Morandi X. Osteomyelitis of the skull vault induced by self-inflicted dermatitis of the scalp. Acta Neurochir (Wien). 2001;143(7):737–8.
120. Onoue S, Matsubara I, Nishizaki O, Kumon Y, Sakaki S. A case of cranial osteomyelitis after head injury with exaggeration and remission for thirty years. No Shinkei Geka. 1997;25(6):543–7. Japanese.
121. Gross T, Kaim AH, Regazzoni P, Widmer AF. Current concepts in posttraumatic osteomyelitis: a diagnostic challenge with new imaging options. J Trauma. 2002;52(6):1210–9.
122. Tudor RB, Carson JP, Pulliam MW, Hill A. Pott's puffy tumor, frontal sinusitis, frontal bone osteomyelitis, and epidural abscess secondary to a wrestling injury. Am J Sports Med. 1981;9(6):390–1.

123. Martinez-Diaz GJ, Hsia R. Pott's puffy tumor after minor head trauma. Am J Emerg Med. 2008;26(6):739.e1–3. doi:10.1016/j.ajem.2007.11.038.
124. Qiu Y, Zhang J, Liu G, Zhong X, Deng J, He Z, Jing B. Retrospective analysis of 14 cases of disseminated Penicillium marneffei infection with osteolytic lesions. BMC Infect Dis. 2015;15:47. doi:10.1186/s12879-015-0782-6.
125. Morris BS, Varma R, Garg A, Awasthi M, Maheshwari M. Multifocal musculoskeletal tuberculosis in children: appearances on computed tomography. Skeletal Radiol. 2002;31 (1):1–8.
126. Panos GZ, Karydis I, Velakoulis SE, Falagas ME. Multi-skeletal Pneumocystis jiroveci (carinii) in an HIV-seropositive patient. Int J STD AIDS. 2007;18(2):134–7.
127. Baddley JW, Cobbs CS, Pappas PG. Surgical treatment of multiple skull abscesses associated with coccidioidomycosis. Mycoses. 2004;47(1–2):69–71.
128. Senegor M, Lewis HP. Salmonella osteomyelitis of the skull base. Surg Neurol. 1991;36 (1):37–9.
129. Park KH, Lee MS, Hong IK, Sung JY, Choi SH, Park SO, Shin MJ, Chung HW, Lee SH. Bone involvement in secondary syphilis: a case report and systematic review of the literature. Sex Transm Dis. 2014;41(9):532–7. doi:10.1097/OLQ.0000000000000164.
130. Prasad A, Madan VS, Suri ML, Buxi TB. Cryptogenic osteomyelitis of the skull and intracerebral abscess. Childs Nerv Syst. 1992;8(3):142–3.
131. Blom NA, Vreede WB. Infected cephalhematomas associated with osteomyelitis, sepsis and meningitis. Pediatr Infect Dis J. 1993;12(12):1015–7.

Chapter 3
Different Pathogens Involved

Contents

Abbreviations

AFB Acid fast bacillus
MRSA Methicillin resistant *Staphylococcus aureus*

Collection and Sample Processing

The correct collection and transport of specimens is critical for the isolation, identification, and characterization of microorganisms that cause skull osteomyelitis. Pus, bone and debrided material should be sent for histopathological and for routine microbiological studies including aerobic and anaerobic bacteria, acid-fast bacillus (AFB) and fungal culture as well as sensitivity testing. In order to avoid loss of viability of the etiological agents, clinical specimens should be obtained before administration of antimicrobial therapy. However, in daily practice, many cases of cranial osteomyelitis have already been pre-treated with antibiotics by the referring physician. It is also important to collect as much material as possible from fluid, purulent material and tissue specimens (Figs. 3.1 and 3.2). However, bacterial cultures should be obtained using tissue specimens rather than swabs. Additionally, cultures from the sinus tracts may be misleading because of contamination with bacteria or fungi from skin. Ideally, both culture and histological examination should be done together and transported to the laboratories as soon as possible (Fig. 3.3). The possibility of polymicrobial infections with a mixture of aerobic and

A. Akhaddar, *Cranial Osteomyelitis*, DOI 10.1007/978-3-319-30268-3_3

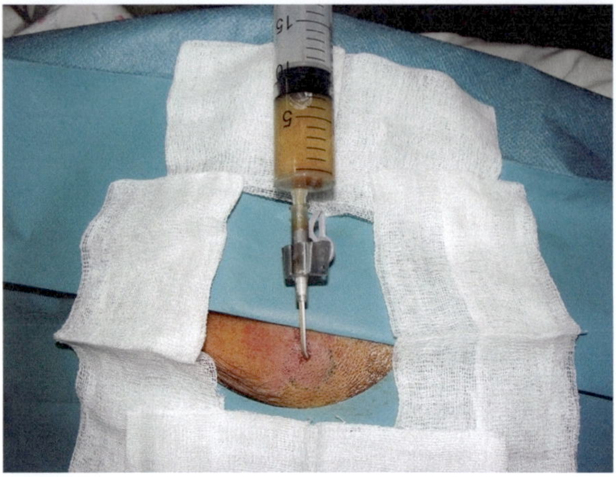

Fig. 3.1 Percutaneous collection of extracranial purulent fluid

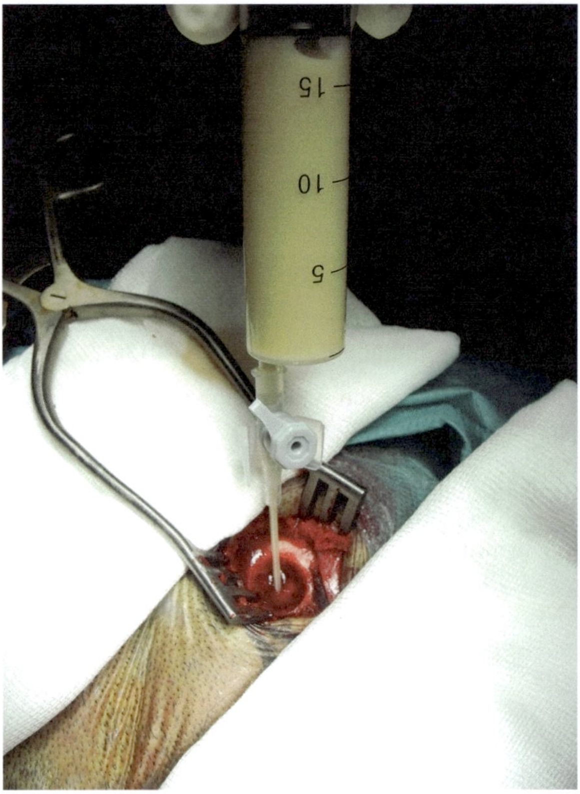

Fig. 3.2 Operative view. A thick yellowish green pus drained from the subdural space through a burr hole craniotomy

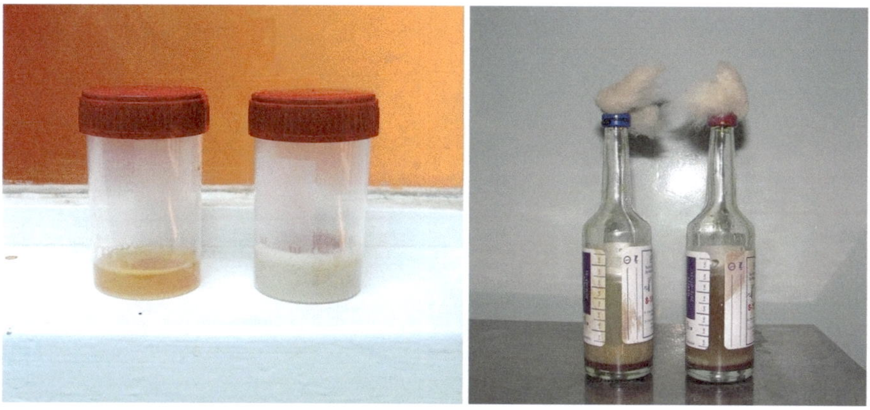

Fig. 3.3 Samples and purulent material are collected and transported to the laboratories as soon as possible in dedicated collection tubes (*left*) and/or adapted transport medium (*right*)

anaerobic organisms must be always taken in consideration [1–3]. In the same way, associations between bacteria and fungi are also possible [4–6] as well as mycobacteria and pyogenic bacteria [7, 8]. For this reason, special anaerobic and fungi transport must be used without introducing air during direct injection of liquid samples. Properly Gram-stained preparation and analysis is a simple and fast method to give preliminary information to the clinicians. Anyway, specially suspected bacteria, fungi or parasites must be communicated to the laboratory. After isolation and identification of microorganisms (Fig. 3.4), antimicrobial susceptibility testing is performed in vitro to predict in vivo success or failure of antibiotic therapy (Fig. 3.5). Small colony variants of bacteria must be taken into account. These slow-growing subpopulations of bacteria have distinctive phenotypic and pathogenic traits. Phenotypically, small colony variants have a slow growth rate, atypical colony morphology and unusual biochemical characteristics, making them a challenge for clinical microbiologists to identify. Clinically, small colony variants are better able to persist in mammalian cells and are less susceptible to antibiotics than their wild-type counterparts, and can cause latent or recurrent infections on emergence from the protective environment of the host cell [9, 10].

The results of antimicrobial susceptibility testing should be combined with clinical information and experience when selecting the most appropriate antibiotic for the patient. With this in mind, clinicians and biologists must work together closely.

Pathogens in Cranial Osteomyelitis

The skull may be infected by various microorganisms, including non-specific and specific bacteria (Fig. 3.6), fungi (Fig. 3.7), and parasites (Fig. 3.8). These causative agents vary according to age of onset, pathogenesis (spread from an otorhinogenic

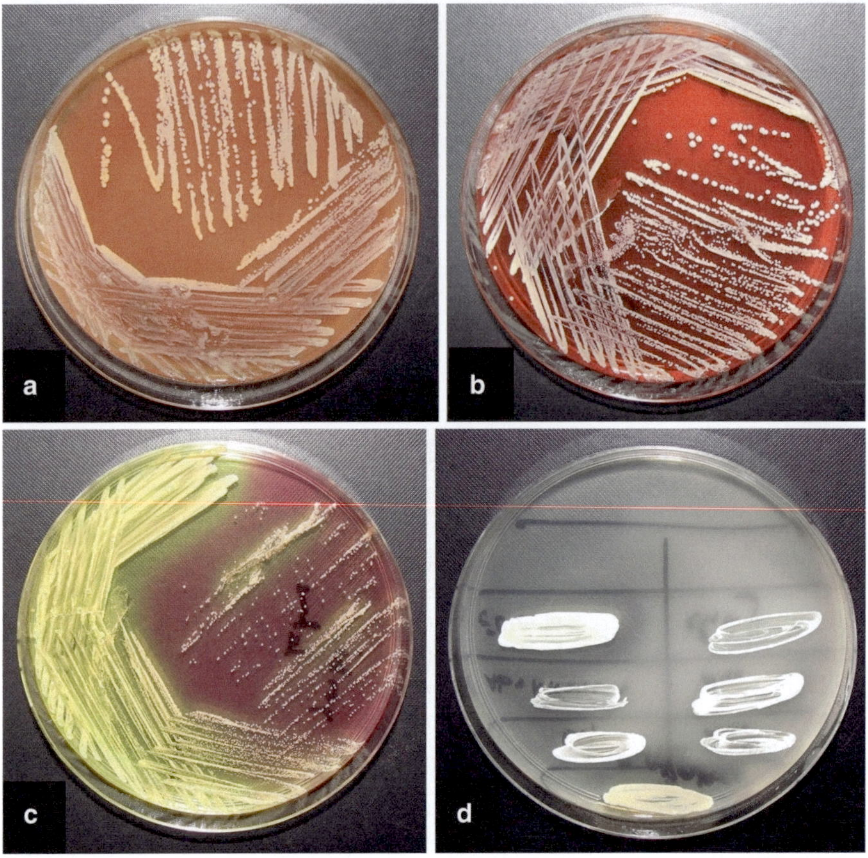

Fig. 3.4 Culture of colonies of *Staphylococcus aureus* on chocolate agar + PolyViteX (**a**), blood agar (**b**), mannitol salt agar (Chapman medium) (**c**), and on DNAse agar (**d**) of a per-surgical bone sample from a patient with osteomyelitis

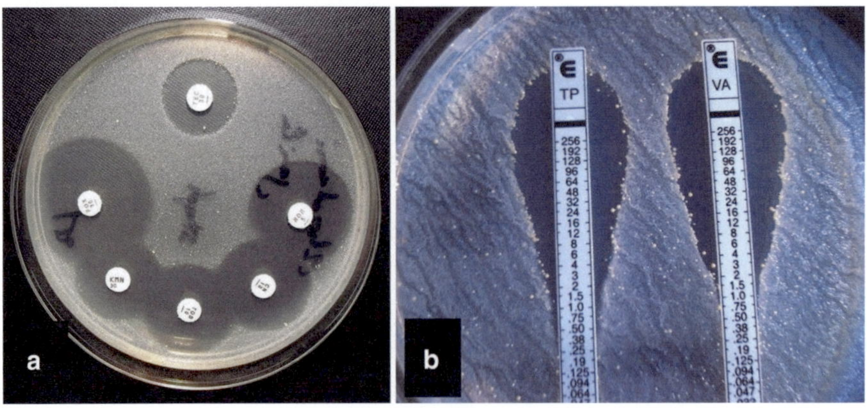

Fig. 3.5 Antibiogram of *Staphylococcus aureus* on Mueller-Hinton agar (**a**). E-test (Epsilometer test) on *Staphylococcus aureus* for teicoplanin (*left*) and vancomycin (*right*) (**b**)

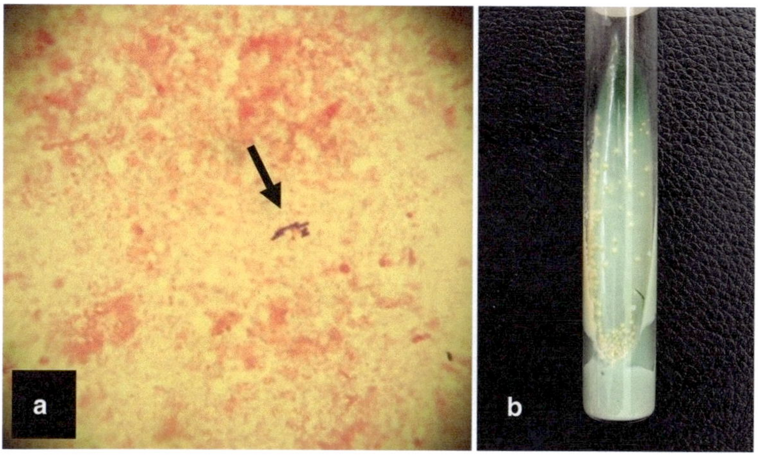

Fig. 3.6 Positive Acid Fast Bacilli (AFB) smear results following Zeil-Neelsen staining (**a**). Formation of *Mycobacterium tuberculosis* colonies on Löwenstein-Jensen medium (**b**)

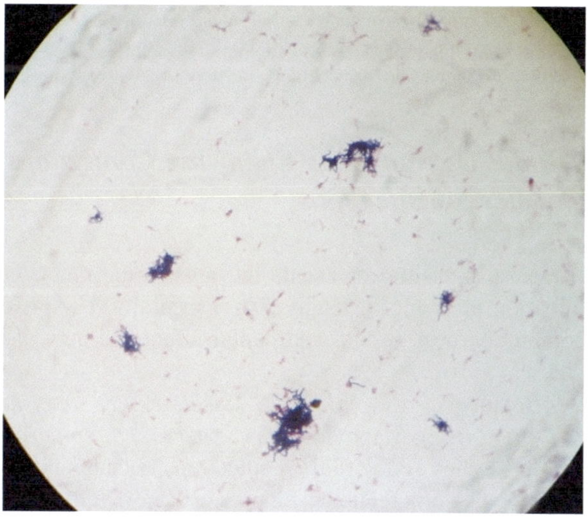

Fig. 3.7 Gram-positive filamentous branching bacillary forms consistent with *Actinomyces species*

disease, contiguous source following head injuries or cranial surgeries, and hematogenous spread), anatomic location (cranial vault, skull base), and underlying medical status. It is important to recognize that many cranial osteomyelitis are polymicrobial and can even contain both anaerobic and aerobic bacteria [2, 5]. Culture-negative cases are not insignificant. Efforts should be undertaken to identify more and more pathogens. The types of microorganisms found within skull bone infections have evolved over the past few decades [11, 12]. For examples, the predominance of *Staphylococcus aureus* has decreased and identification of anaerobes has increased. This is in part due to improvements in the microbiological identifications of microorganisms and the early diagnosis and treatment of skull osteomyelitis.

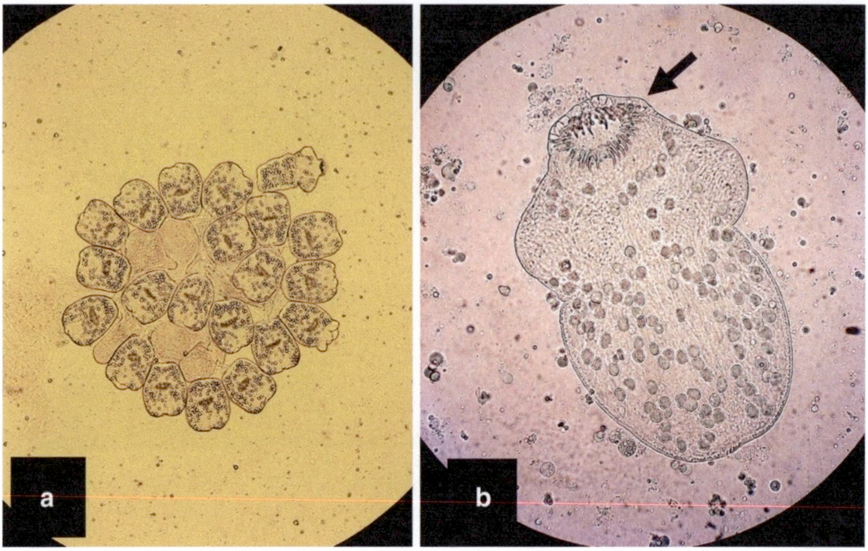

Fig. 3.8 Various protoscoleces being released from a hydatid cyst (**a**). Inside, a line of hooklets is observed, grouped around elongated axis in the superior extremity of the protoscolex and forming a crown (*arrow*) (**b**) (Courtesy of B. Lmimouni MD, Rabat, Morocco)

Cranial Osteomyelitis Following Contiguous Source of Adjacent Infections

Paranasal sinusitis represents the most important contiguous source of adjacent infection in cranial osteomyelitis, especially it is proximity to frontal bone. Less commonly, oral, orbital and dental infections may also spread directly to cranial bones [13–16].

Streptococci (*S. milleri*, *S. viridians*, *S. intermedius*, *S. constellatus* and *S. pneumoniae*), Staphylococci (S. *aureus*, *S. epidermidis* and *S. saccharolyticus*) and anaerobes (Bacteroids, Peptostreptococcus and Fusobacterium) are the most common bacteria related to sinogenic osteomyelitis and reflect the bacterial species responsible for sinusitis (Table 3.1) [17]. Less frequently Gram-negative organisms (such as *Klebsiella pneumoniae* and *Proteus mirabilis*), *Haemophilus influenza*, and *Enterococcus spp*. [18–21]. Anaerobic bacteria may be more common in frontal sinusitis, compared to other ear and nose infections, because of the relatively lower oxygen concentration in the frontal sinus caused by compromised patency of the sinus ostium [22–25]. In addition, when intracranial complications occur, anaerobes are the predominant pathogens [26–28]. Unlike skull base osteomyelitis, the reports of sinogenic frontal osteomyelitis related to *Pseudomonas aeruginosa* infection are scarce [26, 29, 30].

Cultures from patients with Pott's puffy tumor often reveal polymicrobial involvement in up to two-third of the cases in which culture is positive [17, 19,

Table 3.1 Associated source of infection and most common pathogens of cranial osteomyelitis

Source of infection	Common pathogens
Paranasal sinuses	Aerobes: *Streptococcus spp.* *Staphylococcus spp.* *Haemophilus spp.* *Enterobacteriaceae* Anaerobes: *Bacteroids spp.* *Peptostreptococcus spp.* *Fusobacterium spp.*
Otogenic	*Streptococcus spp.* *Staphylococcus spp.* Gram-negative bacteria (*Klebsiella pneumoniae, Proteus mirabilis*) *Enterobacteriaceae* *Bacteroids spp.* *Pseudomonas aeruginosa* (skull base) *Aspergillus spp.* (skull base)
Previous scalp infectious diseases	*Staphylococcus aureus* *Escherichia coli* *Streptococcus spp.* *Proteus mirabilis*
Postneurosurgical Post-traumatic	*Staphylococcus spp.* (*S. aureus, MRSA, coagulase-negative*) *Acinetobacter baumanii* *Enterobacteriaceae* *Streptococcus spp.* (*S. epidermidis*) *Pseudomonas aeruginosa* *Propionibacterium acnes* *Corynebacterium spp.*
Hematogenous spread	Depends on source and immunologic status Usually monomicrobial (bacteria or fungi)
Acquired immune deficiency syndrome	*Salmonella spp.* *Treponema pallidum* *Aspergillus spp.* *Mycobacterium spp.*

28, 31–33]. Sterile cultures were common, probably because most patients received antibiotics before surgery [17].

Until recently involvement of *Staphylococcus aureus* and *Streptococcus species* were still discussed as the major pathogens in cases of sinogenic cranial bone osteomyelitis. More recent studies favor the concept of a polymicrobic infection with several responsible pathogens including anaerobes agents. This change may be explained by modern, sophisticated culture methods, especially involving anaerobic media, which enable identification of possible pathogens more accurately. Consequently, many pathogens, which are mostly found in the healthy oral cavity or skin, have been associated with cases of skull osteomyelitis [13].

Other rare organisms that have been described following oro-odonto-sinogenic source of cranial osteomyelitis are too numerous to list completely, but include *Mycobacterium tuberculosis* [7, 34, 35], *Aspergillus species* [36, 37], *Candida species* [38], *Prevotella species* [39], *Pasteurella multocida* [40, 41], *Burkholderia pseudomallei* (Melioidosis) [42], *Actinomyces species* [43], and *Lactococcus lactis* [13]. These pathogens generally occur in patients with specific risk factors, such as endemic exposure or immunosuppression.

In our experience, cranial osteomyelitis secondary to paranasal sinusitis or odontogenic infection was seen in eight patients. The most frequently isolated pathogen was *Streptococcus species* (37.5 %), followed by *Staphylococcus aureus* (12.5 %), *Peptostreptococcus species* (12.5 %) and *Actinomyces species* (12.5 %). Polymicrobial infections and culture-negative cases account for 12.5 % and 37.5 % of cases, respectively.

Skull base osteomyelitis is principally seen in otorhinolaryngology practice mostly from infections of the external auditory canal and less frequently from sinonasal infections. Classically, *Pseudomonas aeruginosa* is the most common pathogenic microorganism especially in elderly diabetic patients. Less frequently skull base osteomyelitis is attributed to fungal pathogens such as *Aspergillus species* [36, 44, 45]. Malnutrition, malignant disease, immunodeficiency and diabetes mellitus predispose to infection of the base of the skull [46]. In comparison to mastoiditis which commonly seen organisms are *Streptococcus pneumoniae*, *Haemophilus influenza*, *Moraxella (Branhamella) catarrhalis*, *Streptococcus pyogenes*, and *Staphylococcus species* [35].

Pseudomonas aeruginosa is a Gram-negative aerobic bacillus of low virulence which is an uncommon commensal of the external auditory meatus. It causes opportunistic otitis externa following minor trauma or water exposure, but in an immunocompromised host, it can cause coagulative necrosis of soft tissues by production of endotoxin, collagenase and elastase [47, 48]. Classically, Pseudomonas spreads along vascular channels, and for that reason the infection may not be in bony continuity, unlike typical acute mastoiditis, which spreads along pneumatized tracts [49]. International reports of Pseudomonas resistance to fluoroquinolones are currently emerging [50, 51].

In recent literature, a changing is observed in epidemiology and microbiology of skull base osteomyelitis. This affection is not always related to malignant otitis externa and it should be considered in non-diabetic, immunocompetent and older patients. Moreover, Pseudomonas infections seem to be less important than commonly expected [11]. Other infectious organisms such as *Staphylococcus aureus* (with or without methicillin-resistance), *Proteus mirabilis*, *Klebsiella pneumonia*, *Streptococcus milleri*, and *Mycobacterium species* also play an important role in the past decade [11, 35, 49, 52–55]. More rarely, *Enterococcus species*, *Moxarella catarrhalis*, *Haemophilus influenzae*, *Eikenella corrodens*, *Entamoeba coli*, *Corynebacterium jeikeium*, and *Fusobacterium necrophorum* [4, 5, 15, 53, 54].

In human immunodeficiency virus infection and acquired immunodeficiency syndrome presenting with skull base osteomyelitis, multiple species of organisms have been cultured such as *P. aeruginosa*, *S. aureus*, *S. viridans*, *S. pneumoniae*, *Proteus mirabilis*, and *Aspergillus fumigatus* [46, 56, 57] (see also Chap. 15).

Interestingly, a recent study of 42 patients with a central skull base osteomyelitis (unrelated to otologic etiology) found that *Staphylococcus aureus* (21 %) are the most frequent pathogens, followed by *Pseudomonas aeruginosa* (19 %) and *Mycobacterium chelonae* (9.5 %). Overall, 17 % presented with involvement of fungi: *Aspergillus species* (7 %) and *Mucor species* (5 %). Fungal pathogens are mixed to bacteria in two patients (5 %) [58].

In the literature and apart from *Aspergillus species*, other fungi are seen such as Zygomycetes (*Scedosporium species*), *Candida species*, *Rhizopus oryzae* and mucormycosis [4, 5, 44, 53, 59–62].

Osteomyelitis of the temporal bone can be an uncommon complication of acute mastoiditis, which in turn is a complication of acute otitis media. An important fact is that, microbiology of mastoiditis and osteomyelitis are different. Commonly seen agents in mastoiditis are *Streptococcus pneumoniae*, *Haemophilus influenzae*, *Moraxella (Branhamella) catarrhalis*, *Streptococcus pyogenes*, *P. aeruginosa*, and *Staphylococcus spp*. Although, classically and as seen above, osteomyelitis of the temporal bone is predominantly caused by *P. aeruginosa* [63]. Temporal bone osteomyelitis may be caused by fungi following chronic otitis media. Farr et al. reported a patient with a temporal bone osteomyelitis caused by *Blastomyces dermatitidis*, which presented as a chronic serous otitis media. The presenting serous otitis media was refractory to conventional medical and surgical management and progressed to a temporal bone osteomyelitis prior to diagnosis [64].

Among our four patients (13.8 %) with central skull base osteomyelitis, an 11-year-old girl presented with an ethmoidal osteomyelitis associated with an orbital abscess due to *Peptostreptococcus species*. Three men had a sphenoidal osteomyelitis: two had an intrasellar extension but no pathogens were isolated and *Aspergillus terreus* was found in the last patient who presented with intraorbital and intracranial extension.

The scalp is a common location for a variety of infectious diseases. Previous scalp lesions over the skull can direct to osteomyelitis. Classically, *Staphylococcus aureus* is most usually isolated [65–68] among a wide range of organisms including *Escherichia coli* [69], *Streptococcus species* [70, 71] and *Proteus mirabilis* [70]. Unusual organisms, such as *Cryptococcus species* [72] and Actinomycosis [73], are occasionally detected. Additionally, infection may be polymicrobial [70].

Cranial Osteomyelitis Secondary to Direct Inoculation

The most frequent organisms isolated in surgical site infections after neurosurgical procedures are gram-positive cocci, particularly *Staphylococcus aureus*, *Staphylococcus epidermidis* and other Coagulase-Negative Staphylococci indicating contamination from the skin. A variety of other bacteria, such as *Acinitobacter baumanii*, *Enterobacter*, Pneumococcus, *Pseudomonas aeruginosa*, *Propionibacterium acnes* and *Escherichia coli* are also seen less frequently [74–80]. Overall, the spectrum of causative organisms secondary to postoperative cranial osteomyelitis is poorly described. Classically, they do not differ greatly from cutaneous organisms mentioned above. In the prospective analysis by Korinek in 2005, 83 microorganisms were identified in 77 patients with postoperative cranial osteomyelitis. *S. aureus* was most commonly isolated (30 %) followed by *Propionibacterium acnes* (24 %) and coagulase negative staphylococci (23 %). Enterobacteriaceae (12 %) and other Gram positive cocci (1 %) were also recognized. In 10 % of the patients, the cultures remained negative. An alarming frequency of cases (9.6 %) was caused by methicillin-resistant *Staphylococcus aureus* (MRSA) [78]. This major community of nosocomial gram-positive pathogens is problematic because of recalcitrance to antibiotic therapy [77, 81].

In 2002, Larsson et al. reported a series of 31 consecutive patients with postoperative bone flap infections treated with hyperbaric oxygen therapy. The most common organisms isolated were *Staphylococcus aureus* (25.8 %) and *Staphylococcus epidermidis* (19.3 %). Various other microorganisms were also identified, such as *Propionibacterium, Streptococcus milleri, Klebsiella*, and *Corynebacterium* [82].

In general, delayed infections occurring several months after surgery are usually caused by more indolent bacteria such as *Propionibacterium acnes, Corynebacterium* species and *S. epidermidis.*

A decrease in the percentage of *Staphylococcus aureus* osteomyelitis in recent reports is attributable to the use of more sophisticated culture methods that result in more accurate identification of responsible organisms [77, 83, 84]. The previous estimate of anaerobic involvement for all instances of osteomyelitis was <1 %. The number of sterile cultures from many series of patients with osteomyelitis was significant [77, 78]. On the contrary, anaerobes now are associated frequently with aerobic organisms in osteomyelitis, and anaerobic osteomyelitis also may occur alone [12].

Propionibacterium acnes is a pleomorphic gram-positive anaerobic rod usually isolated as a contaminant from skin. The notable presence of *Propionibacterium acnes* may relate to its prevalence in the skin of the upper body due to the increased density of sebaceous glands in that location. Historically this bacterium was an unusual cause of post-neurosurgical infection. While it has most frequently been isolated from infected neurosurgical shunts [21, 85]. However, *Propionibacterium acnes* is increasingly recognized as a cause of neurosurgical site infection [83, 86, 87]. Nisbet et al. reported an important series of 28 patients with *Propionibacterium acnes* neurosurgical infection over 6.5 years. Interestingly, 21 patients (75 %) have a bone flap infection. The authors highlight the need for routine anaerobic culture for 10 days for all neurosurgical specimens [12].

Few cases of polymicrobial skull osteomyelitis after a craniotomy were reported [2, 83, 84]. However, 6 of the 12 patients reported by Kshettry et al. have more than one bacterium and three bacteria were isolated in 2 patients [84]. Unusual organisms, such as corynebacteria, mycetoma, tuberculosis and candidiasis, are occasionally detected in postcraniotomy bone flap osteomyelitis [84, 88–92]. In our series of 13 patients with a postoperative osteomyelitis, *Salmonella enteritidis* was isolated in one case which has a cranial bone flap osteomyelitis with subgaleal abscess. According to Uhari and colleagues, a 12-year-old girl developed a chronic *Salmonella typhimurium* osteitis in her calvarium at the site of operation for hypophyseal adenoma [93].

Pathogens isolated from cranial bone infections secondary to direct injuries do not differ greatly from those in bone flap osteomyelitis excepting *Escherichia coli*. The latter is the most common etiologic agents associated with infected cephalhematomas and this infection may be relevant as nosocomial [6, 94, 95]. The systemic approach includes cultures of blood and CSF, as sepsis, meningitis or osteomyelitis can be associated with infected cephalhematomas [96, 97]. In osteomyelitis with cranial halo-pin traction *Staphylococcus aureus* is the most commonly isolated organism [1, 98, 99]. *Escherichia Coli, Staphylococcus aureus, Pseudomonas aeruginosa, Propionibacterium* and *Streptococcus pneumoniae* are encountoured in the rest of varieties of skull osteomyelitis secondary to scalp injuries [26, 67, 100–103]. Fungus may also isolated in post-traumatic cranial osteomyelitis [104, 105]. In 2001, Rodriguez-Hernandez et al. reported a unique case of cranial infection caused by *Aspergillus fumigatus* following a traumatic wound infection in an immunocompetent patient [104]. More recently, a case of frontal supraorbital bone tuberculosis was described 3 months after a head injury with a lacerated wound in the frontal area [106]. Finally, two cases of cranial osteomyelitis were presented as chronic non-healing ulcers of the scalp after trauma encountered after 4 and 50 years, respectively. *Nocardia spp.* was isolated in the first patient [107]. In the second case, *Streptococcus parasanguis* was isolated from the skin culture, and *Proteus mirabilis* and *Peptostreptococcus spp.* were identified in the cultures from the bone [70].

Cranial Osteomyelitis via Hematogenous Bloodborne Route

Unlike long bones, hematogenous spread due to bacteremia or fungemia becomes very unusual in skull osteomyelitis. There have been occasional case reports where the infection is typically monobacterial. Camargo et al. report a case of *Aspergillus spp.* osteomyelitis of the lumbar spine complicated with right orbital apex syndrome due to orbital and sphenoid wing involvement [108]. Yocum and Seligson report a case of septic arthritis of the knee combined with osteomyelitis of the skull vault following arthroscopy. A concomitant cavitary lung lesion was found caused by Blastomycosis [109]. Recently, Hayashi et al. reported a patient with septicemia and recurrent meningitis complicated by skull base osteomyelitis. A secondary septic pulmonary embolism was highly suspected [110]. Few other cases were reported particularly with *Salmonella species* [111, 112], *Mycobacterium tuberculosis* [113], *Escherichia coli* [96, 97], secondary syphilis [114–117], coccidiodomycosis agents [118], *Penicillium marneffei* [119], *Gemella haemolysans* [110], and *Cryptococcus spp.* [120].

References

1. Uppal HS, Issa F, Byren I, Johnson D. A case of pancalvarial osteomyelitis: diagnosis and management. J Plast Reconstr Aesthet Surg. 2010;63(2):e159–60. doi:10.1016/j.bjps.2009.05.015.
2. Calcagno SW, Graves RM, Baum SE, Teff RJ. Polymicrobial skull osteomyelitis: a rare complication of subdural hematoma evacuation. Surg Infect (Larchmt). 2007;8(4):483–90.
3. Adams JR, Bryant DG. Cranial osteomyelitis: a late complication of a dental infection. Br J Oral Maxillofac Surg. 2008;46(8):673–4. doi:10.1016/j.bjoms.2008.03.025.
4. Ridder GJ, Breunig C, Kaminsky J, Pfeiffer J. Central skull base osteomyelitis: new insights and implications for diagnosis and treatment. Eur Arch Otorhinolaryngol. 2015;272(5):1269–76. doi:10.1007/s00405-014-3390-y.
5. Ganhewa AD, Jafri KJ. A diagnostic dilemma of central skull base osteomyelitis mimicking neoplasia in a diabetic patient. BMJ Case Rep. 2013;2013:bcr2012007183. doi:10.1136/bcr-2012-007183.
6. Tutela JP, Banta JC, Boyd TG, Kelishadi SS, Chowdhry S, Little JA. Scalp reconstruction: a review of the literature and a unique case of total craniectomy in an adult with osteomyelitis of the skull. Eplasty. 2014;14, e27. eCollection 2014.
7. Akhaddar A, Baallal H, Elouennass M, Elgharbaoui H, Mahi M, Boucetta M. Combined Serratia liquefaciens and Mycobacterium tuberculosis in temporal osteitis with brain extension. Surg Infect (Larchmt). 2011;12(4):329–31. doi:10.1089/sur.2010.100.
8. Sethi A, Sethi D, Mrig S, Passey JC, Srivastav N. Coexistent acute pyogenic and tubercular petrous apicitis: a diagnostic dilemma. J Laryngol Otol. 2006;120(10):875–8.
9. Sendi P, Rohrbach M, Graber P, Frei R, Ochsner PE, Zimmerli W. Staphylococcus aureus small colony variants in prosthetic joint infection. Clin Infect Dis. 2006;43(8):961–7.
10. Neut D, van der Mei HC, Bulstra SK, Busscher HJ. The role of small-colony variants in failure to diagnose and treat biofilm infections in orthopedics. Acta Orthop. 2007;78(3):299–308.
11. Chen JC, Yeh CF, Shiao AS, Tu TY. Temporal bone osteomyelitis: the relationship with malignant otitis externa, the diagnostic dilemma, and changing trends. ScientificWorldJournal. 2014;2014:591714. doi:10.1155/2014/591714.
12. Nisbet M, Briggs S, Ellis-Pegler R, Thomas M, Holland D. Propionibacterium acnes: an under-appreciated cause of post-neurosurgical infection. J Antimicrob Chemother. 2007;60(5):1097–103.
13. Akhaddar A, El Mostarchid B, Gazzaz M, Boucetta M. Cerebellar abscess due to Lactococcus lactis. A new pathogen. Acta Neurochir (Wien). 2002;144(3):305–6.
14. Hayek BR, Sitole S, Andreoli M, Banich A, Ahmad AZ. Bilateral eyelid edema and orbital cellulitis associated with Pott's puffy tumor. Ophthal Plast Reconstr Surg. 2007;23(2):163–5.
15. He J, Lam JC, Adlan T. Clival osteomyelitis and hypoglossal nerve palsy-rare complications of Lemierre's syndrome. BMJ Case Rep. 2015;2015:pii: bcr2015209777. doi:10.1136/bcr-2015-209777.
16. Chandy B, Todd J, Stucker FJ, Nathan CO. Pott's puffy tumor and epidural abscess arising from dental sepsis: a case report. Laryngoscope. 2001;111(10):1732–4.
17. Nisa L, Landis BN, Giger R. Orbital involvement in Pott's puffy tumor: a systematic review of published cases. Am J Rhinol Allergy. 2012;26(2):e63–70. doi:10.2500/ajra.2012.26.3746.
18. Bambakidis NC, Cohen AR. Intracranial complications of frontal sinusitis in children: Pott's puffy tumor revisited. Pediatr Neurosurg. 2001;35(2):82–9.
19. Kombogiorgas D, Solanki GA. The Pott puffy tumor revisited: neurosurgical implications of this unforgotten entity. Case report and review of the literature. J Neurosurg. 2006;105(2 Suppl):143–9.
20. Karaman E, Hacizade Y, Isildak H, Kaytaz A. Pott's puffy tumor. J Craniofac Surg. 2008;19(6):1694–7. doi:10.1097/SCS.0b013e31818b432e.

21. Brook I. Recovery of anaerobic bacteria from clinical specimens in 12 years at two military hospitals. J Clin Microbiol. 1988;26:1181–8.
22. Baker AS. Role of anaerobic bacteria in sinusitis and its complications. Ann Otol Rhinol Laryngol Suppl. 1991;154:17–22.
23. Blackman SC, Schleiss MR. Forehead swelling caused by Pott's puffy tumor in a 9-year-old boy with sinusitis. Pediatr Int. 2005;47(6):704–7.
24. Feder Jr HM, Cates KL, Cementina AM. Pott puffy tumor: a serious occult infection. Pediatrics. 1987;79(4):625–9.
25. Salomão JF, Cervante TP, Bellas AR, Boechat MC, Pone SM, Pone MV, de A Pereira B. Neurosurgical implications of Pott's puffy tumor in children and adolescents. Childs Nerv Syst. 2014;30(9):1527–34.
26. Wu CT, Huang JL, Hsia SH, Lee HY, Lin JJ. Pott's puffy tumor after acupuncture therapy. Eur J Pediatr. 2009;168(9):1147–9.
27. Clark JR, Lim JK, Poole M. Pott's puffy tumour: a clinical variant. Aust N Z J Surg. 1999;69 (10):759–62.
28. Verbon A, Husni RN, Gordon SM, Lavertu P, Keys TF. Pott's puffy tumor due to Haemophilus influenzae: case report and review. Clin Infect Dis. 1996;23(6):1305–7.
29. Ibarra S, Aguirrebengoa K, Pomposo I, Bereciartúa E, Montejo M, González de Zárate P. Osteomyelitis of the frontal bone (Pott's puffy tumor). A report of 5 patients. Enferm Infecc Microbiol Clin. 1999;17(10):489–92. Spanish.
30. Canbaz B, Tanriverdi T, Himi Kaya A, Tüzgen S. Pott's puffy tumour: a rare clinical entity. Lancet Infect Dis. 2003;3(11):721.
31. Babu RP, Todor R, Kasoff SS. Pott's puffy tumor: the forgotten entity. Case report. J Neurosurg. 1996;84(1):110–2.
32. Tsai BY, Lin KL, Lin TY, Chiu CH, Lee WJ, Hsia SH, Wu CT, Wang HS. Pott's puffy tumor in children. Childs Nerv Syst. 2010;26(1):53–60.
33. Wang WH, Hwang TZ. Extensive subgaleal abscess and epidural empyema in a patient with acute frontal sinusitis. J Formos Med Assoc. 2003;102(5):338–41.
34. Shahat AH, Rahman NU, Obaideen AM, Ahmed I, Zahman Au A. Cranial-epidural tuberculosis presenting as a scalp swelling. Surg Neurol. 2004;61(5):464–6.
35. Prasad KC, Prasad SC, Mouli N, Agarwal S. Osteomyelitis in the head and neck. Acta Otolaryngol. 2007;127(2):194–205.
36. Akhaddar A, Gazzaz M, Albouzidi A, Lmimouni B, Elmostarchid B, Boucetta M. Invasive Aspergillus terreus sinusitis with orbitocranial extension: case report. Surg Neurol. 2008;69 (5):490–5. discussion 495.
37. Panda NK, Ekambar Eshwara Reddy C. Primary frontal sinus aspergillosis: an uncommon occurrence. Mycoses. 2005;48(4):235–7.
38. Patel SA, Chatterjee A, Simonsen K. Recurrent midline frontal mass in a patient with sinusitis. Clin Pediatr (Phila). 2011;50(3):266–8.
39. Tacon LJ, Parkinson JF, Hudson BJ, Brewer JM, Little NS, Clifton-Bligh RJ. Headache of a diagnosis: frontotemporal pain and inflammation associated with osteolysis. Med J Aust. 2008;189(10):591–2.
40. Skomro R, McClean KL. Frontal osteomyelitis (Pott's puffy tumour) associated with Pasteurella multocida—a case report and review of the literature. Can J Infect Dis. 1998;9 (2):115–21.
41. Per H, Kumandaş S, Gümüş H, Oztürk MK, Coşkun A. Meningitis and subgaleal, subdural, epidural empyema due to Pasteurella multocida. J Emerg Med. 2010;39(1):35–8.
42. Kumar GS, Raj PM, Chacko G, Lalitha MK, Chacko AG, Rajshekhar V. Cranial melioidosis presenting as a mass lesion or osteomyelitis. J Neurosurg. 2008;108(2):243–7.
43. Akhaddar A, Elmostarchid B, Boulahroud O, Elouennass M, Boucetta M. Actinomycotic brain abscess with osteomyelitis arising from frontal sinusitis. Intern Med. 2009;48 (8):619–20.

44. Kountakis SE, Kemper Jr JV, Chang CY, DiMaio DJ, Stiernberg CM. Osteomyelitis of the base of the skull secondary to Aspergillus. Am J Otolaryngol. 1997;18(1):19–22.
45. Stodulski D, Kowalska B, Stankiewicz C. Otogenic skull base osteomyelitis caused by invasive fungal infection. Case report and literature review. Eur Arch Otorhinolaryngol. 2006;263(12):1070–6.
46. Rothholtz VS, Lee AD, Shamloo B, Bazargan M, Pan D, Djalilian HR. Skull base osteomyelitis: the effect of comorbid disease on hospitalization. Laryngoscope. 2008;118 (11):1917–24. doi:10.1097/MLG.0b013e31817fae0d.
47. Chandler JR. Malignant external otitis: further considerations. Ann Otol Rhinol Laryngol. 1977;86:417–28.
48. Slattery WH, Brackmann DE. Skull base osteomyelitis: malignant external otitis. Otolaryngol Clin North Am. 1996;29:795–806.
49. Spielmann PM, Yu R, Neeff M. Skull base osteomyelitis: current microbiology and management. J Laryngol Otol. 2013;127 Suppl 1:S8–12.
50. Bernstein JM, Holland NJ, Porter GC, Maw AR. Resistance of pseudomonas to ciprofloxacin: implications for the treatment of malignant otitis externa. J Laryngol Otol. 2007;121:118–23.
51. Berenholz L, Katzenell U, Harell M. Evolving resistant pseudomonas to ciprofloxacin in malignant otitis externa. Laryngoscope. 2002;112:1619–22.
52. Laurens MB, Becker RM, Johnson JK, Wolf JS, Kotloff KL. MRSA with progression from otitis media and sphenoid sinusitis to clival osteomyelitis, pachymeningitis and abducens nerve palsy in an immunocompetent 10-year-old patient. Int J Pediatr Otorhinolaryngol. 2008;72(7):945–51.
53. Chang PC, Fischbein NJ, Holliday RA. Central skull base osteomyelitis in patients without otitis externa: imaging findings. AJNR Am J Neuroradiol. 2003;24(7):1310–6.
54. Clark MP, Pretorius PM, Byren I, Milford CA. Central or atypical skull base osteomyelitis: diagnosis and treatment. Skull Base. 2009;19(4):247–54.
55. Suchanda B, Alugolu R, Purohit A, Lakshmi V, Sundaram C. A rare concomitant tubercular and Fonsecaea pedrosoi fungal infection of the skull base. J Neurosci Rural Pract. 2012;3 (2):189–91. doi:10.4103/0976-3147.98237.
56. Ress BD, Luntz M, Telischi FF, Balkany TJ, Whiteman ML. Necrotizing external otitis in patients with AIDS. Laryngoscope. 1997;107(4):456–60.
57. Rubin Grandis J, Branstetter IV BF, Yu VL. The changing face of malignant (necrotising) external otitis: clinical, radiological, and anatomic correlations. Lancet Infect Dis. 2004;4 (1):34–9.
58. Johnson AK, Batra PS. Central skull base osteomyelitis: an emerging clinical entity. Laryngoscope. 2014;124(5):1083–7. doi:10.1002/lary.24440.
59. Blyth CC, Gomes L, Sorrell TC, da Cruz M, Sud A, Chen SC. Skull-base osteomyelitis: fungal vs. bacterial infection. Clin Microbiol Infect. 2011;17(2):306–11. doi:10.1111/j.1469-0691.2010.03231.x.
60. Weber ML, Abela A, de Repentigny L, Garel L, Lapointe N. Myeloperoxidase deficiency with extensive candidal osteomyelitis of the base of the skull. Pediatrics. 1987;80(6):876–9.
61. Wilkinson EP, Robinson RA, Trask DK. Skull base thrombotic mycosis. Ear Nose Throat J. 2007;86(3):137.
62. Alvernia JE, Patel RN, Cai DZ, Dang N, Anderson DW, Melgar M. A successful combined endovascular and surgical treatment of a cranial base mucormycosis with an associated internal carotid artery pseudoaneurysm. Neurosurgery. 2009;65(4):733–40. doi:10.1227/01.NEU.0000351773.74034.5E.
63. Prasad SC, Prasad KC, Kumar A, Thada ND, Rao P, Chalasani S. Osteomyelitis of the temporal bone: terminology, diagnosis, and management. J Neurol Surg B Skull Base. 2014;75(5):324–31. doi:10.1055/s-0034-1372468.
64. Farr RC, Gardner G, Acker JD, Brint JM, Haglund LF, Land M, Schweitzer JB, West BC. Blastomycotic cranial osteomyelitis. Am J Otol. 1992;13(6):582–6.

65. Haines SJ, Chou SN. Infections of the scalp and osteomyelitis of the skull. In: Wilkins RH, Rengachary SS, editors. Neurosurgery. New York: McGraw-Hill; 1985.
66. Ramasastry SS, Granick MS, Boyd JB, Futrell JW. Severe perifolliculitis capitis with osteomyelitis. Ann Plast Surg. 1987;18(3):241–4.
67. Raja V, Low C, Sastry A, Moriarty B. Pott's puffy tumor following an insect bite. J Postgrad Med. 2007;53(2):114–6.
68. Yuen JC, Puri SK, Feng Z. Scalp necrotizing fasciitis with osteomyelitis of the skull from Aspergillus. J Craniofac Surg. 2002;13(6):762–4.
69. Chang HY, Chiu NC, Huang FY, Kao HA, Hsu CH, Hung HY. Infected cephalohematoma of newborns: experience in a medical center in Taiwan. Pediatr Int. 2005;47(3):274–7.
70. Valerón-Almazán P, Gómez-Duaso AJ, Rivero P, Vilar J, Dehesa L, Santana N, Carretero G. Extensive, non-healing scalp ulcer associated with trauma-induced chronic osteomyelitis. Ann Dermatol. 2011;23 Suppl 3:S364–7. doi:10.5021/ad.2011.23.S3.S364.
71. Lamoreau KP, Fanciullo LM. Pott's puffy tumour mimicking preseptal cellulitis. Clin Exp Optom. 2008;91(4):400–2. doi:10.1111/j.1444-0938.2007.00234.x.
72. Rerolle JP, Szelag JC, Diaconita M, Paraf F, Aldigier JC, Le Meur Y. Intracranial granuloma and skull osteolysis: complication of a primary cutaneous cryptococcosis in a kidney transplant recipient. Am J Kidney Dis. 2005;46(6):e113–7.
73. Nugent NF, Murphy M, Kelly J. Scalp abscess—a cautionary tale. J Plast Reconstr Aesthet Surg. 2010;63(8):e619–21. doi:10.1016/j.bjps.2010.02.011.
74. Borges LF. Infections in neurologic surgery. Host defenses. Neurosurg Clin N Am. 1992;3 (2):275–8.
75. Syrmos N, Patiakas S, Iliadis C, Grigoriou K, Valadakis V, Chatzinasiou F, Arvanitakis D. Craniotomy infections: the Venizeleio hospital experience. Ann Gen Psychiatry. 2010;9 Suppl 1:S98.
76. McClelland 3rd S, Hall WA. Postoperative central nervous system infection: incidence and associated factors in 2111 neurosurgical procedures. Clin Infect Dis. 2007;45(1):55–9.
77. Dashti SR, Baharvahdat H, Spetzler RF, Sauvageau E, Chang SW, Stiefel MF, Park MS, Bambakidis NC. Operative intracranial infection following craniotomy. Neurosurg Focus. 2008;24(6):E10. doi:10.3171/FOC/2008/24/6/E10.
78. Korinek AM, Golmard JL, Elcheick A, Bismuth R, van Effenterre R, Coriat P, Puybasset L. Risk factors for neurological site infections after craniotomy: a critical reappraisal of antibiotic on 4578 patients. Br J Neurosurg. 2005;19(2):155–62.
79. Bhaskar IP, Inglis TJ, Lee GY. Clinical, radiological, and microbiological profile of patients with autogenous cranioplasty infections. World Neurosurg. 2014;82(3–4):e531–4. doi:10.1016/j.wneu.2013.01.013.
80. Rasmussen S, Ohrström JK, Westergaard L, Kosteljanetz M. Post-operative infections of osteoplastic compared with free bone flaps. Br J Neurosurg. 1990;4(6):493–5.
81. Nam JR, Kim MS, Lee CH, Whang DH. Linezolid treatment for osteomyelitis due to Staphylococcus epidermidis with reduced vancomycin susceptibility. J Korean Neurosurg Soc. 2008;43(6):307–10.
82. Larsson A, Engström M, Uusijärvi J, Kihlström L, Lind F, Mathiesen T. Hyperbaric oxygen treatment of postoperative neurosurgical infections. Neurosurgery. 2002;50(2):287–95.
83. Abu Hamdeh S, Lytsy B, Ronne-Engström E. Surgical site infections in standard neurosurgery procedures—a study of incidence, impact and potential risk factors. Br J Neurosurg. 2014;28(2):270–5. doi:10.3109/02688697.2013.835376.
84. Kshettry VR, Hardy S, Weil RJ, Angelov L, Barnett GH. Immediate titanium cranioplasty after debridement and craniectomy for postcraniotomy surgical site infection. Neurosurgery. 2012;70(1 Suppl Operative):8–14. doi:10.1227/NEU.0b013e31822fef2c. discussion 14–5.
85. Beeler B, Crowder J, Smith J, White A. Propionibacterium acnes: pathogen in central nervous system shunt infection. Am J Med. 1976;61:935–8.

86. Levitt MR, Gabikian P, Pottinger PS, Silbergeld DL. Propionibacterium acnes osteomyelitis occurring 23 years after craniotomy: case report and review of literature. Neurosurgery. 2011;69(3):E773–9. doi:10.1227/NEU.0b013e31821964ba.
87. Ghosh M, Talwani R, Gilliam BL. Propionibacterium skull osteomyelitis treated with daptomycin. Clin Neurol Neurosurg. 2009;111(7):610–2. doi:10.1016/j.clineuro.2009.04.003.
88. Kaplan K, Weinstein L. Diphtheroid infections of man. Ann Intern Med. 1969;70:919–29.
89. Wilson IF, Candia GJ, Worthington MG, Sullivan JG. Chronic osteomyelitis due to corynebacteria in a postcraniotomy bone flap. Clin Infect Dis. 1999;28(6):1323–4.
90. Fernández-Guerrero ML, Ruiz Barnés P, Alés JM. Postcraniotomy mycetoma of the scalp and osteomyelitis due to Pseudallescheria boydii. J Infect Dis. 1987;156(5):855.
91. Pandey AS, Surana A. Tuberculous osteomyelitis of the bone flap following craniotomy. Indian J Tuberc. 2011;58(3):129–31.
92. Biniwale SN, Rajshekhar V. Tuberculous osteomyelitis of bone flap following craniotomy for a glioma. Neurol India. 2000;48:91–2.
93. Uhari M, Rantala H, Herva E. Perioperative dissemination of Salmonella. Arch Dis Child. 1987;62(10):1079–80.
94. Vale B, Morais S, Resende C, Taborda A. Neonatal meningitis associated with osteomyelitis and epidural empyema. BMJ Case Rep. 2013;2013:pii: bcr2013009149. doi:10.1136/bcr-2013-009149.
95. Miedema CJ, Ruige M, Kimpen JL. Primarily infected cephalhematoma and osteomyelitis in a newborn. Eur J Med Res. 1999;4(1):8–10.
96. Blom NA, Vreede WB. Infected cephalhematomas associated with osteomyelitis, sepsis and meningitis. Pediatr Infect Dis J. 1993;12:1015–7.
97. Nakwan N, Nakwan N, Wannaro J, Dissaneevate P, Kritsaneepaiboon S, Chokephaibulkit K. Septicemia, meningitis, and skull osteomyelitis complicating infected cephalhematoma caused by ESBL-producing Escherichia coli. Southeast Asian J Trop Med Public Health. 2011;42(1):148–51.
98. Garfin SR, Botte MJ, Waters RL, Nickel VL. Complications in the use of the halo fixation device. J Bone Joint Surg Am. 1986;68(3):320–5.
99. Hayes VM, Silber JS, Siddiqi FN, Kondrachov D, Lipetz JS, Lonner B. Complications of halo fixation of the cervical spine. Am J Orthop (Belle Mead NJ). 2005;34(6):271–6.
100. Phillips NI, Robertson IJ. Osteomyelitis of the skull vault from a human bite. Br J Neurosurg. 1997;11(2):168–9.
101. Riffaud L, Morandi X. Osteomyelitis of the skull vault induced by self-inflicted dermatitis of the scalp. Acta Neurochir (Wien). 2001;143(7):737–8.
102. Listinsky JL, Wood BP, Ekholm SE. Parietal osteomyelitis and epidural abscess: a delayed complication of fetal monitoring. Pediatr Radiol. 1986;16(2):150–1.
103. Barry J, Fridley J, Sayama C, Lam S. Infected subgaleal hematoma following blunt head trauma in a child: case report and review of the literature. Pediatr Neurosurg. 2015;50(4):223–8. doi:10.1159/000433442.
104. Rodríguez-Hernández MJ, Jiménez-Mejías ME, Montero JM, Regordan C, Ferreras G. Aspergillus fumigatus cranial infection after accidental traumatism. Eur J Clin Microbiol Infect Dis. 2001;20(9):655–6.
105. Fortún J, Cobo J, Cañal J, Martínez-San MJ. Post-traumatic cranial mucormycosis in an immunocompetent patient. J Oral Maxillofac Surg. 1995;53(9):1099–102.
106. Sundar VI, Shekhawat J, Gupta A, Sinha VD. Post traumatic tubercular osteomyelitis of skull vault. J Neurosci Rural Pract. 2013;4 Suppl 1:S138–41. doi:10.4103/0976-3147.116471.
107. Kulkarni V, Rajshekhar V. Chronic non-healing ulcers of the scalp after trauma. Postgrad Med J. 2000;76(897):437, 450–1.
108. Camargo JF, Seriburi V, Tenner M, El Khoury MY. Aspergillus osteomyelitis of the lumbar spine complicated with orbital apex syndrome: A potential role of the Batson's plexus in

disease propagation. Med Mycol Case Rep. 2012;1(1):9–12. doi:10.1016/j.mmcr.2012.02.004.

109. Yocum J, Seligson D. Blastomycosis of the knee and skull after arthroscopy. Am J Sports Med. 1991;19(6):670–2.

110. Hayashi T, Uchiumi H, Yanagisawa K, Ogawa Y, Handa H, Tsukamoto N, Nojima Y. Recurrent Gemella haemolysans meningitis in a patient with osteomyelitis of the clivus. Intern Med. 2013;52(18):2145–7.

111. Bhooshan P, Shivaprakasha S, Dinesh KR, Kiran M, Karim P. Chronic subdural empyema and cranial vault osteomyelitis due to Salmonella paratyphi A. Indian J Med Microbiol. 2010;28(1):60–2. doi:10.4103/0255-0857.58733.

112. Senegor M, Lewis HP. Salmonella osteomyelitis of the skull base. Surg Neurol. 1991;36(1):37–9.

113. Morris BS, Varma R, Garg A, Awasthi M, Maheshwari M. Multifocal musculoskeletal tuberculosis in children: appearances on computed tomography. Skeletal Radiol. 2002;31(1):1–8.

114. Park KH, Lee MS, Hong IK, Sung JY, Choi SH, Park SO, Shin MJ, Chung HW, Lee SH. Bone involvement in secondary syphilis: a case report and systematic review of the literature. Sex Transm Dis. 2014;41(9):532–7. doi:10.1097/OLQ.0000000000000164.

115. Son C, Samples D, Brenner A, Floyd J. Osteolytic calvarial lesions as initial presentation of latent neurosyphilis. J Clin Neurosci. 2015;22(5):909–10. doi:10.1016/j.jocn.2014.11.014.

116. Elopre L, Morell V, Bosshardt C, Geisler WM. A case of syphilitic osteitis in a patient with HIV infection. Int J STD AIDS. 2014;25(10):765–7. doi:10.1177/0956462414522031.

117. Kang SH, Park SW, Kwon KY, Hong WJ. A solitary skull lesion of syphilitic osteomyelitis. J Korean Neurosurg Soc. 2010;48(1):85–7.

118. Baddley JW, Cobbs CS, Pappas PG. Surgical treatment of multiple skull abscesses associated with coccidioidomycosis. Mycoses. 2004;47(1–2):69–71.

119. Qiu Y, Zhang J, Liu G, Zhong X, Deng J, He Z, Jing B. Retrospective analysis of 14 cases of disseminated Penicillium marneffei infection with osteolytic lesions. BMC Infect Dis. 2015;15:47. doi:10.1186/s12879-015-0782-6.

120. Prendiville S, Bielamowicz SA, Hawrych A, Deeb ZE. Isolated cryptococcal sphenoid sinusitis with septicemia, meningitis, and subsequent skull base osteomyelitis in an immunocompetent patient. Otolaryngol Head Neck Surg. 2000;123(3):277–9.

Chapter 4
Histopathologic Changes

Contents

Abbreviations

H&E Hematoxylin and eosin
PAS Periodic Acid-Schiff
PCR Polymerase chain reaction

Role of Histopathologic Examination

Pathology plays an important role for confirming the diagnosis of osteomyelitis if clinical findings, biological studies and diagnostic imaging investigations are not conclusive. It is also an important tool for identifying some "specific" osteomyelitis such as *Mycobacteria*, fungi and parasites. However, histopathology of cranial osteomyelitis should always be interpreted in combination with clinical, biological and radiological findings and should not be used independently. Moreover, pathology has also been regarded as valuable in excluding other diseases of the bone (differential diagnoses). Interestingly, one patient with chronic osteomyelitis of the skull had a concomitant localized squamous carcinoma diagnosed only on pathological examination [1]. On the other hand, cranial osteomyelitis can occur in the setting of a primary tumor such as fibrous dysplasia or meningioma [2, 3].

Against this background and in order to facilitate the diagnosis, it is recommended to send all bone and adjacent soft tissues removed such as biopsies, curettage, and

A. Akhaddar, *Cranial Osteomyelitis*, DOI 10.1007/978-3-319-30268-3_4

resection specimens for microbiological culture and histopathological examination [4]. At least three samples each should be taken, numbered and labeled with the anatomic localization during harvesting. Bone tissue is best fixed in formalin, carefully decalcified in a chelating agent such as Ethylenediaminetetraacetic acid and then paraffin embedded. Decalcification is a long procedure, as bone pieces have to be left in a chelator for several days or even weeks, depending on the size of the bone. For a diagnosis of osteomyelitis, routine stains are applied: hematoxylin-eosin (H&E); van Gieson; Giemsa; and Periodic Acid-Schiff stain (PAS). Usually routine diagnosis of osteomyelitis is made by conventional histology on an H&E slide alone. Subsequently, particular stains are applied to look for possible microbial organisms.

Macroscopic Appearance

Macroscopy of specimens removed for osteomyelitis is determined by the type of surgery and depends on the extent and duration of disease.

The pathologic anatomic appearances of the lesions vary with the stage of the disease. In the early stage, the bone presents no abnormalities evident to the naked eye. Occasionally, the diploë may show some congestion. In the next stage, the diploë appears distinctly hyperemic and scattered with droplets of pus. This is followed by the conversion of the medullary tissue of the diploë into granulation tissue with drops of pus. Thrombosed veins may be seen within the diploë. In the third stage, the purulent secretions extend to the outer and inner surfaces of the bony cranium by the vascular channels or through small cortical opening in the cranial skull tables. Paraosseous abscesses form between the outer table and the pericranium and between the inner table and the dura. The extracranial abscesses tend to be positioned in the subcutaneous tissues of the scalp: this appearance is known as puffy swellings of the scalp. A small, draining skin sinus is often the outlet of an infected sequestered deep infection [5].

Intracranially, the dura mater becomes covered with small granulations. However, it seems resistant for a significant long time. When extradural abscess becomes sufficiently large, intracranial contents may be compressed. The fourth stage of the lesion is marked by more or less extensive destruction of the skull tables. By this time necrotic bone fragments appear with a pale whitish-gray coloration (Fig. 4.1). These are followed by sequestra which usually show an irregular outline. Osteolytic and osteosclerotic foci may alternate. Therefore, the eroded tables of the skull appear “rotten” or “corroded with acid” or like a “lacework” [6] (Fig. 4.2).

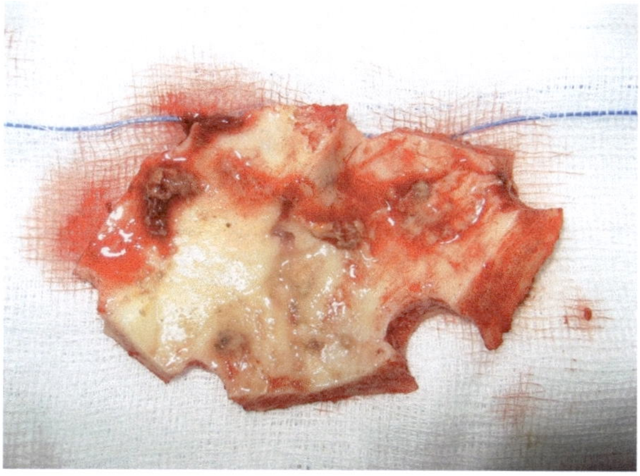

Fig. 4.1 Fronto-parietal bone flap removed (about 6 weeks after the initial surgical intervention) in a case of chronic osteomyelitis with adjacent granulation tissue

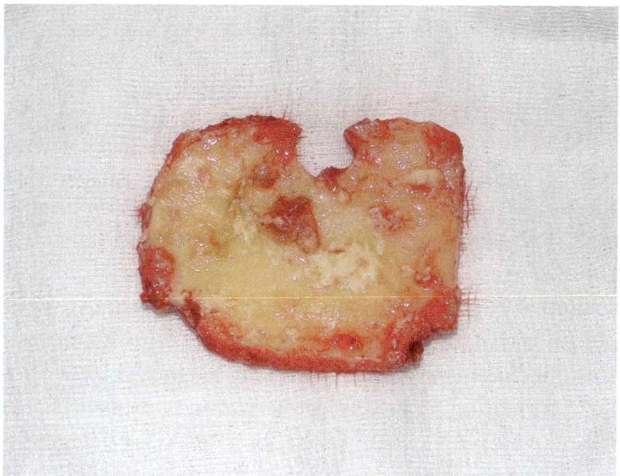

Fig. 4.2 Post-surgical chronic osteomyelitis in a patient with previously irradiated area. The eroded inner table of the devitalized frontal bone flap appears "rotten" or "corroded with acid"

Microscopic Study

Acute Osteomyelitis

Acute osteomyelitis is characterized by an inflammatory exudate composed of fibrin, polymorphonuclear leucocytes, and macrophages (Fig. 4.3). The inflammation is located primarily in the medullary spaces of the diploë but secondarily involves the skull tables (most frequently the external table followed by the internal one) and attains the periosteum. Bone marrow spaces are highly oedematous and replaced by inflammatory exudate, necrotic debris, and microorganisms. Multiple microabscess formations may occur late. Pressure in the diploë is increased and blood vessels are destroyed. As a result, compromised vascular perfusion leads to necrosis of diploë and skull tables. The lamellar bone appears devitalized with

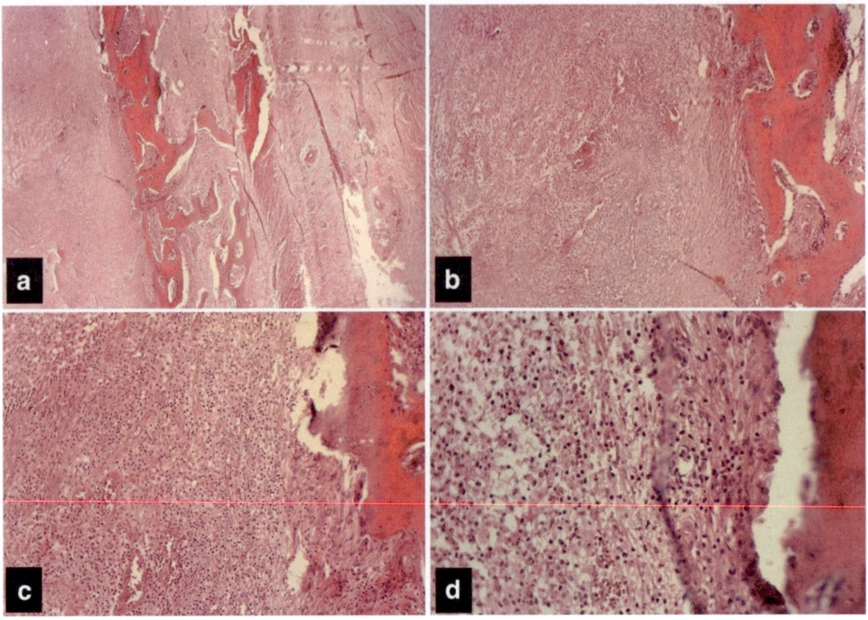

Fig. 4.3 Acute cranial osteomyelitis. Bone trabeculae show irregular contour with congestion and inflammatory exudates composed of fibrin, polynuclear neutrophils and macrophages. Low (**a**), medium (**b**, **c**) and high power magnification (**d**) (H&E stain)

scalloped edges and absence of stainable osteocytes and osteoblasts. The surrounding soft tissues are also oedematous with granulocytic infiltration. Thereafter, specimens show lymphocytes and plasma cells with bone necrosis, reactive new bone formation, capillary proliferation and fibrosis (Fig. 4.4). Sequester formation may develop and some osteoclasts are also detectable together with neutrophilic granulocytes on the irregular trabecular surface [7, 8]. The sequestrum will frequently be colonized with biofilmforming microorganisms that then perpetuate the inflammation and lead to secondary chronic suppurative osteomyelitis for further than a 1-month duration [9]. Late complications include fistula formation and intracranial invasion. The microorganism most frequently responsible for osteomyelitis is *Staphylococcus aureus* which may be demonstrable in the paraffin section by a Gram stain or PAS staining. Microorganisms preferably colonize necrotic bone and form large colonies that spread within lacunae and channels on bone surfaces.

Chronic Osteomyelitis

Acute osteomyelitis becomes "secondary chronic" after a variable duration of 1–2 months. Chronic osteomyelitis is characterized by irregular fragments of devitalized bone surrounded by dense fibrous tissue (bone sequester) heavily

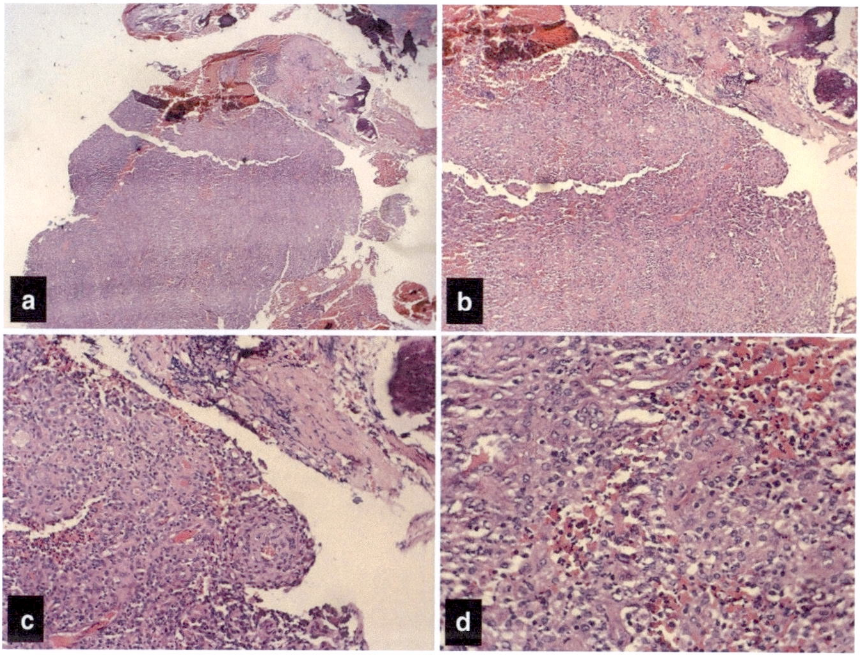

Fig. 4.4 Subacute form of cranial osteomyelitis. Bone necrosis with lymphoplasmocytic inflammatory infiltrates, together with neutrophilic granulocytes. Low (**a**), medium (**b**, **c**) and high power magnification (**d**) (H&E stain)

infiltrated by plasma cells, lymphocytes, and only a few granulocytes [10] (Fig. 4.5). The blood vessels contain thrombi more or less infiltrated with pus cells, and signs of perivascular inflammation accompany the thrombosis [6]. In cases of chronic osteomyelitis with significant suppuration, specimens demonstrate similar features as cases of acute osteomyelitis with large amounts of polymorphonuclear leucocytes, macrophages, and plasma cells, accompanied by a variable degree of marrow fibrosis and reactive bone formation. Some patients may present with little pus, fistula, and sequester formation, or may even lack these symptoms at a later stage of disease. This category of patients has a less fulminate course of chronic osteomyelitis with predominance of marrow fibrosis and reactive bone scleroses [8]. Occasionally, bacteria may be identified.

Osseous changes demonstrate mostly bone neogenesis. The spongy osseous tissue is accompanied by reactive network bone neogenesis and the bone surface is bordered by osteoblasts. The diploic space tissue shows fibrosing with granulation tissue formation. The surrounding soft tissues are also fibrosed with granulation tissue formation containing a few neutrophilic granulocytes [7].

When intracranial extension occurs, the dura mater becomes thickened and granular throughout the complete extent of the skull bones. If the lesions do not evolve too rapidly, the arachnoid will be adhesive and the brain is protected against encephalitis. However, once the natural resistance is overcome, the infection may

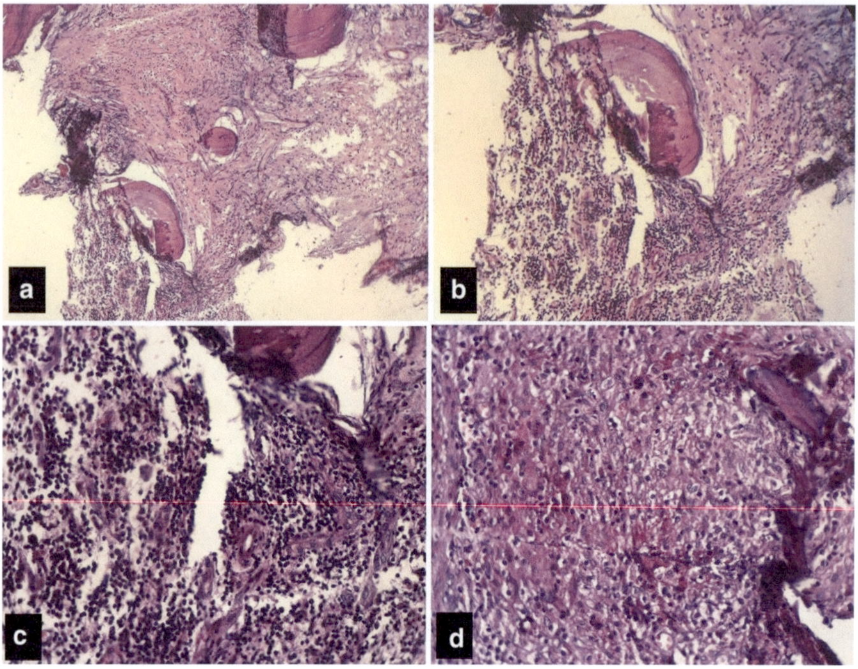

Fig. 4.5 Chronic cranial osteomyelitis. Irregular fragments of devitalized bone surrounded by dense fibrous tissue heavily infiltrated with lymphocytes, plasmocytes and only a few granulocytes. Low (**a**), medium (**b**, **c**) and high power magnification (**d**) (H&E stain)

reach the pia mater and cause variable forms of meningitis, intracranial suppurations, encephalitis and thrombophlebitis [6]. It is also common to have mixed forms of intracranial complications [11, 12].

Specific Osteomyelitis of the Skull

Some "specific" osteomyelitis such as *Mycobacteria*, fungi and parasites, may be identified on histopathologic study. This section focuses on the most pertinent specific osteomyelitis of the skull. Please refer to Chap. 14 about "Unusual pathogens" for more diagnosis details.

Tuberculosis

Histopathology is essential for identifying tuberculosis of the skull. The causative pathogen is usually *Mycobacterium tuberculosis*. Tubercular osteomyelitis is caused by hematogenous or by lymphatic dissemination of bacilli from an active

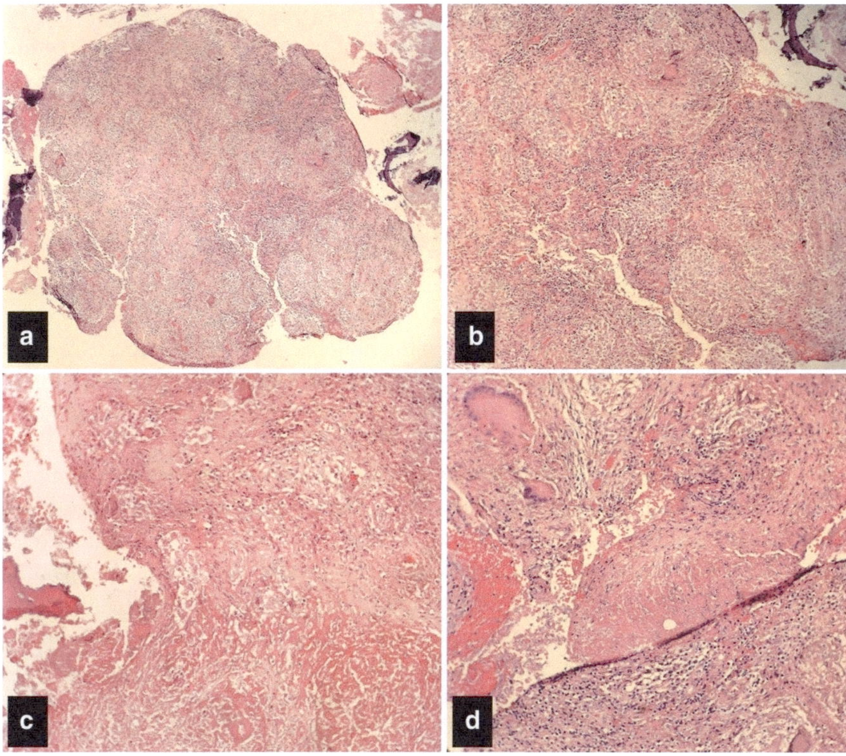

Fig. 4.6 Tuberculous cranial osteomyelitis. Irregular bone trabeculae with specific inflammatory exudates composed by epitheloid giant cell granulomas and areas of caseating necrosis. Low (**a**) and medium power magnification (**b–d**) (H&E stain)

focus, generally in the lungs. The relative paucity of lymphatic systems in the skull has been considered to explain the rare tuberculosis infections of the skull bones. The setting of the bacillus in the diploë marks the onset of acute inflammation surrounded by fibroblasts. Granulation tissue takes place in the bone trabeculae, and Langhans giant cells and epithelioid histiocytes appear. Because the dura is extremely resistant to calvarial tuberculosis, concomitant meningitis is rare. With further development, cold abscess formation appears. Cases of tubercular osteomyelitis have been diagnosed on the basis of pathological evaluation of fine needle aspirates or deep tissue biopsies from the infected bones or the adjacent soft tissues. The key diagnostic finding for mycobacterial infection is a specific inflammatory response with Epithelioid-giant cell granulomas with caseating necrosis (Fig. 4.6). On conventional histology, microorganisms may be rare and may not be shown; for that reason, more sensitive special techniques have been developed such as polymerase chain reaction (PCR) performed on DNA extracted from paraffin-embedded tissue [13, 14]. PCR is a rapid and inexpensive technique with high sensitivity and specificity. However, as a result from formalin fixation and decalcification, the quality of DNA extracted from such tissue may not be optimal and the PCR consequently false negative. In such cases, microbial culture from fresh tissue remains the gold standard of identification of the responsible mycobacterial agent.

Actinomycosis

Actinomycosis is a chronic granulomatous disease that can occurs anywhere in the body especially the cervicofacial region. Actinomycosis is not due to a fungus as the name suggests but to a gram-positive branching bacillus. *Actinomyces israelii* is the most prevalent species isolated in human infections and is found in most clinical forms of actinomycosis [15]. The portal of entry is generally the oral cavity. If the lesion progresses slowly, little suppuration takes place. However, in more acute forms, abscesses are formed and discharge pus containing yellow granules (or sulfur granules) through multiple skin sinuses. Histopathologic aspects are described as indurated masses or single or multiple abscesses. Typical microscopic findings include necrosis with yellowish sulfur granules and filamentous Gram-positive fungal-like pathogens. Yellowish sulfur granules (average 300 μm in diameter) are constituted by conglomeration of bacteria trapped in biofilm. A typical abscess has an outer zone of granulations around soft central loculations containing white or yellow pus where typical granules are seen [16]. Sinus tracts extend from abscesses to the skin surface or other tissues [17]. Bacteriological examination is often difficult because *Actinomyces species* usually grows in anaerobic culture and it is frequently associated with other organisms [18, 19].

Nocardia

Nocardia is a Gram-positive bacteria (bacteria-like fungus) found in the environment. It causes a wide spectrum of diseases in humans depending on immune status of the host. Nocardiosis is chiefly an opportunistic infection either localized or disseminated. *Nocardia asteroides* accounts for 80 % of cases of noncutaneous invasive disease. This primary infection is the most commonly acquired through respiratory tract. Subsequent hematogenous spread may lead to involvement of central nervous system and other tissues. Bone involvement is rare especially in the skull skeleton [20, 21]. Histology shows dense chronic inflammatory cell collections comprising lymphocytes and histiocytes filling the marrow spaces and destroying skull bone. Within the inflammatory centre, bluish colonies were seen surrounded by multinucleate giant cells, which revealed tightly packed slender branching hyphae highlighted by periodic acid-Schiff and methenamine silver stains suggestive of *Nocardia species* [21–23].

Fungi

The incidence of fungal infections involving the central nervous system and the cranial bones has increased in recent years because of the increasing number of patients with compromised immune systems. This is in great part due to increased use of immunosuppressive agents, which are commonly given to treat malignancies, some inflammatory conditions, acquired immunodeficiency syndrome (AIDS) and transplant recipients. Administrations of corticosteroids and broad-spectrum antibiotics are also at risk of fungal infections. The diagnosis of fungi encountered in the skull bones often requires the histopathologic examination of deep surgical biopsied lesion or debrided necrotic tissue. The role of histology is also to differentiate fungal infections from malignant tumors especially in the skull base (see Chap. 9).

The most frequent etiologic agents for invasive fungal osteomyelitis of the skull are Aspergillosis. These opportunistic pathogens have a tendency for invading blood vessels walls, circulatory disorders, resulting in coagulative necrosis caused by fungal toxins such as aflatoxin [24]. Mucosa of paranasal sinuses and upper airways become necrotic and the skull base progressively involved, which create an ideal environment for fungal proliferation and more dissemination [25]. *Aspergillus fumigatus* is the most causative agent isolated in humans and less commonly *A. flavus* [26]. Histopathologic examination shows vascular thrombosis that is surrounded by extensive coagulative necrosis and hemorrhage. Granulomatous inflammation with septate hyphae with acute-angle, dichotomous branching at regular intervals indicate aspergillus infection [27, 28] (Fig. 4.7). In contrast, irregular hyphea with right-angle branching and absence of septa are seen with mucormycosis.

Mucormycosis (also called zygomycosis) refers to several different diseases caused by infection with fungi in the order of Mucorales. *Rhizopus species* are the most common causative organisms [29]. Infection typically results from direct extension of an infectious focus involving the deep facial soft-tissue, paranasal

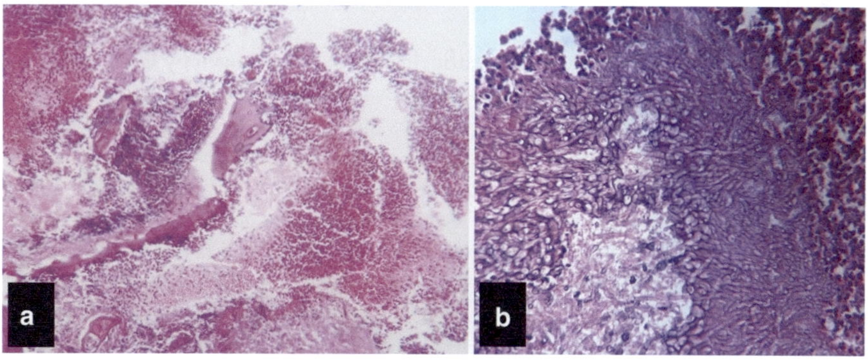

Fig. 4.7 Cranial bone aspergillosis. Chronic osteomyelitis with histologic findings of septate, densely clustered fungal hyphea (**a**). The septate hyphae with acute-angle and dichotomous branching designate *Aspergillus species* (**b**) (H&E stain)

sinus, orbit or nasopharynx. Mucormycosis infection is characterized by deep extension of the infection through perivascular channels causing vasculitis, thrombosis and infarcts leading to cavernous sinuses thrombosis which precede obvious bony destruction. Histopathological analysis revealed fibro-collagenous tissue with granulomas, necrotic foci with aseptate irregular fungal hyphae with 90° branching, sheets of foamy macrophages areas of hemorrhage [30]. Bony changes demonstrate necrotic osseous trabaculae mixed with osteoclast cells [31].

Cryptococcosis is a disseminated infection of men and animals mainly caused by *Cryptococcus neoformans* [32]. This yeast-like fungus is widely distributed and found especially in the pigeon droppings and eucalyptus trees. Cryptococcosis can rarely affect the skeletal system and the skull is the less frequent target [33]. Mechanisms involving Cryptococcal infections of the skull include disseminated infections, skull trauma, and embolic phenomena involvement of the temporal bone [34]. Histologic study shows chronic granulomatous inflammation and the presence of numerous yeast-like organisms using H&E stain, periodic acid methenamine silver stain, and Alcian Blue stain [35]. PAS-stained bone sample may reveal same granulomatous reaction with spherical PAS-positive fungi within the cytoplasm of large macrophages [36, 37].

Blastomycosis is found in soil and decaying wood in its hyphal form. But it forms spherical yeasts in infected tissue. This systemic fungal infection affects primarily the lungs. *Blastomyces dermatitis* is the most causative agent isolated in humans. Head and neck involvement has been reported most commonly in the larynx as well as oral and nasal mucosa. Cranial bone involvement is extremely rare and difficult to diagnose [38–40]. Hematoxylin and eosin staining usually reveals pseudoepitheliomatous hyperplasia, dense granulomatous infiltration, microabscesses, or giant cells. Granulomatous reaction with central suppuration is highly suggestive for the diagnosis. However, definitive diagnosis requires culture on enriched agars [39, 41].

Hydatidosis

Hydatidosis is a rare cosmopolite parasitic disease usually caused by the larval cysts of *Echinococcus granulosis*. Cranial hydatid cyst may involve the cranial vault and skull base when one or multiples larva reaches the bone via the bloodstream [42]. In the beginning, it invades the diploe, and as it grows it enlarges the diploic space with no development of the fibrous adventitious layer or pseudocapsule (pericyst) found in other locations. The external layer (ectocyst) is an acellular membrane that allows the transfer of nutrients. The internal layer (or germinal layer) usually forms multiple compartments containing clear hydatid fluid and protoscoleces. The parasite replaces the osseous tissue between trabeculae due to the slow growth of multiple vesicles which remain attached to the germinal layer (Fig. 4.8). Bone vesicles expand slowly and usually have a multilocular growth through the external layer of the main cyst. Enlargement is achieved by local erosion of skull bone, and the pressure on the blood vessels of the diploë may result in a vascular necrosis.

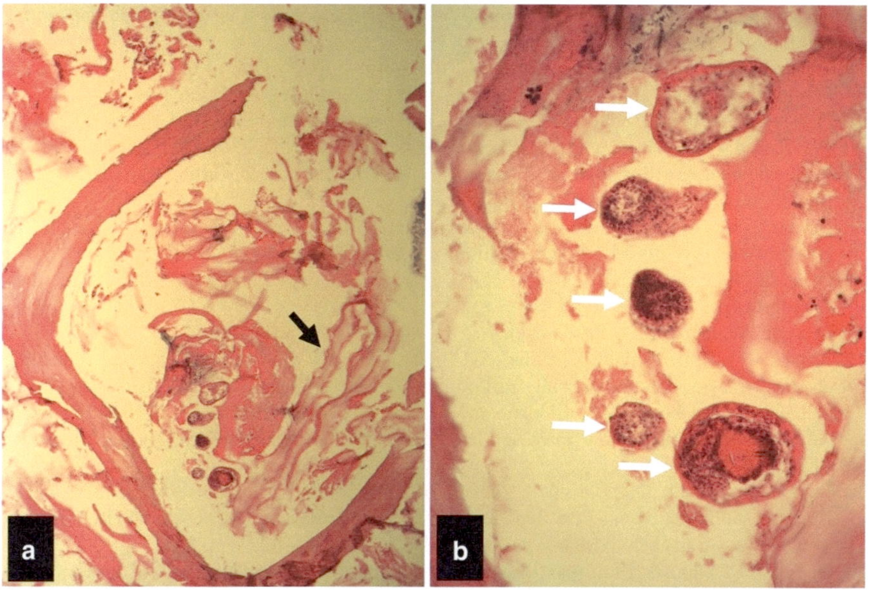

Fig. 4.8 Bone hydatidosis. Devitalized and eroded bone trabeculae by the growth of cysts. Medium power view showing hydatid membranes (*black arrow*) (**a**). High power view showing free protoscoleces of *Echinococcus granulosus* (*white arrows*) (**b**) (H&E stain)

With time, trabecular destruction is complete and the parasite reaches and destroys the skull tables, with subsequent spread of the disease to surrounding tissues extracranially and intracranially [42, 43]. If both outer table and inner table are destroyed, intra-cranial and extra-cranial spaces may communicate. Extraosseous hydatid cysts may calcify, while intraosseous hydatid cysts rarely present calcification [44, 45].

If bone lesions become infected by bacteria, severe bone necrosis and inflammatory reaction may appear forming granulomas with lymphocytes, eosinophils, polymorphonuclears, and giant cells mimicking a granulomatous infection.

References

1. Lu Y, Cen Y, Qing Y, Wang H. Surgical treatment of chronic osteomyelitis of the skull. Zhongguo Xiu Fu Chong Jian Wai Ke Za Zhi. 2011;25(5):558–61. Chinese.
2. Williams GT, Anderson W, Bryce DP. Osteomyelitis complicating fibrous dysplasia of the skull. Arch Otolaryngol. 1972;96(3):278–81.
3. Qureshi A, Quinones-Hinojosa A, Ziai W. A rare infectious presentation of a temporal bone meningioma. J Neurooncol. 2014;116(3):633–4. doi:10.1007/s11060-013-1319-8.
4. Valerón-Almazán P, Gómez-Duaso AJ, Rivero P, Vilar J, Dehesa L, Santana N, Carretero G. Extensive, non-healing scalp ulcer associated with trauma-induced chronic osteomyelitis. Ann Dermatol. 2011;23 Suppl 3:S364–7. doi:10.5021/ad.2011.23.S3.S364.

5. Boeckx WD, van der Hulst RR, Nanhekhan LV, De Lorenzi F. The role of free flaps in the treatment of persistent scalp osteomyelitis. Neurosurgery. 2006;59(1 Suppl 1):ONS64–7.
6. Wilensky AO. Osteomyelitis of the skull. Arch Surg. 1933;27(1):83–158.
7. Schmidt HG, Tiemann AH, Braunschweig R, Diefenbeck M, Bühler M, Abitzsch D, Haustedt N, Walter G, Schoop R, Heppert V, Hofmann GO, Glombitza M, Grimme C, Gerlach UJ, Flesch I. Arbeitsgemeinschaft septische Chirugie der DGOUC10 [Definition of the diagnosis osteomyelitis-osteomyelitis diagnosis score (ODS)]. Z Orthop Unfall. 2011;149 (4):449–60. doi:10.1055/s-0030-1270970. German.
8. Bruder E, Jundt G, Eyrich G. Pathology of osteomyelitis. In: Baltensperger MM, Eyrich GK, editors. Osteomyelitis of the jaws. Berlin: Springer; 2009.
9. Chandler JR, Grobman L, Quencer R, Serafini A. Osteomyelitis of the base of the skull. Laryngoscope. 1986;96(3):245–51.
10. Lew DP, Waldvogel FA. Osteomyelitis. Lancet. 2004;364(9431):369–79.
11. Akhaddar A, Elmostarchid B, Boulahroud O, Elouennass M, Boucetta M. Actinomycotic brain abscess with osteomyelitis arising from frontal sinusitis. Intern Med. 2009;48(8):619–20.
12. Akhaddar A, Albouzidi A, Elouennas M, Elmostarchid B, Boucetta M. Nonsuppurative calvarial thickening: a new form of Garré disease? J Neurosurg. 2009;110(4):808. doi:10.3171/2008.3.17458.
13. Ikonomopoulos JA, Gorgoulis VG, Zacharatos PV, Manolis EN, Kanavaros P, Rassidakis A, Kittas C. Multiplex polymerase chain reaction for the detection of mycobacterial DNA in cases of tuberculosis and sarcoidosis. Mod Pathol. 1999;12(9):854–62.
14. Gopinath K, Singh S. Multiplex PCR assay for simultaneous detection and differentiation of Mycobacterium tuberculosis, Mycobacterium avium complexes and other Mycobacterial species directly from clinical specimens. J Appl Microbiol. 2009;107(2):425–35. doi:10.1111/j.1365-2672.2009.04218.x.
15. Könönen E, Wade WG. Actinomyces and related organisms in human infections. Clin Microbiol Rev. 2015;28(2):419–42. doi:10.1128/CMR.00100-14.
16. Valour F, Sénéchal A, Dupieux C, Karsenty J, Lustig S, Breton P, Gleizal A, Boussel L, Laurent F, Braun E, Chidiac C, Ader F, Ferry T. Actinomycosis: etiology, clinical features, diagnosis, treatment, and management. Infect Drug Resist. 2014;7:183–97. doi:10.2147/IDR.S39601.
17. Vannier JP, Schaison G, George B, Casin I. Actinomycotic osteomyelitis of the skull and atlas with late dissemination. A case of transient neurosurgical syndrome. Eur J Pediatr. 1986;145 (4):316–8.
18. Akhaddar A, Elouennass M, Baallal H, Boucetta M. Focal intracranial infections due to Actinomyces species in immunocompetent patients: diagnostic and therapeutic challenges. World Neurosurg. 2010;74(2–3):346–50. doi:10.1016/j.wneu.2010.05.029.
19. Nugent NF, Murphy M, Kelly J. Scalp abscess—a cautionary tale. J Plast Reconstr Aesthet Surg. 2010;63(8):e619–21. doi:10.1016/j.bjps.2010.02.011.
20. Ambrosioni J, Lew D, Garbino J. Nocardiosis: updated clinical review and experience at a tertiary center. Infection. 2010;38:89–97. doi:10.1007/s15010-009-9193-9.
21. Kulkarni V, Rajshekhar V. Chronic non-healing ulcers of the scalp after trauma. Postgrad Med J. 2000;76(897):437, 450–1.
22. Nalini A, Saini J, Mahadevan A. Central nervous system norcardiosis with granulomatous pachymeningitis and osteomyelitis of skull vault. Indian J Pathol Microbiol. 2014;57:332–4. doi:10.4103/0377-4929.134735.
23. Shin KH, Lee WS, Son YK, Lee K, Chong Y. Nocardia osteomyelitis in a pachymeningitis patient: an example of a difficult case to treat with antimicrobial agents. Yonsei Med J. 1998;39(6):604–10.
24. Miyabe S, Koizuka I, Ochi K, Tanaka K, Kuroda H, Kenmochi M, Okada T, Tomisawa H, Sugiyama Y. Two cases of Aspergillus sinusitis with bone destruction. Auris Nasus Larynx. 2003;30:S115.

25. Akhaddar A, Gazzaz M, Albouzidi A, Lmimouni B, Elmostarchid B, Boucetta M. Invasive Aspergillus terreus sinusitis with orbitocranial extension: case report. Surg Neurol. 2008;69(5):490–5. doi:10.1016/j.surneu.2007.02.059.
26. Segal BH. Aspergillosis. N Engl J Med. 2009;360(18):1870–84. doi:10.1056/NEJMra0808853.
27. Panda NK, Ekambar Eshwara Reddy C. Primary frontal sinus aspergillosis: an uncommon occurrence. Mycoses. 2005;48(4):235–7.
28. Kountakis SE, Kemper Jr JV, Chang CY, DiMaio DJ, Stiernberg CM. Osteomyelitis of the base of the skull secondary to Aspergillus. Am J Otolaryngol. 1997;18(1):19–22.
29. Kwon-Chung KJ. Taxonomy of fungi causing mucormycosis and entomophthoramycosis (zygomycosis) and nomenclature of the disease: molecular mycologic perspectives. Clin Infect Dis. 2012;54 Suppl 1:S8–15. doi:10.1093/cid/cir864.
30. Fortún J, Cobo J, Cañal J, Martínez-San MJ. Post-traumatic cranial mucormycosis in an immunocompetent patient. J Oral Maxillofac Surg. 1995;53(9):1099–102.
31. Devireddy SK, Kumar RVK, Gali R, Kanubaddy SR, Dasari MR, Akheel M. Mucormycotic skull base osteomyelitis: a case report. J Oral Maxillofac Surg Med Pathol. 2014;26(3):336–9.
32. Amit A, Sudish K, Pople IK. Primary calvarial cryptococcal osteomyelitis in a patient with idiopathic lymphopenia. Acta Neurochir (Wien). 2008;150(7):713–4. doi:10.1007/s00701-008-1608-8.
33. Prendiville S, Bielamowicz SA, Hawrych A, Deeb ZE. Isolated cryptococcal sphenoid sinusitis with septicemia, meningitis, and subsequent skull base osteomyelitis in an immunocompetent patient. Otolaryngol Head Neck Surg. 2000;123(3):277–9.
34. Armonda RA, Fleckenstein JM, Brandvold B, Ondra SL. Cryptococcal skull infection: a case report with review of the literature. Neurosurgery. 1993;32(6):1034–6.
35. Kong QT, Zhou WQ, Feng J, Sang H, Deng DQ, Wang Z, Li J, Shi QL, Wu B, Liu WD. Isolated skull cryptococcosis in an immunocompetent patient. Mycopathologia. 2013;175(1–2):187–91. doi:10.1007/s11046-012-9609-9.
36. Corral JE, Lima S, Quezada J, Samayoa B, Arathoon E. Cryptococcal osteomyelitis of the skull. Med Mycol. 2011;49(6):667–71. doi:10.3109/13693786.2011.558124.
37. Agadi JB, Madni NA, Nanjappa V, Govindaiah HK. Cryptococcal osteomyelitis of the skull in a patient with transient lymphopenia. Neurol India. 2010;58(2):300–2. doi:10.4103/0028-3886.63798.
38. Devgan BK, Devgan M, Gross CW. Blastomycosis of fronto-ethmoid complex. South Med J. 1978;71(2):191–4.
39. Makary CA, Roberts TD, Wetmore SJ. Disseminated blastomycosis presenting as mastoiditis and epidural abscess. W V Med J. 2014;110(1):46–7.
40. Yocum J, Seligson D. Blastomycosis of the knee and skull after arthroscopy. Am J Sports Med. 1991;19(6):670–2.
41. Farr RC, Gardner G, Acker JD, Brint JM, Haglund LF, Land M, Schweitzer JB, West BC. Blastomycotic cranial osteomyelitis. Am J Otol. 1992;13(6):582–6.
42. Limaiem F, Bellil S, Bellil K, Chelly I, Mekni A, Kallel J, Haouet S, Zitouna M, Kchir N. Hydatid cyst of the cranial vault. J Infect Dev Ctries. 2009;3(10):807–10.
43. Aydin Y, Aydin F, Ture U. Intradiploeic and cerebral hydatidosis: a case report and review of literature. Clin Neurol Neurosurg. 1992;94(3):229–33.
44. Ciurea AV, Vasilescu G, Nuteanu L, Carp N. Cerebral hydatid cyst in children. Experience of 27 cases. Childs Nerv Syst. 1995;11(12):679–85.
45. Polat P, Kantarci M, Alper F, Suma S, Koruyucu MB, Okur A. Hydatid disease from head to toe. Radiographics. 2003;23(2):475–94.

Chapter 5
Pathophysiology and Anatomical Spreads of Infection

Contents

Over the years, major changes and modifications have been introduced to improve the diagnosis accuracy and treatment of cranial osteomyelitis. Many of these changes have been based on a better understanding of the pathophysiologic basis of skull bone infection. Pathogens may reach the skull bone using various conceivable portals of entry and mechanisms of spread in order to establish infection. The most usual possibilities are secondary to direct inoculation (by trauma or surgical manipulation), following contiguous source of adjacent infection (mainly paranasal sinusitis) or via hematogenous bloodborne route. We must highlight that cranial osteomyelitis is often the transitional point between a primary extracranial infection and its secondary intracranial extension.

Applied Anatomy of Neurocranium

Skull osteomyelitis develops as a logical consequence of the anatomic relationships of the skull structures and the infectious organisms. A brief review of these unique anatomic relationships is fundamental to understand the pathogenesis, varieties of clinico-pathological presentations and potential complications associated with this

A. Akhaddar, *Cranial Osteomyelitis*, DOI 10.1007/978-3-319-30268-3_5

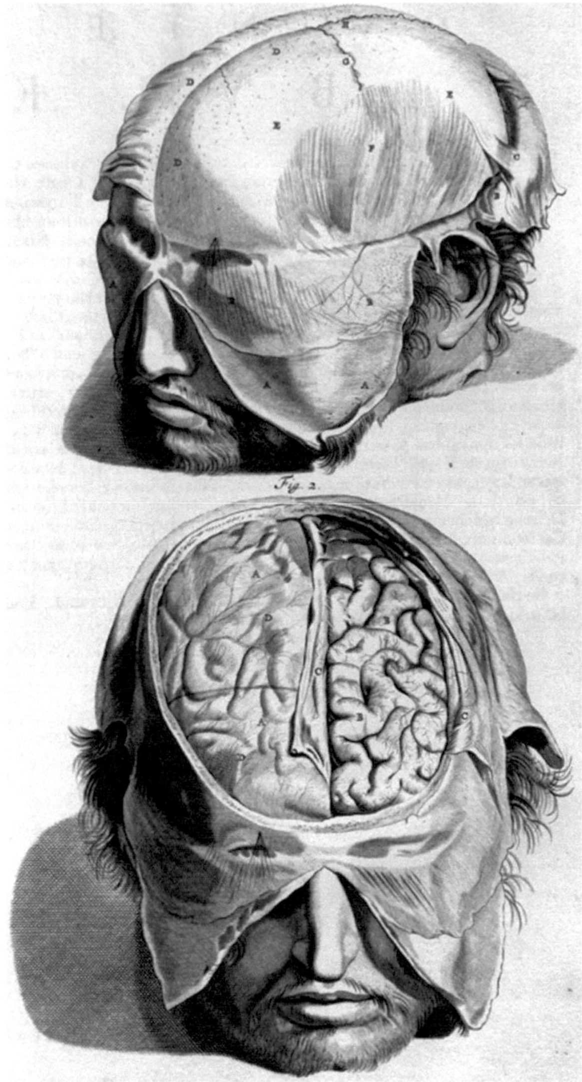

Fig. 5.1 Illustration from *Bidloo's Anatomia humani corporis (1685)*. Table 5 showing a dissection of the skull and scalp in the first figure (*up*) and the dura mater and cerebrum in the second (*down*) [1]

disease. Classically, the neurocranium has significant proximity with extracranial structures (scalp and facial formations) and intracranial spaces (meninges and brain parenchyma) which largely explain risk factors and complications related to cranial osteomyelitis (Figs. 5.1, 5.2, 5.3, and 5.4). Also, extracranial, cranial and intracranial areas may communicate with an important venous network which allows extension of infection.

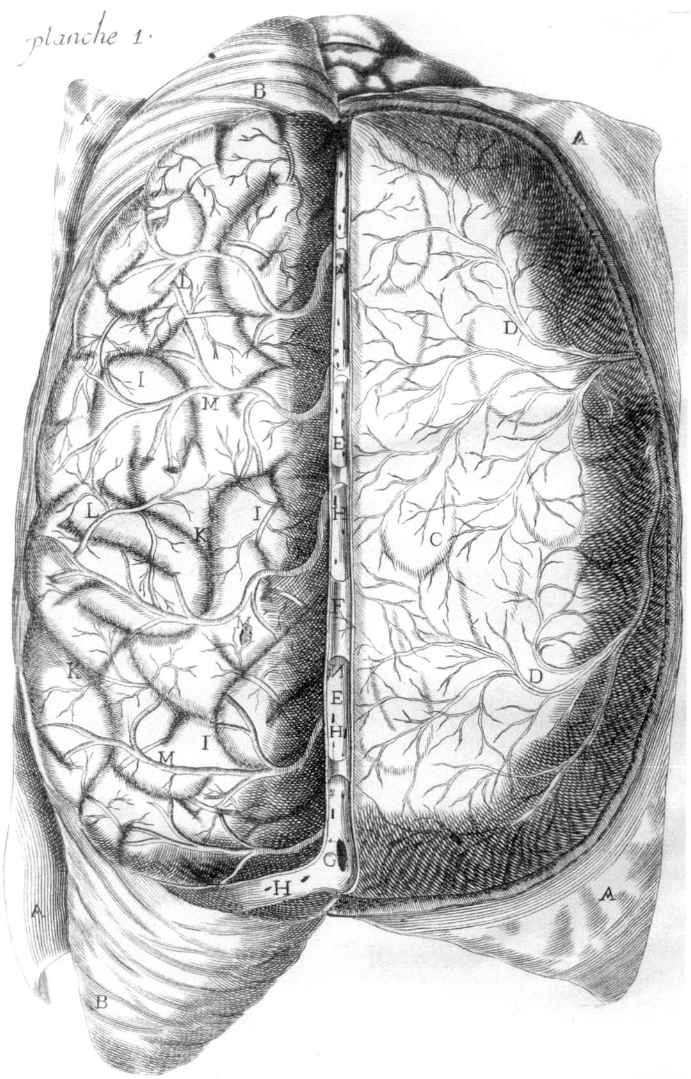

Fig. 5.2 Illustration from *Bonhomme's Anatomie (1748)*. Board 1 showing the internal part of the cranial vault: the exposed dura mater and brain cortex [2]. (From the personal collection of A. Akhaddar, Marrakech, Morocco)

Extracranial Structures

The scalp represents the soft tissues which cover the cranial vault. It is usually described as having five layers (Fig. 5.5), which can be memorized by the simple mnemonic acronym "**SCALP**" from superficial to deep [3–5]:

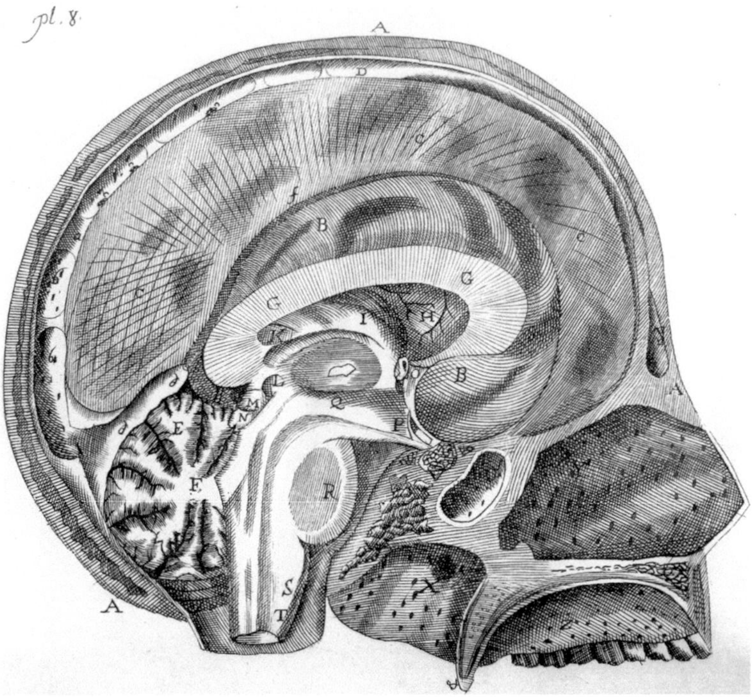

Fig. 5.3 Illustration from *Bonhomme's Anatomie (1748)*. Board 8 showing the intracranial content of the neurocranium and its relationships with the cavities of the face [2]. (From the personal collection of A. Akhaddar, Marrakech, Morocco)

- S: **Skin** (epidermis + dermis) is thick and subdivided into the epiderm and derm with numerous hairs, sebaceous and sweat glands. Aesthetically, it is the most important structure in any repair.
- C: **Connective tissue**. It is a dense subcutaneous layer of fat and fibrous tissue (a thickness of 4–7 mm) that attaches the skin to the underlying galea. All large blood vessels, nerves of the scalp and lymphatic system are located in this layer.
- A: **Aponeurosis** (also called epicranium or galea layers) which separates the underlying bone and the overlying layers. It is a tough layer of dense fibrous tissue (fascial plane) which runs from the frontalis muscle anteriorly to the occipitalis muscle posteriorly and the temporalis fascia laterally.
- L: **Loose connective tissue** (subgaleal space). This thin layer accounts for the mobility of the scalp on the underlying skull. It provides a plane of access in neurosurgery via a scalp flap. This layer is often called the "dangerous area of scalp" because of the ease by which infectious agents can spread through it to emissary veins which then drain into intracranial sinuses.
- P: **Pericranium** which is the external periosteum of the skull. It can be separated from the skull, except near the sutures. The pericranium provides nutrition to the bone and the capacity for repair.

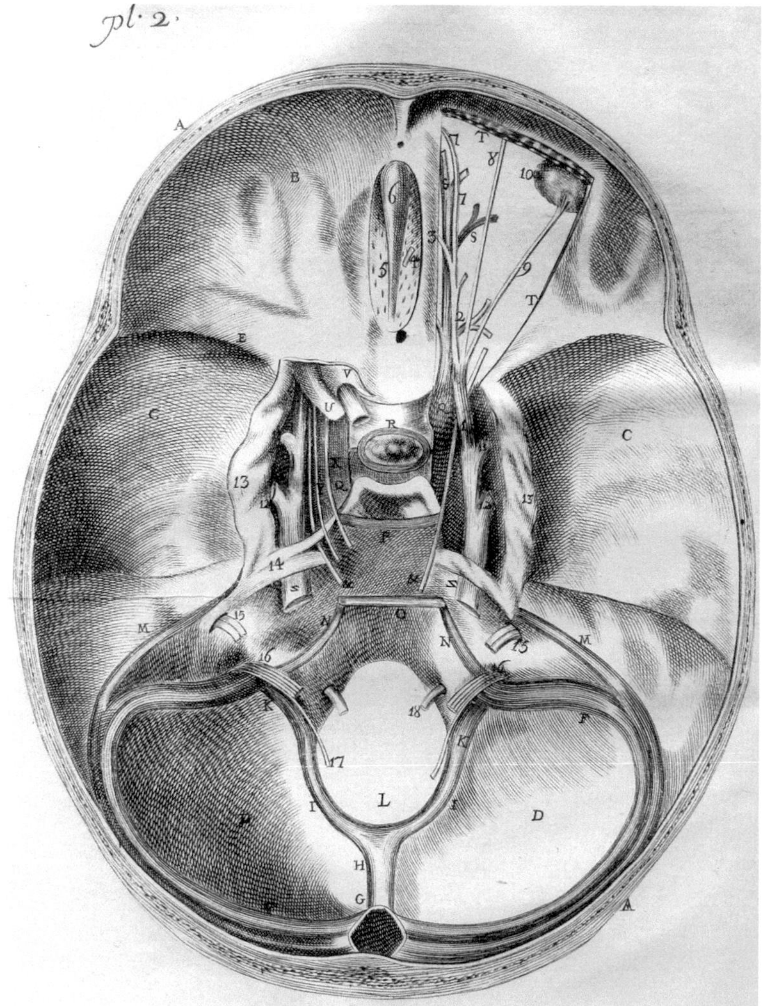

Fig. 5.4 Illustration from *Bonhomme's Anatomie (1748)*. Board 2 showing the intracranial content of the skull base [2]. (From the personal collection of A. Akhaddar, Marrakech, Morocco)

According to Hyman et al., the mentioned anatomic layers can be regrouped into three clinically useful coverings that are distinct on modern imaging (magnetic resonance imaging and computed tomography-scan): skin, fatty subcutaneous space and the galea/subgalea/periosteal complex that blend with the outer table of the skull [4].

The blood supply of the scalp depends on five main vessels including the superficial temporal, the supraorbital, the frontal, the posterior auricular and the occipital arteries. These arterial pedicles form an extensive interconnecting network with a multiplicity of anastomoses and collateral circulation across the vertex of the cranial vault that connect the circulation on both sides [6].

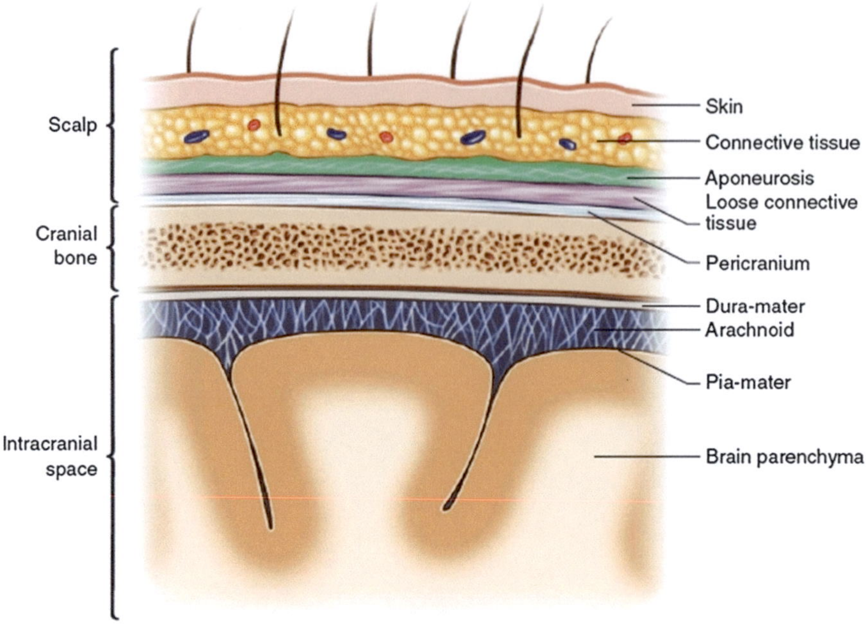

Fig. 5.5 Schematic drawing showing the different layers of the scalp, cranial bones, meninges and brain parenchyma

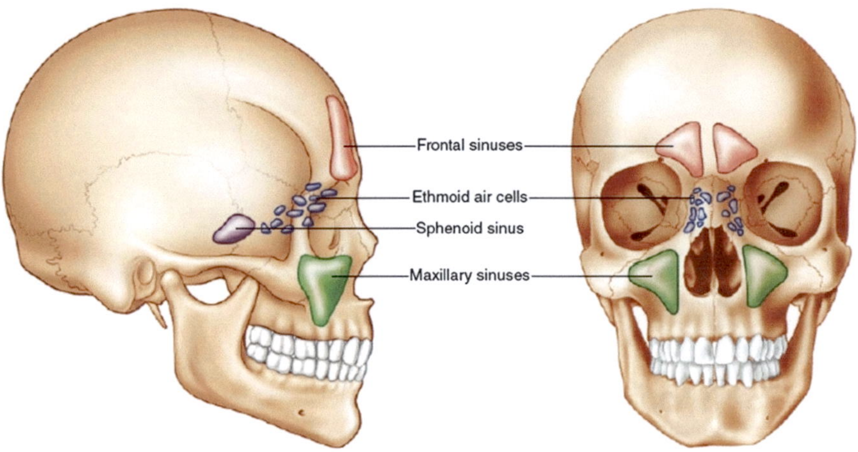

Fig. 5.6 Schematic drawing showing the different types of paranasal sinuses

Beside the scalp, the aerated sinus cavities of the skull (frontal, ethmoidal, maxillary and sphenoidal sinuses) are a source for cranial infection (Fig. 5.6). Due to their anatomic proximity, sinus and middle ear infections may spread to the cranial vault and skull base structures. The frontal sinus cavity is an enlargement within the marrow medullary cavity of the frontal bone. Frontal sinuses develop from the ethmoid air cells, with pneumatization starting during the first years of life. However frontal sinuses are not radiographically apparent until nearly 6–7 years of age. By age 12–13 years, the frontal sinuses are close to adult size [7–9]. The maxillary sinuses are anterior to the middle cranial fossa and are separated from the orbit laterally by the perpendicular plate of the ethmoid bone. The nasal cavities are positioned inferior to the anterior cranial fossa separated by the cribriform plate of the ethmoid. The sphenoid sinus is situated below the cavernous sinuses and anterior to the prepontine cistern and brainstem. These paranasal sinuses are lined by ciliated epithelium and are usually sterile; however transient colonization from mouth and nasal flora may occur [10].

The middle and inner ear are within the aerated mastoid air cells. There is essentially a pre-existing pathway through the internal acoustic meatus to the dura and potentially the subarachnoid space. On the other hand, to prevent meningeal extension, there is only a thin cartilaginous sheet between the squamous and the petrous portion of the temporal bone [11].

Enlargement and tenderness of the regional lymph nodes may signify an unrecognized scalp infection.

Cranial Bone Formations

The skull is the skeletal structure of the head that supports the face (viscerocranium) and protects the brain (neurocranium). The neurocranium consists of two parts: the cranial vault (calvaria) and the skull base. The cranial vault is formed by the frontal, parietal, and occipital bones, as well as a small portion formed by the temporal bones (squamous parts) (Fig. 5.7). The skull base is composed of portions of a variety of different bones including the occipital bone, temporal bones (mastoid and petrous portions, tympanic part and styloïd process), sphenoid bone, orbital plate of the frontal bone and the ethmoid cribriform plate. This complex anatomical structure can be divided into three areas: a more elevated anterior part (anterior cranial fossa), a middle part (middle cranial fossa) which contains in its center the central skull base, and finally a lower posterior part (posterior cranial fossa) (Fig. 5.8). The bones of the calvaria are plat, regular and formed of two cortical layers of compact bone: the inner and outer tables with spongious bony tissue between them known as diploë. The thickness of diploic space varies greatly between the site and the age of the subject [3, 12] (Fig. 5.9). All the bones of the cranial vault are developed from membrane, and with age, vascularity and periosteal propensity to new bone formation diminishes. However, the blood flow through the emissary channels in the diploë persists. The diploë in the calvarial bones are important, especially in the parietal, frontal and occipital bones. The temporal bone with the attached temporalis muscle and the occipital bone with the attached occipitalis are somewhat vascular, with important flow rates. Therefore, the septic nidus cannot establish a foothold in these bones. The frontalis muscle has no attachment to bone, so the

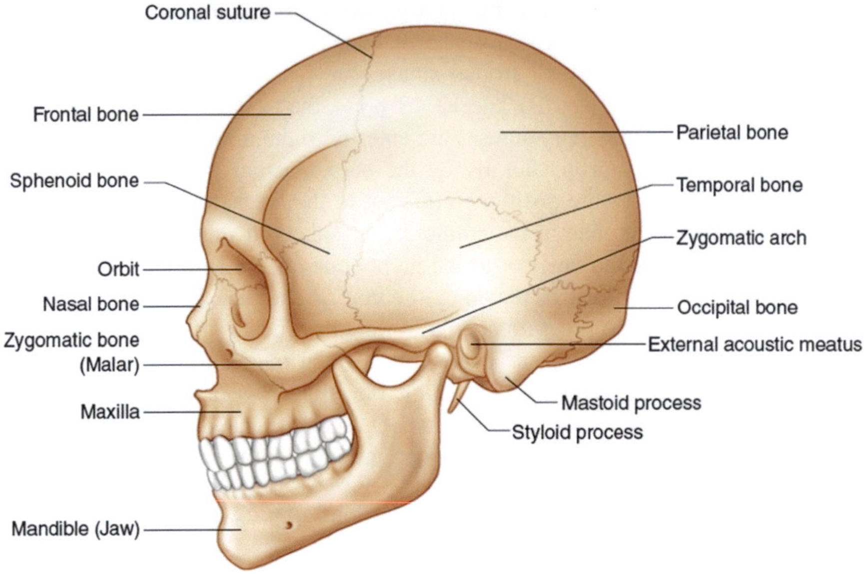

Fig. 5.7 Schematic design showing the lateral extracranial view of the skull bone

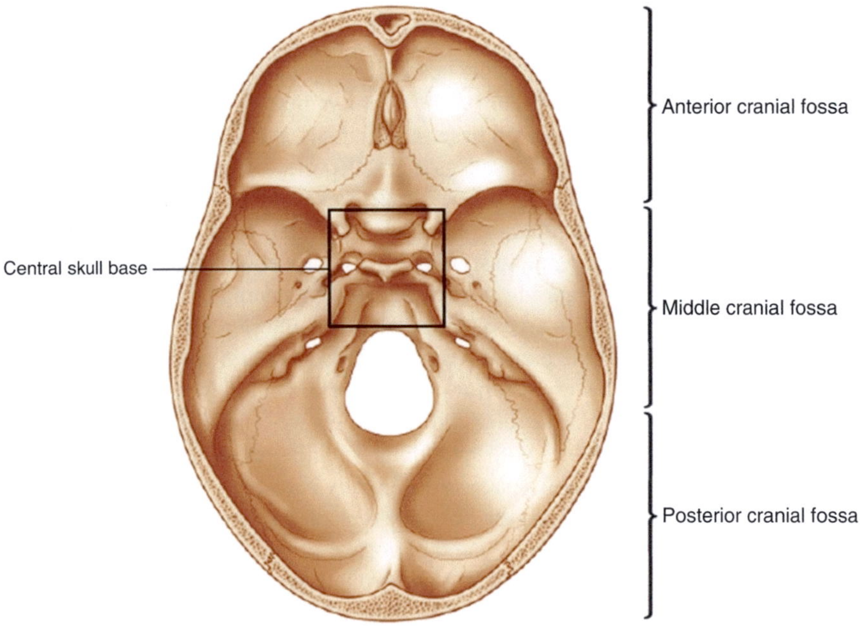

Fig. 5.8 Schematic design showing the superior intracranial view of the skull base and its 3 anatomic divisions

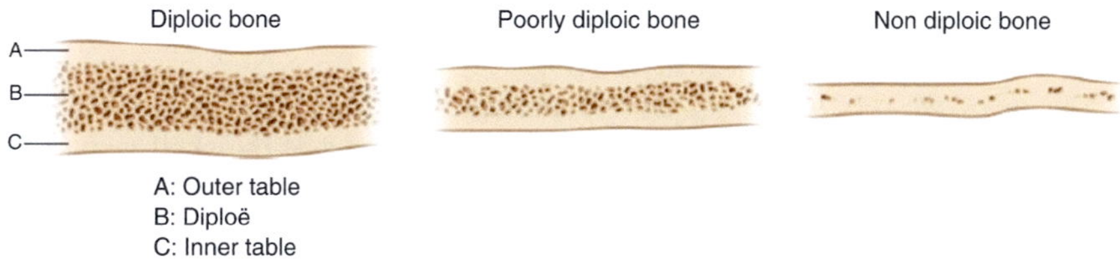

Fig. 5.9 Schematic drawing showing the various types of thickness of cranial bones

frontal and parietal bones are less vascular and only have the diploic emissary circulation. The flow in this area is of the "ebb and flow" type, allowing a septic nidus to establish a focus. This is one among other explanations for the predilection of cranial osteomyelitis to develop in the frontal and parietal bones [13].

The bones of the skull base are dense, irregulars, nondiploics and the spongious bony tissue may be very little represented or absent (Fig. 5.9). This is also one reason for the rarity of skull base osteomyelitis. In addition, there are some openings in the skull base (foramina and fissures), through which nerves or vessels pass. Infection tends to invade via these openings. The pterygopalatine fossa communicates with the middle cranial fossa via foramen rotundum, nasal cavity via sphenopalatine foramen, oral cavity via palatine foramen, foramen lacerum, and infra temporal fossa via pterygomaxillary fissure. The occipital bone forms the foramen magnum which communicates with the superior spinal canal and its content [14].

Intracranial Spaces

The meninges are the membranes that envelop and protect the brain. They consist of three layers: the dura mater, the arachnoid mater, and the pia mater (Fig. 5.5). The dura mater or pachymeninge (the outermost of the three meningeal layers) is attached to the internal surface of the inner table and forms the falx cerebri and the tentorium cerebelli and also delineates the dural veinous sinuses intracranially. In addition, the internal periosteum of the skull bone is included in the dura. The cranial dura is closely adhered to the skull at the cranial sutures, at the cranial base, and at the neural foramina where the dura becomes adjacent with the epineurium of the cranial nerves. Over the cranial vault, the dura mater is relatively less adherent, particularly in adolescents and young adults; therefore it is more predisposed to separation, resulting in a true space [11]. The arachnoid membrane is thin and avascular with trabeculae that reaches the pia mater. The pia mater itself is a thin membrane of connective tissue that firmly adheres to the cerebral surface. This last meningeal layer is pierced by blood vessels to the brain and its capillaries nourish the brain.

The extradural space (also known as epidural) is outside the dura. The subdural space is inside the dura. The cerebrospinal fluid flows in the subarachnoids spaces between the arachnoid membrane and the pia mater. More deeply we find the complex elements of brain parenchyma (Figs. 5.1 and 5.2).

The blood vessels which supply the meninges, of which the largest are the middle meningeal artery and vein, groove the inner aspect of the skull vault and lie between the bone and the dura. In addition to supplying the meninges, theses vessels also supply the overlying bone and the diploë [5].

Venous Communications

Beside classic arterial supply and venous drainage of the scalp, many sets of emissary veins are usually encountered in the scalp. This special venous system connects the classic extracranial venous system with the intracranial venous sinuses. They drain from the scalp, through the skull by diploic veins, into the larger meningeal veins and dural venous sinuses. They also serve as routes where infections are carried into the cranial cavity from the extracranial veins to the intracranial veins and produce a septic thrombosis within it. There are several types of emissary veins including posterior condyloid, mastoid, occipital, and parietal emissary veins. There are also emissary veins passing through the foramen ovale, jugular foramen, foramen lacerum and hypoglossal canal in the skull base [15–18].

In addition to such venous channels, there is a giant emissary system formed by the diploic veins. The latter are positioned between the inner and outer tables of the cranial vault, communicate with one another, traverse the sutures and they may drain into the dural venous sinuses intracranially. The four major types of diploic veins found on each side of the head are frontal, anterior temporal, posterior temporal, and occipital diploic veins. The parietal bone contained the most diploic vessels and no diploic veins were found in the area delimited by the temporal squama. Major anterior diploic system connects the superior sagittal sinus with the sphenoparietal veinous sinus. The posterior diploic system connects the superior sagittal sinus with the transverse and sigmoid sinuses. The diploic system develops fully by 2 years after birth and it is proportionally larger and more active in adolescents and young adults than in young children [15, 16, 19]. Some communicating veins may connect the emissary veins with the diploic system. Historically, Sir Victor Horsley in 1892 was the first user of bone wax as a practical solution to skull bones bleeding from diploic veins [20].

Because emissary veins, diploic veins, and dural sinuses have no valves, any infectious material that penetrates a small vein of the face, scalp, or nasal cavity may flow through an emissary vein into one of the dural sinuses and produce a septic thrombosis within it. Such a state can progress to bacteremia, meningitis, encephalitis or brain abscess [15, 16, 21]. Particular attention should be given to the frontal sinus area. Communications with the veins in the muco-periosteum of the frontal sinus are normally extremely fine. The frontal diploic veins allow frontal sinus muco-periosteum capillaries to communicate with the marrow cavity of the frontal bone and dural sinuses intracranially. It is via this disposition that purulent infections in the frontal sinuses occasionally give rise to osteomyelitis and intracranial infections [10, 22–24]. It is also important to know that the original composition of this complex venous channels and their anatomic disposition offer a unique way by which infection my travel from the frontal sinus or the scalp directly to the intracranial structures, without an intervening cranial bone infections [25–27]. Pearson et al. reported two cases of septic lateral sinus thrombosis in adults presenting with extracranial head and neck abscesses without previous otological history nor apparent cranial osteomyelitis [28].

Development and Progression of the Disease

The development and progression of infection in the skull bone requires some important factors including virulence and number of the infecting organisms, patients predisposing causes and comorbidities and lastly, the type and location of the skull bones [29–31]. Close interaction of these factors determine the pathological pathway of disease formation. Spread of infections may be disastrous, not only locally and regionally but possibly even systemically. Sadly, there is always a chance of a lethal complication from cranial osteomyelitis.

Virulence of the Pathogens

According to the anatomical structures discussed above, healthy bones are generally highly resistant to microbial invasion. However, when microorganisms are introduced into bone from surrounding structures, from direct inoculation related to surgery or trauma or hematogenously (via the bloodstream), osteomyelitis can occur. Bacteria may have various factors that can contribute to the development of osteomyelitis such as bacterial adherence, resistance to host defense mechanism, and proteolytic activity [30]. Bacteria must be able to subsequently adhere to components of the bone matrix in order to start the infection. *Staphylococcus aureus* has been known to bind fibrinogen for a long time. Bacteria clump together and are covered in a layer of fibrinogen, thus protected from host defense mechanisms and antibiotics [32]. In addition, Bacteria (principally *Staphylococcus aureus* and *Staphylococcus epidermidis*) adhere to bone matrix and foreign bodies via receptors to fibronectin, collagen and laminin and to other structural proteins [33]. They subsequently elude host defenses and antibiotics by "hiding" intracellularly, by developing a slimy coat (biofilm formation) or by acquiring a very slow metabolic rate [34–36]. The presence of a bony implant also causes a local polymorphonuclear cell defect, with decreased ability to kill phagocytosed bacteria [31, 37]. For all these reasons, antibiotic resistance increases more and more, antimicrobial treatment needs broad spectrum antibiotics with longer course of therapy and operative treatment should be considered whenever possible.

Normal osseous remodeling needs the synchronized interaction of osteoblasts and osteoclasts [38]. Osteolysis is determined locally by the interaction of bacterial surface components with immune system cells and subsequent cytokine production (such as interleukin-1, interleukin-6, interleukin-11, and tumor necrosis factor). Numerous soluble mediators are involved; the end result being both increased osteoclastic activity and decreased new bone formation by osteoblasts [39–42]. Streptococcal surface protein can stimulate bone resorption and inhibit protein synthesis in cultured mouse calvariae by a prostaglandin independent mechanism [43].

Gradually pus is formed and spreads into vascular channels, increasing the intraosseous pressure and impairing blood flow. This process will cause an intense inflammatory response, thrombosis, with subsequent purulent dissection of the periosteum from the skull bone and subperiosteal abscess formations that leads to devascularized bony fragments and bone infarcts. Microorganisms, infiltrations of neutrophils, and congested or thrombosed blood vessels are then the principal histologic findings in acute osteomyelitis [31]. A slower indolent infection will produce a mild to moderate inflammatory response and little or no ischemic necrosis as seen in subacute or intermediate osteomyelitis. In chronic osteomyelitis, a balance will be achieved between bone resorption and new bone formation, and sequestra are less likely to develop [29]. One of the distinguishing features of chronic osteomyelitis is necrotic bone, which can be recognized by the absence of living osteocytes [31].

On another side, chronic osteomyelitis may develop from 4.4 to 30 % of acute osteomyelitis [29, 44–47]. These chronic forms have less marked inflammatory cell reactions and there is a variable amount of necrotic tissue which protects organisms from antibiotics. Then the infection while self perpetuate and sequestra may also form in some cases. Because these are avascular, levels of antibiotics sufficient to eradicate the bacteria may not be achieved during treatment. For that reason, some cases may present as a recurrent or intermittent disease and bacteria may remain indolent for a long time (inactive disease) with period of quiescence of variable duration following by late reactivation of the disease after the initial acute episode (active disease). This phenomenon may require several years [29]. It is also important to know that in postoperative osteomyelitis, proposed mechanisms for cranial bone involvement include direct extension of a superficial infection and intraoperative contamination.

Patients Predisposing Causes and Comorbidities

Some local or general predisposing factors were frequently involved in cranial osteomyelitis (Table 5.1) such as vulnerability due to metabolic states (as diabetes mellitus), unbalanced nutritional states (obesity and malnutrition), smoking,

Table 5.1 Patients comorbidities and risk factors in cranial osteomyelitis

Systemic conditions	Obesity and malnutrition Diabetes mellitus Renal or hepatic failure Chronic hypoxia Compromised immune function Malignancy Long period of hospitalization Extremes of age Tobacco abuse
Local conditions	Extensive scarring Radiation fibrosis Small vessel disease Heavy contamination Presence of foreign body Bone necrosis

tobacco and cocaine use, specific exposure risks (prolonged preoperative stay, colonization with *Staphylococcus aureus)*, compromised immune function (defective immune system, human immunodeficiency virus infection, use of immunosuppressive medications or chronic systemic corticosteroids, irradiation of the head), malignancy, hemodialysis and age (especially newborn and advanced age) [48–52]. Patients with sickle cell disease are susceptible to acute skeletal infections mostly by *Salmonella species* [53, 54]. Moreover, the presence of devitalized bone fragments, bone necrosis, heavy contamination or implanted devices promote the development of the disease [55]. Foreign materials mistakenly left behind during cranial operations (named textilomas or gossypibomas) cause foreign body reaction in the surrounding tissue and may cause abscess formation and/or osteomyelitis in the early stage, whereas others remain clinically silent for many years [56].

Type and Location in the Skull Bones

Cranial bones have a singular osseous composition and vascular supply. These characteristics give not only a natural resistance to bony infection in the skull, but also provide a potential route for hematogenous seeding from other locations. Furthermore, the extensive anastomosis of vessels of the scalp, cranial bones, face and neck permits retrograde extension of infections. Generally, cranial diploic tissue is more vulnerable against the infectious process than the cortical tables.

Frontal sinusitis can directly cause frontal osteomyelitis by the erosion of bone by the microorganisms. If the outer table of the skull is involved, then the suppuration is subgaleal (under the aponeurosis). Similar erosion of the inner table results in suppuration that is subperiosteal, causing cranial epidural abscess or extradural empyema (Table 5.2). Expansion of this epidural process is by lateral progression of the osteomyelitic bone and by the suppuration dissecting the periosteum from the

Table 5.2 Localization of cranial, extracranial, and intracranial infections

Level	Anatomic space	Disease
Scalp		Subgaleal abscess Subcutaneous abscess Draining sinus tract
Skull	Bone	Osteomyelitis
	Extradural space	Extradural abscess
Dura matter		
	Subdural space	Subdural empyema
	Dural sinus	Dural thrombophlebitis
Arachnoid matter		
	Subarachnoid space	Meningitis
Pia matter/brain parenchyma	Pia matter	Cortical venous thrombosis
	Brain parenchyma	Brain abscess Cerebritis
	Ventricle	Intraventricular abscess Ventriculitis
Orbit	Orbital space	Orbital abscess
Spine	Craniocervical junction	Prevertebral abscess Osteoarticular infection Spondylodiscitis

bone at the lateral margins of the abscess. This mass grows slowly due to the rigidity of the pachymeninges and bone, has a convex or lentiform shape, and does not significantly deform underlying brain parenchyma unless it is quite large [57]. Ethmoid and sphenoid sinusitis can result in the same cranial invasion with anterior and central skull base osteomyelitis but are a less frequent source of complications [58–60].

More frequently infection spreads via septic thrombophlebitis or emboli [61]. The frontal sinus mucosa is drained by small diploic veins travelling through both the anterior and posterior bony borders of the sinus. As seen above, these veins are valveless and go along with venous plexuses draining the dura, periorbita and cranial periosteum. Therefore, thrombophlebitis may spread infection to the cranial diploe, periorbita, or intracranially [62, 63] (Table 5.2). A skull osteomyelitis on either the forehead or the scalp may result because thrombophlebitic infection crosses the scalp's suture lines via venous connections. Once a cranial osteomyelitis is established, infection may spread below the periosteum to cause an abscess. Such a subperiosteal abscess associated with an underlying cranial osteomyelitis of either the forehead or scalp is the classic Pott's puffy tumor [64] (see Chap. 15). Most of the diffuse forms of osteomyelitis of the skull occur after frontal sinusitis. The general tendency is to spread from anterior to posterior regions of the cranium: from the frontal bone to the parietal and temporal regions and finally to the occipital bone [63, 65]. The disease is not limited to one side of the skull; the opposite side may be involved by contiguity [48, 66–68]. However, there is no tendency for the cranial vault to spread into the skull base.

The diploic system is proportionally larger and more active in adolescents and young adults (particularly in men) and this might explain the higher risk of cerebral complications in patients of that age group with frontal bone osteomyelitis [24, 69–74]. Additionally, adolescents have a rapid growth of the frontal sinuses which sometimes have aberrant development [8]. For Ruf and Pancherz, the sinus enlargement pattern is similar to that of body height development, and its peak takes place at the mean age of 15 years [75].

Subdural empyema forms following bacterial seeding to the subdural space. An important inflammatory response occurs and usually the process progresses rapidly [76]. The leptomeninges offer little resistance to the expansion of the suppuration and subdural empyemas can become quite large over the brain convexity, the falx cerebri or tentorium cerebella and can extend bilaterally along dural septa [77]. Local meningeal irritation is present that becomes diffuse meningitis if a breach to the subarachnoid space occurs [78]. Septic thrombosis of involved bridging cortical veins creates cortical inflammation and vascular congestion, causing ischemia and edema within the brain parenchyma. All these effects are responsible for clinical signs and deficits that are observed and may accelerate the already rapid clinical decline [10]. However, it is important to keep in mind that sinogenic intracranial involvement is possible with or without direct erosion of the cranial bone [21, 25, 72, 79]. Interestingly, when subdural empyema occurs as a post-operative complication, the progress and presentation of this infectious collection are often less aggressive [80]. This is attributed to the postoperative formation of membranes that protect the cortex and limit the extension of the empyema [81].

Osteomyelitis of the skull base is much less frequent than that of the cranial vault: firstly, because the blood supply appears more extensive. Secondly, thin cortical plates and a relative paucity of diploic space (Fig. 5.9) in the skull base prevent confinement of infections within bone and permit the dissipation of edema and pus into the soft tissues and mastoid cells. In the skull base, osteomyelitis is frequently related to temporal bone infection.

As mentioned in Chap. 1, two types of osteomyelitis in the temporal bone can be recognized: one developing in the mastoid and the middle ear cleft (lateral temporal bone) and the other developing in the petrous apex (medial temporal bone). Lateral temporal osteomyelitis is predominantly caused by malignant external otitis, acute mastoiditis, and suppurative otitis media. Whereas medial temporal osteomyelitis is caused not only by malignant external otitis, but also by sphenoid sinusitis and other skull base infections (such as clivus). Nevertheless, it is important to note that the term "malignant external otitis" was improperly used by many otorhinolaryngologists to describe skull base osteomyelitis [65, 82, 83]. This term must be used to describe features limited to lateral temporal osteomyelitis which is a less serious condition than medial temporal osteomyelitis. Malignant external otitis can rarely progress to true skull base osteomyelitis [84]. More specifically, central skull base osteomyelitis is centered on the clivus rather than the temporal bones and presumably arises in most cases from paranasal sinus inflammatory disease rather than otitis or mastoiditis, although it may also be hematogenous in origin.

Skull base osteomyelitis originates from a chronic infection that has been inadequately treated, including chronic otitis media, chronic otitis externa, or any infection near the skull base. The infection may extend anteriorly to involve the parotid gland, temporomandibular joint, or the VIIth cranial nerve at its exit of the stylomastoid foramen. It may also extend posteriorly to the mastoid and vertical portion of VIIth cranial nerve or inferomedially to the skull base, including the carotid artery, jugular bulb, and sigmoid sinus [85, 86]. Facial nerve paralysis typically results when the extratemporal segment of the facial nerve becomes surrounded by infection at the stylomastoid foramen. Palsy can occur in cranial nerve IX, X, or XI when the jugular foramen becomes involved [87, 88]. Spread to the contralateral petrous apex, in opposite side, may also occurs in advanced disease through the basisphenoid [67, 84].

As described by Prasad et al., acute otomastoiditis may be complicated by temporal osteomyelitis. The evolution of acute mastoiditis begins when the mucosal lining of the pneumatized cells becomes inflamed and produces an exudate. Serosanguinous fluid eventually becomes mucopurulent. Spontaneous perforation of the tympanic membrane (myringotomy) would stop the process at this point. If the infection continues to progress, the cellular walls of the pneumatized cells then become demineralized. This demineralization occurs because of increased osteoclastic activity, pressure of the purulent exudate on the thin bony septae, and ischemia of the septae secondary to reduced blood flow. As the bony septae break down, small abscess cavities form, leading to coalescence. Lastly, the coalescent cells form an empyema, which then extends to surrounding areas. Acute mastoiditis becomes clinically significant when infection spreads through the periosteum (periostitis). When the blood vessels get involved, bony destruction occurs and a sequestrum is formed in the mastoid, leading to chronic osteomyelitis [65]. About 5 % of patients with acute mastoiditis developed osteomyelitis of the temporal bone as a complication [89]. Several serious complications have been described in the literature occurring from skull base osteomyelitis such as cranial nerve palsies, cavernous sinus involvement (inducing suppurative intracranial thrombophlebitis), meningitis, intrasellar infection and brain parenchyma extension [90, 91]. Cranial nerve neuropathy arises secondary to proximity to the brain stem, basal cisterns, cavernous sinus, and foramina of the skull base [92]. Other complications of skull base osteomyelitis reported in the literature have included epidural abscess of the cervical spine as a result from spread of infection through the prevertebral space [93] and petroclival abscess [94].

In lateral temporal osteomyelitis, diabetes mellitus seems to be a predisposing factor in the development of malignant otitis externa due to defects in chemotaxis and phagocytosis of polymorphonuclear leukocytes, monocytes, and macrophages, in addition to an increase in the cerumen pH. The oxidative burst and killing function of polymorphonuclear leukocytes has also been shown to be decreased in the diabetic population [82, 85].

The mechanical disruption that is caused by trauma or neurosurgical intervention can, as expected, result in cranial osteomyelitis mainly when frontal sinus is opened. The majority of postoperative infections result from skin organisms acquired at the time of surgery such as *Staphylococcus aureus* and *Staphylococcus epidermidis* as well as gram-negative rods including *Pseudomonas species*. Their common physiopathology is suggested by their frequent association in a single patient and by the predominance of saprophyte skin flora microorganisms [95]. Recently, Chiang et al. reported that operative factors such as the way the skin is prepared before the incision rather than the skin flora contaminants on the bone flaps may play an important role in the pathogenesis of surgical site infections after craniotomy/craniectomy [96].

Rarely there are cases that are apparently from hematogenous dissemination. In these cases, infectious agents are determined by the source of infection [97–99]. Sometimes, no pre-existing infections are found [100]. Hematogenous spread is also suspected on infected cephalhematoma with cranial vault osteomyelitis in newborns. Indeed, many cases manifested with septicemia, and meningitis [101, 102].

Towards a New Classification

Skull osteomyelitis is believed to be a difficult and challenging entity to diagnose and manage correctly. Most cases occur as a consequence of paranasal sinusitis, otomastoiditis or secondary to surgical site infections. In addition, and as mentioned above, the skull has important and complex anatomic relationships with extracranial and intracranial structures. So, the problem of cranial osteomyelitis is likely to get worse when intracranial suppurations occur with their potentially life-threatening consequences.

Due to the scarce presentations in the literature of cranial bone infections, there is no specific classification for cranial osteomyelitis. Current classifications are applied to osteomyelitis of tubular bones and some others for osteomyelitis of the jaws. Most of these classifications were established by orthopedic surgeons and infectious disease specialists [103–110]. This is mainly due to the reality that osteomyelitis principally involves long bones and foreign devices are widely used. The two most commonly used classifications for osteomyelitis are Waldvogel classification [103] (Table 5.3) and Cierny-Mader Staging [104] (Table 5.4). Although these two classifications describe the infection, they do not apply for special situations such as skull osteomyelitis. The topic of cranial osteomyelitis differs considerably from osteomyelitis of the long bones and at other skeletal sites, so the previous classifications do not seem appropriate to the skull.

Table 5.3 Waldvogel classification system for osteomyelitis [103]

Hematogenous osteomyelitis	
Osteomyelitis secondary to contiguous focus of infection	No generalized vascular disease
Osteomyelitis secondary to contiguous focus of infection	Generalized vascular disease
Chronic osteomyelitis (necrotic bone)	

Table 5.4 Cierny-Mader staging system for osteomyelitis [104]

Classification	Description
Anatomic type	
Stage 1	Medullary osteomyelitis
Stage 2	Superficial osteomyelitis
Stage 3	Localized osteomyelitis
Stage 4	Diffuse osteomyelitis
Physiological class	
A host	Normal host
B host	Systemic compromise (Bs), local compromise (Bl), or systemic and local compromise (Bls)
C host	Treatment worse than the disease

Dissatisfaction with existing classifications encouraged us to develop a new one to allow specialists to speak a uniform language globally related to different anatomic stages of skull osteomyelitis. Computed tomography scan is often needed for the diagnosis. However, in the early stage, computed tomography scan may not reveal an osteomyelitis and in such cases, a radionuclide bone scanning or magnetic resonance imaging are quite helpful. However, the gold standard for diagnosis of osteomyelitis is bone biopsy.

According to this simple new classification (staging system for skull osteomyelitis or **3SO**), cranial osteomyelitis is classified into five main types based on the location of skull involved and its extension (Fig. 5.10). Type 0 (initial cranial bone involvement), type I (limited to cranial bone), type II (extracranial extension), type III (intracranial extension), and type IV (cranial, extracranial and intracranial involvement).

The above classification is very simple, easy to remember, useful as a teaching tool and it is practical. It will reflect the complexity of skull osteomyelitis; provide conclusions for the treatment and prevention of progression of the disease. This classification must also prognosticate and compare the results of treatment.

Concerning our 29 patients with cranial osteomyelitis, type I had 2 patients (6.9 %), type II with 4 patients (13.8 %), type III had 11 patients (37.9 %) while type IV with 12 patients (41.4 %).

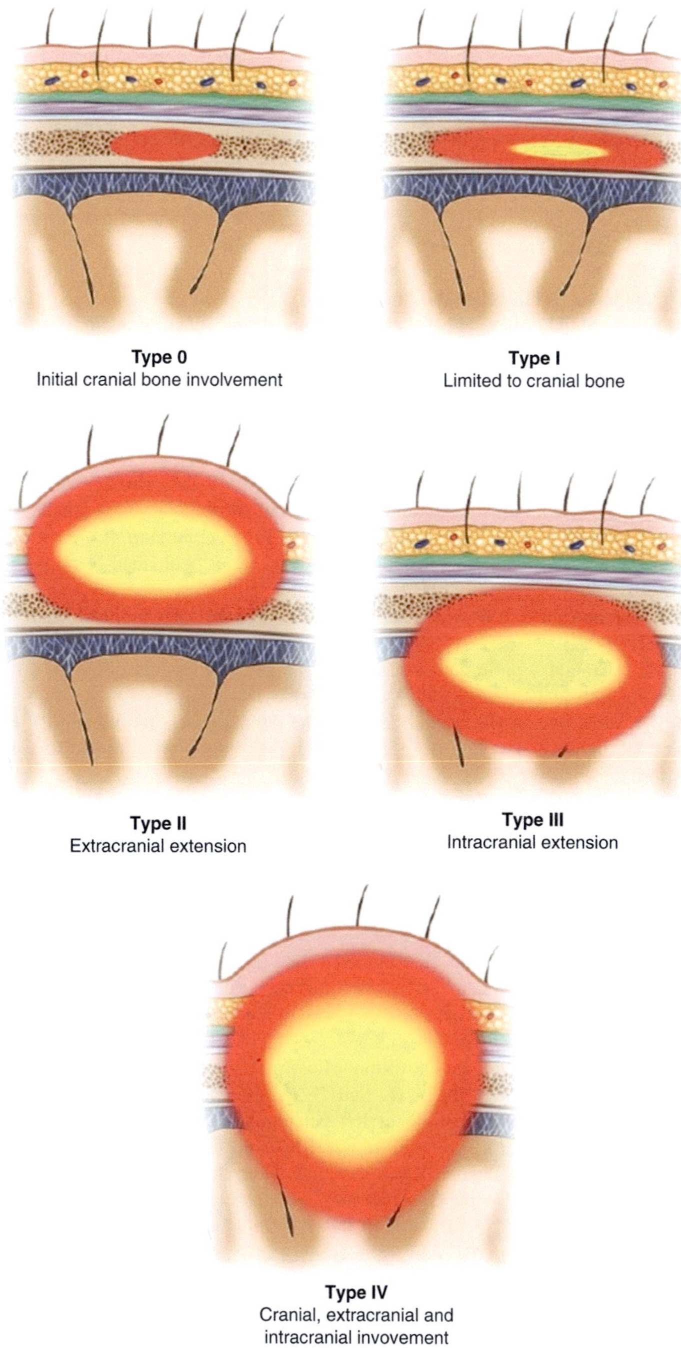

Fig. 5.10 Illustration showing the author's classification of cranial osteomyelitis (staging system for skull osteomyelitis or **3SO**) into five main types based on the location of infection and its extension

References

1. Bidloo G. Medicinae Doctoris & Chirurgi, Anatomia Hvmani Corporis: Centum & quinque Tabvlis Per artificiosiss. G. De Lairesse ad vivum delineatis, Demonstrata, Veterum Recentiorumque Inventis explicata plurimisque, hactenus non detectis, Illvstrata. Amsterdam (Netherlands): Sumptibus Viduae Joannis à Someren, Haeredum Joannis à Dyk, Henrici & Viduae Theodori Boom; 1685.
2. Bonhomme J. Traité de la céphalotomie ou description anatomique des parties que la tête renferme. Avignon, France: François Girard Edition; 1748.
3. Agur AMR, Dalley II AF. Grant's atlas of anatomy. 13th ed. Philadelphia: Wolters Kluwer Health/Lippincott Williams & Wilkins; 2012.
4. Hayman LA, Shukla V, Ly C, Taber KH. Clinical and imaging anatomy of the scalp. J Comput Assist Tomogr. 2003;27(3):454–9.
5. Ellis H, Mahadevan V. The surgical anatomy of the scalp. Surgery—Oxford International Edition. 2014;32(Supp 1):e1–5. doi:http://dx.doi.org/10.1016/j.mpsur.2013.04.02
6. Dingman RD, Argenta LC. The surgical repair of traumatic defects of the scalp. Clin Plast Surg. 1982;9:131–3.
7. Huijssoon E, Woerdeman PA, van Diemen-Steenvoorde RA, Hanlo PW, Plötz FB. An 8-year-old boy with a Pott's puffy tumor. Int J Pediatr Otorhinolaryngol. 2003;67(9):1023–6.
8. Germiller JA, Monin DL, Sparano AM, Tom LW. Intracranial complications of sinusitis in children and adolescents and their outcomes. Arch Otolaryngol Head Neck Surg. 2006;132 (9):969–76.
9. Vidić B. The morphogenesis of the lateral nasal wall in the early prenatal life of man. Am J Anat. 1971;130(2):121–39.
10. Bartt RE. Cranial epidural abscess and subdural empyema. Handb Clin Neurol. 2010;96:75–89. doi:10.1016/S0072-9752(09)96006-7.
11. Smith BH. Infections of the cranial dura and the dural sinuses. In: Vinken PJ, Bruyn GW, Klawans HL, editors. Handbook of clinical neurology, infections of the nervous system part I. Amsterdam: Elsevier; 1978.
12. Standring S. Gray's anatomy: the anatomical basis of clinical practice. 40th ed. Churchill-Livingstone: Elsevier; 2008.
13. Mukherjee KK, Kaushik R, Nada R, Khosla VK, Khandelwal N, Kak VK. Calvarial tuberculosis. Surg Neurol. 2002;57(3):195–202.
14. Casselman JW. The skull base: tumoral lesions. Eur Radiol. 2005;15(3):534–42.
15. Stern Jr JT. Essentials of gross anatomy. Philadelphia: FA Davis Company; 1988.
16. San Millán Ruíz D, Gailloud P, Rüfenacht DA, Delavelle J, Henry F, Fasel JH. The craniocervical venous system in relation to cerebral venous drainage. AJNR Am J Neuroradiol. 2002;23(9):1500–8.
17. Saleh E, Naguib M, Aristegui M, Cokkeser Y, Sanna M. Lower skull base: anatomic study with surgical implications. Ann Otol Rhinol Laryngol. 1995;104(1):57–61.
18. Chauhan NS, Sharma YP, Bhagra T, Sud B. Persistence of multiple emissary veins of posterior fossa with unusual origin of left petrosquamosal sinus from mastoid emissary. Surg Radiol Anat. 2011;33(9):827–31. doi:10.1007/s00276-011-0822-x.
19. García-González U, Cavalcanti DD, Agrawal A, Gonzalez LF, Wallace RC, Spetzler RF, Preul MC. The diploic venous system: surgical anatomy and neurosurgical implications. Neurosurg Focus. 2009;27(5), E2. doi:10.3171/2009.8.FOCUS09169.
20. Horsley V. Antiseptic wax. Br Med. 1892;1(1639):1165.
21. Akhaddar A, Zalagh M, Gazzaz M, Boucetta M. Brain abscess as a complication of intranasal ethmoidectomy for sinonasal polyposis. Surg Infect (Larchmt). 2010;11(5):483–5. doi:10.1089/sur.2009.031.
22. McLaughlin Jr RB, Rehl RM, Lanza DC. Clinically relevant frontal sinus anatomy and physiology. Otolaryngol Clin North Am. 2001;34(1):1–22.

23. Kombogiorgas D, Solanki GA. The Pott puffy tumor revisited: neurosurgical implications of this unforgotten entity. Case report and review of the literature. J Neurosurg. 2006;105 (2 Suppl):143–9.
24. Kombogiorgas D, Seth R, Athwal R, Modha J, Singh J. Suppurative intracranial complications of sinusitis in adolescence. Single institute experience and review of literature. Br J Neurosurg. 2007;21(6):603–9.
25. Fountas KN, Duwayri Y, Kapsalaki E, Dimopoulos VG, Johnston KW, Peppard SB, Robinson JS. Epidural intracranial abscess as a complication of frontal sinusitis: case report and review of the literature. South Med J. 2004;97(3):279–82.
26. Fernández LM, Domínguez J, Callejón A, López S, Pérez-Avila A, Martín V. Intracranial epidural abscess in a newborn secondary to skin catheter. Neurocirugia (Astur). 2001;12 (4):338–41. Spanish.
27. Lefkowitz MA, Chin LS, Couldwell WT. Pediatric intracranial epidural abscess secondary to an infected scalp vein catheter. Pediatr Neurosurg. 1998;29(6):297–9.
28. Pearson CR, Riden DK, Garth RJ, Thomas MR. Two cases of lateral sinus thrombosis presenting with extracranial head and neck abscesses. J Laryngol Otol. 1994;108(9):779–82.
29. Ciampolini J, Harding KG. Pathophysiology of chronic bacterial osteomyelitis. Why do antibiotics fail so often? Postgrad Med J. 2000;76(898):479–83.
30. Newman LG, Waller J, Palestro CJ, Schwartz M, Klein MJ, Hermann G. Unsuspected osteomyelitis in diabetic foot ulcers. Diagnosis and monitoring by leukocyte scanning with indium in 111 oxyquinoline. JAMA. 1991;266(9):1246–51.
31. Lew DP, Waldvogel FA. Osteomyelitis. Lancet. 2004;364(9431):369–79.
32. Duthie ES. The action of fibrinogen on certain pathogenic cocci. J Gen Microbiol. 1955;13 (2):383–93.
33. Patti JM, Boles JO, Höök M. Identification and biochemical characterization of the ligand binding domain of the collagen adhesin from Staphylococcus aureus. Biochemistry. 1993;32:11428–35.
34. Hudson MC, Ramp WK, Nicholson NC, Williams AS, Nousiainen MT. Internalization of Staphylococcus aureus by cultured osteoblasts. Microb Pathog. 1995;19:409–19.
35. Vaudaux PE, Waldvogel FA, Morgenthaler JJ, Nydegger UE. Adsorption of fibronectin onto polymethylmethacrylate and promotion of Staphylococcus aureus adherence. Infect Immun. 1984;45(3):768–74.
36. Herrmann M, Vaudaux PE, Pittet D, Auckenthaler R, Lew PD, Schumacher-Perdreau F, Peters G, Waldvogel FA. Fibronectin, fibrinogen, and laminin act as mediators of adherence of clinical staphylococcal isolates to foreign material. J Infect Dis. 1988;158(4):693–701.
37. Zimmerli W, Lew PD, Waldvogel FA. Pathogenesis of foreign body infection. Evidence for a local granulocyte defect. J Clin Invest. 1984;73(4):1191–200.
38. Manolagas SC, Jilka RL. Bone marrow, cytokines, and bone remodeling: emerging insights into the pathophysiology of osteoporosis. N Engl J Med. 1995;332(5):305–11.
39. Nair SP, Meghji S, Wilson M, Reddi K, White P, Henderson B. Bacterially induced bone destruction: mechanisms and misconceptions. Infect Immun. 1996;64(7):2371–80.
40. Nair SP, Meghji S, Wilson M, Nugent I, Ross A, Ismael A, Bhudia NK, Harris M, Henderson B. Clinical isolates of Staphylococcus aureus have osteolytic surface proteins and a proportion of the population have antibodies that block this activity: is this of prognostic significance? Br J Rheumatol. 1997;36(3):328–32.
41. Meghji S, Crean SJ, Nair S, Wilson M, Poole S, Harris M, Henderson B. Staphylococcus epidermidis produces a cell-associated proteinaceous fraction which causes bone resorption by a prostanoid-independent mechanism: relevance to the treatment of infected orthopaedic implants. Br J Rheumatol. 1997;36(9):957–63.
42. Lerner UH, Sundqvist G, Ohlin A, Rosenquist JB. Bacteria inhibit biosynthesis of bone matrix proteins in human osteoblasts. Clin Orthop Relat Res. 1998;346:244–54.
43. Meikle MC, Gowen M, Reynolds JJ. Effect of streptococcal cell wall components on bone metabolism in vitro. Calcif Tissue Int. 1982;34(4):350–64.

44. Craigen MA, Watters J, Hackett JS. The changing epidemiology of osteomyelitis in children. J Bone Joint Surg Br. 1992;74(4):541–5.
45. Jain AKC. A new classification of diabetic foot osteomyelitis. OA Case Reports. 2013;2 (13):121.
46. Nelson JD. Acute osteomyelitis in children. Infect Dis Clin North Am. 1990;4(3):513–22.
47. Kahn DS, Pritzker KP. The pathophysiology of bone infection. Clin Orthop Relat Res. 1973;96:12–9.
48. Richter RW. Infections other than AIDS. Neurol Clin. 1993;11(3):591–603.
49. Panos GZ, Karydis I, Velakoulis SE, Falagas ME. Multi-skeletal Pneumocystis jiroveci (carinii) in an HIV-seropositive patient. Int J STD AIDS. 2007;18(2):134–7.
50. McClelland III S, Hall WA. Postoperative central nervous system infection: incidence and associated factors in 2111 neurosurgical procedures. Clin Infect Dis. 2007;45(1):55–9.
51. Rerolle JP, Szelag JC, Diaconita M, Paraf F, Aldigier JC, Le Meur Y. Intracranial granuloma and skull osteolysis: complication of a primary cutaneous cryptococcosis in a kidney transplant recipient. Am J Kidney Dis. 2005;46(6):e113–7.
52. Amit A, Sudish K, Pople IK. Primary calvarial cryptococcal osteomyelitis in a patient with idiopathic lymphopenia. Acta Neurochir (Wien). 2008;150(7):713–4. doi:10.1007/s00701-008-1608-8.
53. Bansil NH, Kim TY, Tieu L, Barcega B. Incidence of serious bacterial infections in febrile children with sickle cell disease. Clin Pediatr (Phila). 2013;52(7):661–6. doi:10.1177/0009922813488645.
54. Saito N, Nadgir RN, Flower EN, Sakai O. Clinical and radiologic manifestations of sickle cell disease in the head and neck. Radiographics. 2010;30(4):1021–34. doi:10.1148/rg.304095171.
55. Emslie KR, Nade S. Acute hematogenous staphylococcal osteomyelitis. A description of the natural history in an avian model. Am J Pathol. 1983;110(3):333–45.
56. Akhaddar A, Boulahroud O, Naama O, Al-Bouzidi A, Boucetta M. Paraspinal textiloma after posterior lumbar surgery: a wolf in sheep's clothing. World Neurosurg. 2012;77(2):375–80. doi:10.1016/j.wneu.2011.07.017.
57. Kastenbauer S, Pfister HW, Scheld WM. Epidural abscess. In: Scheld WM, Whitley RJ, Marra CM, editors. Infections of the central nervous system. 3rd ed. Philadelphia: Lippincott Williams & Wilkins; 2004.
58. Laurens MB, Becker RM, Johnson JK, Wolf JS, Kotloff KL. MRSA with progression from otitis media and sphenoid sinusitis to clival osteomyelitis, pachymeningitis and abducens nerve palsy in an immunocompetent 10-year-old patient. Int J Pediatr Otorhinolaryngol. 2008;72(7):945–51. doi:10.1016/j.ijporl.2008.02.025.
59. Hoistad DL, Duvall III AJ. Sinusitis with contiguous abscess involvement of the clivus and petrous apices. Case report. Ann Otol Rhinol Laryngol. 1999;108(5):463–6.
60. Ng J, Connolly DJ, Rittey CD, Mordekar SR. Skull base osteomyelitis leading to lateral medullary syndrome in a child. Eur J Paediatr Neurol. 2007;11(2):111–4.
61. Kuczkowski J, Narozny W, Mikaszewski B, Stankiewicz C. Suppurative complications of frontal sinusitis in children. Clin Pediatr (Phila). 2005;44(8):675–82.
62. Ravitch MM. Surgery in 1776. Ann Surg. 1977;186(3):291–300.
63. Wilensky AO. Osteomyelitis of the skull. Arch Surg. 1933;27(1):83–158.
64. Nisa L, Landis BN, Giger R. Orbital involvement in Pott's puffy tumor: a systematic review of published cases. Am J Rhinol Allergy. 2012;26(2):e63–70. doi:10.2500/ajra.2012.26.3746.
65. Prasad SC, Prasad KC, Bhandary R, Abhijith K, Sampath P. Osteomyelitis of the temporal bone in identical twin infants. Ear Nose Throat J. 2011;90(6):E16–21.
66. Emejulu JC, Ekweogwu OC. Complicated Pott's puffy tumour involving both frontal and parietal bones: a case report. J Infect Dis Ther. 2014;2:166. doi:10.4172/2332-0877.1000166.
67. Leventhal D, Willcox TO, Evans JJ, Finden SG. Bilateral skull base osteomyelitis in an immunocompetent patient. Ear Nose Throat J. 2011;90(12):E23–6.

68. Baddley JW, Cobbs CS, Pappas PG. Surgical treatment of multiple skull abscesses associated with coccidioidomycosis. Mycoses. 2004;47(1–2):69–71.
69. Gower DJ, McGuirt WF, Kelly Jr DL. Intracranial complications of ear disease in a pediatric population with special emphasis on subdural effusion and empyema. South Med J. 1985;78:429–34.
70. Herrmann BW, Chung JC, Eisenbeis JF, Forsen Jr JW. Intracranial complications of pediatric frontal rhinosinusitis. Am J Rhinol. 2006;20(3):320–4.
71. Kraus M, Tovi F. Central nervous system complications secondary to oto-rhinologic infections. An analysis of 39 pediatric cases. Int J Pediatr Otorhinolaryngol. 1992;24(3):217–26.
72. Gupta S, Vachhrajani S, Kulkarni AV, Taylor MD, Dirks P, Drake JM, Rutka JT. Neurosurgical management of extraaxial central nervous system infections in children. J Neurosurg Pediatr. 2011;7(5):441–51. doi:10.3171/2011.2.PEDS09500.
73. Forgie SE, Marrie TJ. Pott's puffy tumor. Am J Med. 2008;121(12):1041–2. doi:10.1016/j.amjmed.2008.08.018.
74. Clayman GL, Adams GL, Paugh DR, Koopmann Jr CF. Intracranial complications of paranasal sinusitis: a combined institutional review. Laryngoscope. 1991;101(3):234–9.
75. Ruf S, Pancherz H. Development of the frontal sinus in relation to somatic and skeletal maturity. A cephalometric roentgenographic study at puberty. Eur J Orthod. 1996;18 (5):491–7.
76. Morgan DW, Williams B. Posterior fossa subdural empyema. Brain. 1985;108(Pt 4):983–92.
77. Shapiro S. Cranial epidural abscess and cranial subdural empyema. In: Roos KL, editor. Central nervous system infectious diseases and therapy. New York: Marcel Dekker; 1997.
78. Avasthi G, Parti A, Gupta SN, Goel R. Frontal bone osteomyelitis causing recurrent meningitis. J Assoc Physicians India. 1991;39(5):409–10.
79. Tuon FF, Russo R, Nicodemo AC. Brain abscess secondary to frontal osteomyelitis. Rev Inst Med Trop Sao Paulo. 2006;48(4):233–5.
80. Hlavin ML, Kaminski HJ, Fenstermaker RA, White RJ. Intracranial suppuration: a modern decade of postoperative subdural empyema and epidural abscess. Neurosurgery. 1994;34 (6):974–80.
81. Hlavin ML, Ratcheson RA. Subdural empyema. In: Kaye AH, Black PM, editors. Operative neurosurgery. London, England: Churchill Livingstone; 2000.
82. Rothholtz VS, Lee AD, Shamloo B, Bazargan M, Pan D, Djalilian HR. Skull base osteomyelitis: the effect of comorbid disease on hospitalization. Laryngoscope. 2008;118 (11):1917–24. doi:10.1097/MLG.0b013e31817fae0d.
83. Chen JC, Yeh CF, Shiao AS, Tu TY. Temporal bone osteomyelitis: the relationship with malignant otitis externa, the diagnostic dilemma, and changing trends. ScientificWorldJournal. 2014;2014:591714. doi:10.1155/2014/591714.
84. Nadol Jr JB. Histopathology of Pseudomonas osteomyelitis of the temporal bone starting as malignant external otitis. Am J Otolaryngol. 1980;1(5):359–71.
85. Sreepada GS, Kwartler JA. Skull base osteomyelitis secondary to malignant otitis externa. Curr Opin Otolaryngol Head Neck Surg. 2003;11(5):316–23.
86. Wilkinson EP, Robinson RA, Trask DK. Skull base thrombotic mycosis. Ear Nose Throat J. 2007;86(3):137.
87. Patmore H, Jebreel A, Uppal S, Raine CH, McWhinney P. Skull base infection presenting with multiple lower cranial nerve palsies. Am J Otolaryngol. 2010;31(5):376–80. doi:10.1016/j.amjoto.2009.04.001.
88. Chen CN, Chen YS, Yeh TH, Hsu CJ, Tseng FY. Outcomes of malignant external otitis: survival vs mortality. Acta Otolaryngol. 2010;130(1):89–94. doi:10.3109/00016480902971247.
89. Dudkiewicz M, Livni G, Kornreich L, Nageris B, Ulanovski D, Raveh E. Acute mastoiditis and osteomyelitis of the temporal bone. Int J Pediatr Otorhinolaryngol. 2005;69 (10):1399–405.

90. Soga Y, Oka K, Sato M, Kabata T, Kawasaki T, Kawano H, Hayano M. Cavernous sinus thrombophlebitis caused by sphenoid sinusitis—report of autopsy case. Clin Neuropathol. 2001;20(3):101–5.
91. Taranath A, Prelog K. Sella turcica collection due to skull base osteomyelitis. Pediatr Radiol. 2005;35(4):451.
92. Chang PC, Fischbein NJ, Holliday RA. Central skull base osteomyelitis in patients without otitis externa: imaging findings. AJNR Am J Neuroradiol. 2003;24(7):1310–6.
93. Azizi SA, Fayad PB, Fulbright R, Giroux ML, Waxman SG. Clivus and cervical spinal osteomyelitis with epidural abscess presenting with multiple cranial neuropathies. Clin Neurol Neurosurg. 1995;97(3):239–44.
94. Hoistad DL, Duvall III AJ. Sinusitis with contiguous abscess involvement of the clivus and petrous apices. Case report. Ann Otol Rhinol Laryngol. 1999;108(5):463–6.
95. Korinek AM, Golmard JL, Elcheick A, Bismuth R, van Effenterre R, Coriat P, Puybasset L. Risk factors for neurosurgical site infections after craniotomy: a critical reappraisal of antibiotic prophylaxis on 4,578 patients. Br J Neurosurg. 2005;19(2):155–62.
96. Chiang HY, Steelman VM, Pottinger JM, Schlueter AJ, Diekema DJ, Greenlee JD, Howard III MA, Herwaldt LA. Clinical significance of positive cranial bone flap cultures and associated risk of surgical site infection after craniotomies or craniectomies. J Neurosurg. 2011;114(6):1746–54.
97. Camargo JF, Seriburi V, Tenner M, El Khoury MY. Aspergillus osteomyelitis of the lumbar spine complicated with orbital apex syndrome: a potential role of the Batson's plexus in disease propagation. Med Mycol Case Rep. 2012;1(1):9–12. doi:10.1016/j.mmcr.2012.02.004.
98. Hayashi T, Uchiumi H, Yanagisawa K, Ogawa Y, Handa H, Tsukamoto N, Nojima Y. Recurrent Gemella haemolysans meningitis in a patient with osteomyelitis of the clivus. Intern Med. 2013;52(18):2145–7.
99. Radosavljević R, Zivković V, Mojsilović Z. Chronic recurrent Hematogenous osteomyelitis of the skull bones and other sites. Med Pregl. 1984;37(1–2):47–9. Croatian.
100. Prasad A, Madan VS, Suri ML, Buxi TB. Cryptogenic osteomyelitis of the skull and intracerebral abscess. Childs Nerv Syst. 1992;8(3):142–3.
101. Bléry M, Chagnon S, Picard A, Babin C. Cranial osteitis: a report on four cases, including a Gradenigo-Lannois syndrome (author's transl). J Radiol. 1980;61(11):677–81. French.
102. Blom NA, Vreede WB. Infected cephalhematomas associated with osteomyelitis, sepsis and meningitis. Pediatr Infect Dis J. 1993;12:1015–7.
103. Waldvogel FA, Medoff G, Swartz MN. Osteomyelitis: a review of clinical features, therapeutic considerations and unusual aspects. N Engl J Med. 1970;282(4):198–206.
104. Cierny G, Mader JT. Adult chronic osteomyelitis. Orthopedics. 1984;7(10):1557–64. doi:10.3928/0147-7447-19841001-07.
105. Kelly PJ. Infected nonunion of the femur and tibia. Orthop Clin North Am. 1984;15(3):481–90.
106. McPherson EJ, Woodson C, Holtom P, Roidis N, Shufelt C, Patzakis M. Periprosthetic total hip infection: outcomes using a staging system. Clin Orthop Relat Res. 2002;403:8–15.
107. Bowen TR, Widmaier JC. Host classification predicts infection after open fracture. Clin Orthop Relat Res. 2005;433:205–11.
108. Romanò CL, Romanò D, Logoluso N, Drago L. Bone and joint infections in adults: a comprehensive classification proposal. Eur Orthop Traumatol. 2011;1(6):207–17.
109. Schmidt HG, Diefenbeck M, Krenn V, Abitzsch D, Militz M, Tiemann AH, Haustedt N, Gückel P, Bühler M, Gerlach UJ. Classification of haematogenous and post-traumatic osteomyelitis. Z Orthop Unfall. 2014;152(4):334–42. doi:10.1055/s-0034-1368620. German.
110. Solagberu BA. A new classification of osteomyelitis for developing countries. East Afr Med J. 2003;80(7):373–8.

Part III
Diagnosis of Cranial Osteomyelitis

Chapter 6
Main Clinical Presentations

Contents

Clinical features of cranial osteomyelitis vary greatly according to many factors such as age of onset, duration of disease, route of infection, underlying etiology, causative pathogens, comorbidities, anatomic location of infection and its extension.

In this chapter, the focus will be on the most common bacterial forms of cranial osteomyelitis encountered in clinical practice including (1) direct spread from contiguous infection (mainly otorhinolaryngologic), (2) postoperative or head trauma, and (3) hematogenous (endogenous) spread. These traditional forms must be opposed to those caused by unusual organisms and those with special clinical manifestations, which will be discussed in two separate chapters (Chap. 14 about unusual pathogens and Chap. 15 on special clinical situations in cranial osteomyelitis).

Generally, the patients are referred from the ear-nose-throat service, the emergency service, or from a general practitioner. Defining a typical clinical syndrome of cranial osteomyelitis is not possible. The disease may be asymptomatic or may present with a number of nonspecific manifestations, and the clinical findings are extremely variable. Osteomyelitis of the skull bones requires a detailed history for diagnosis, including information regarding previous otorhinologic, dental or systemic infections, initial injury, immunologic status, underlying disease, previous antibiotic and/or surgical treatment. Usually, five syndromes dominate the presenting clinical manifestations including general and/or regional signs of infection, local cardinal signs of inflammation, local signs of infection, and more rarely

A. Akhaddar, *Cranial Osteomyelitis*, DOI 10.1007/978-3-319-30268-3_6

Table 6.1 Main clinical manifestations of cranial osteomyelitis

Syndromes	Details
General and/or regional signs of infection	Fever, chills, fatigue, lethargy, irritability, headache and lymphadenopathy.
Local signs of inflammation	Redness, heat, swelling (edema) and pain.
Local signs of infection	Swelling (abscess), pus formation, purulent fistula, foul odor discharge and exposed bone.
Meningitis	Nuchal rigidity (neck stiffness), photophobia (intolerance of bright light) and headache.
Neurologic	Cranial nerve palsies, focal neurologic deficits, raised intracranial pressure (headache, vomiting, ocular palsies, altered level of consciousness, back pain and visual disturbances) or seizures.

meningism and neurologic disturbances (Table 6.1). However, we should be aware that clinical symptoms of chronic osteomyelitis may be less or more prominent than in cases of acute form.

Cranial Osteomyelitis Associated with Otorhinologic Disease

Cranial Vault Osteomyelitis

On the calvaria, symptoms of infection can be minimal, but many patients are in poor health at presentation with headache, and/or otalgia (ear pain) and fever. Regional signs of infection as rhinorrhea or otorrhea should be sought. Most patients have a history of untreated or inadequately treated paranasal sinusitis or otitis media. Headache develops in about half of cases, usually in the area of the affected sinus.

Tender fluctuant swelling, reflecting subperiosteal abscess formation, may be present over the involved frontal sinus or more rarely the mastoid (Fig. 6.1). Similar painful swelling with redness and warmth may also present in distant areas of the scalp secondary to spread of suppuration extracranially (Fig. 6.2). In the cases in which the inner table is involved alone, these extracranial local symptoms do not appear. Rarely, a draining fistulous tract with discharge of purulent secretion via the breached scalp develops over the affected cranial bone without prior surgical intervention (Fig. 6.3). However, this extracranial complication is usually a late finding or one that occurs with chronic infection after duration of more than 1 month of onset (Fig. 6.4). A fetid odor caused by anaerobic pyogenic bacteria may often be present [1–3]. In some instances, regional cervical lymphadenopathy is associated.

With spread of infection into the epidural space, headache worsens. In advanced conditions when the abscess increases in seize altered mental state (confusion with or without agitation) and occasionally focal neurologic signs develop with or without signs of raised intracranial pressure. Focal neurologic deficits are according

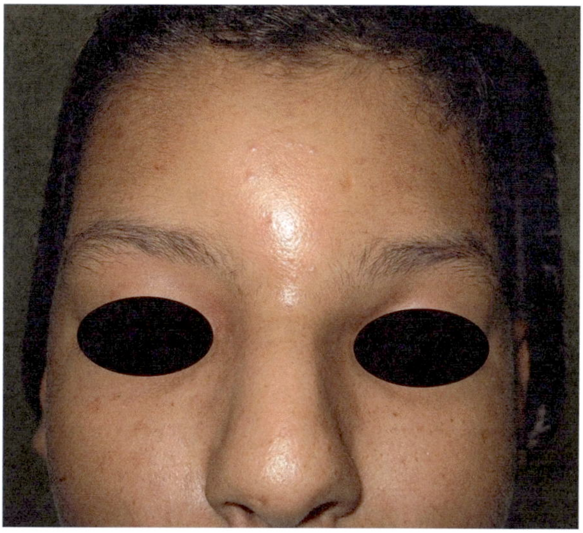

Fig. 6.1 Swelling over the forehead and the frontal sinuses reflecting subperiosteal abscess formation

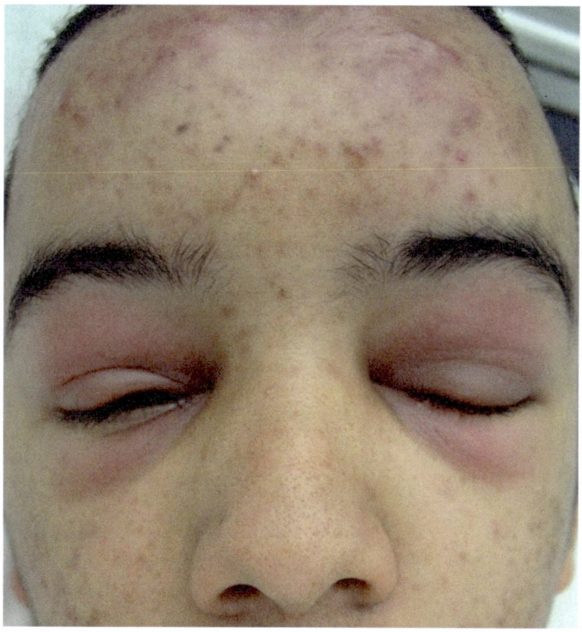

Fig. 6.2 Frontal swelling with bilateral periorbital cellulitis reflecting more extracranial extension of the suppuration (with the patient's signed permission)

to the location of the disease in the cranial vault like hemiparesis, hemisensory deficit, cognitive disorder and visual deficit. Seizures are less common than in the patient with brain abscess and subdural empyema. Meningismus is a rare finding. If infection spread to the orbit, periorbital cellulitis, proptosis, chemosis and ophthalmoplegia may occur (Fig. 6.5).

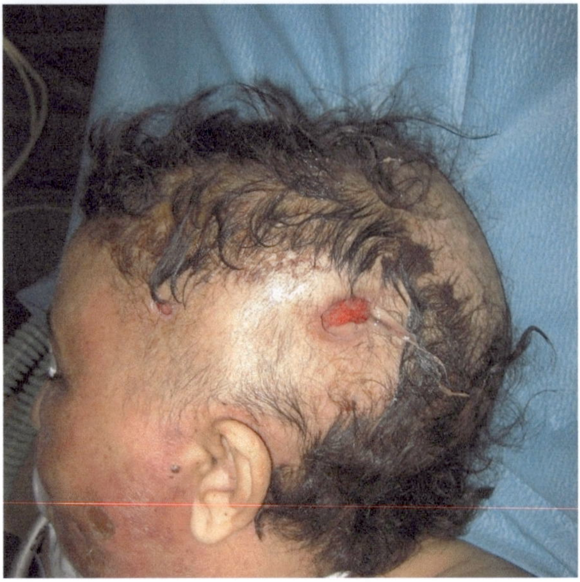

Fig. 6.3 Fronto-parietal osteomyelitis with two fistulous tracts and discharge of purulent secretion via the breached scalp. Note the extensive facial cellulitis on the *left side*

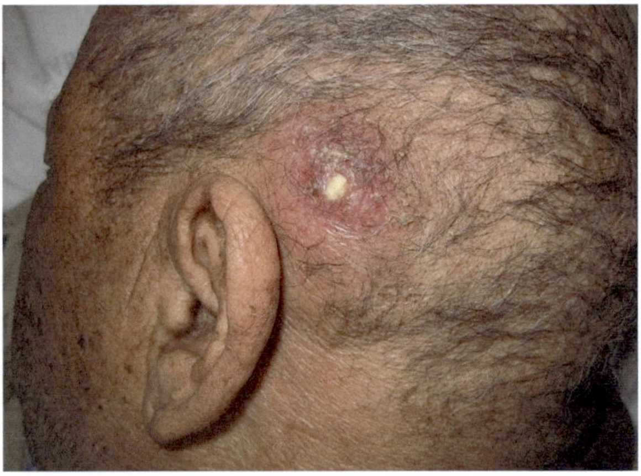

Fig. 6.4 Spontaneous chronic retroauricular purulent fistula developed over the affected cranial bone

Rarely, more severe intracranial complications may arise with rapid neurologic deterioration, respiratory failure, hemodynamic instability, loss of consciousness and death [4–6].

Cranial osteomyelitis associated with extradural abscess present in a more subtle manner (due to the relative isolation of the brain) than other intracranial complications such as subdural empyema and brain abscess, typically with several days of fever, mental status changes and neck pain. Septic thrombosis of the superior sagittal sinus presents with fever, headache, confusion, nausea, vomiting, and seizures. Mental status depression and progression to coma may occur rapidly.

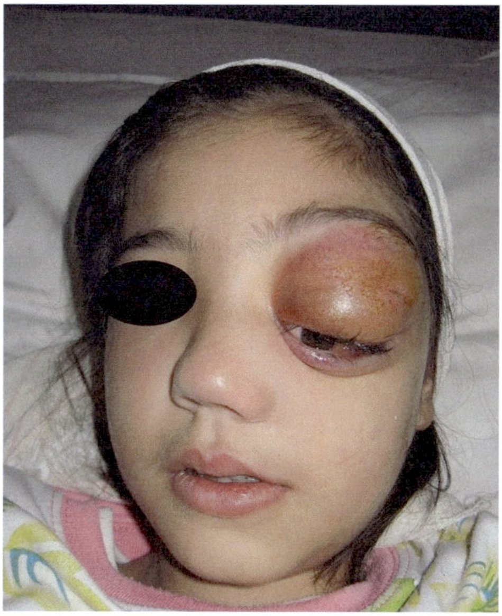

Fig. 6.5 Left orbital abscess with periorbital cellulitis and exophthalmos secondary to fronto-ethmoidal osteomyelitis (with the patient's signed permission)

Upper motor neuron lower extremity weakness or hemiparesis may also be present [7].

The classic forms of chronic osteomyelitis characterized by alternating periods of quiescence and recurrent pain, swelling and sinus tract drainage encountered in long bones, persisting for years despite prolonged antibiotic therapy is not generally described in skull bones [8].

In children, the clinical presentation of cranial osteomyelitis can be challenging for physicians because it can present with only unspecific signs and symptoms such as fatigue, anorexia, irritability, vomiting, indolent presentation and fever of unknown origin.

Also, in cases of a subacute or silent course, the clinical presentation is by definition less impressive. This can make an early diagnosis increasingly difficult, and in many instances these cases are not detected until they have become complicated.

Patients should undergo otorhinologic evaluation to identify possible rhinosinusitis, oral infection, otitis media or mastoiditis. A dental exam should also be performed to detect a potential odontogenic infection. Ophthalmologic examination is recommended to detect probable ocular repercussion of the cranial bone infection, search for orbital and periorbital infections and to exclude other ophthalmologic pathologies [9]. Finally, routine general systems examination should be performed to identify obvious abnormalities and possible other distal source of infection.

Besides otorhinologic diseases, previous primary scalp lesions over the skull can lead to osteomyelitis and should be carefully sought. Non healing ulcerations,

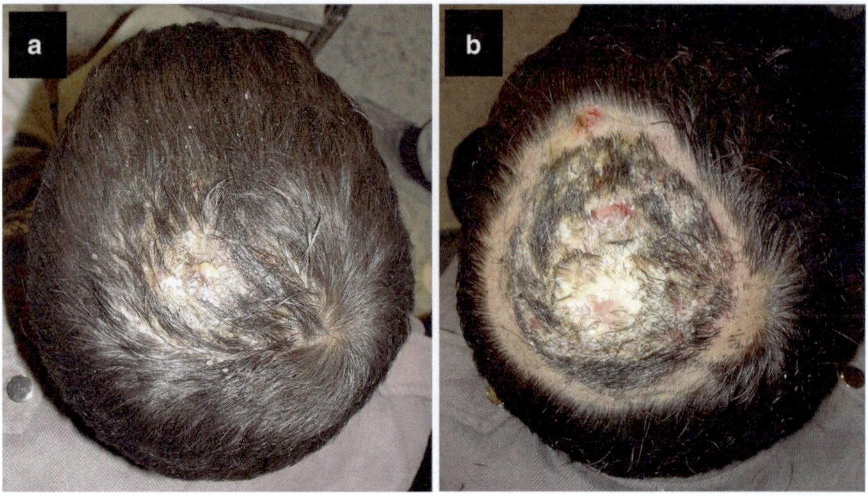

Fig. 6.6 Spontaneous scalp abscess located over the vertex before (**a**) and after shaving (**b**)

spontaneous scalp infections (Fig. 6.6), and chronic sinus tracts (Figs. 6.3 and 6.4), among others, must be suspected.

Patients with cranial vault osteomyelitis can commonly present with signs that mimic other cranial vault and scalp pathologies including: inflammatory cutaneous lesions, vascular malformations, infected hematoma or tumors of the scalp, folliculitis, sebaceous cyst, skin and scalp abscesses, cellulitis, dermoid and epidermoid cysts, encephaloceles, fibrous dysplasia and different benign and malignant tumors of the calvaria (see Chap. 9).

Skull Base Osteomyelitis

Cranial osteomyelitis in the skull base usually remains more silent than in the cranial vault unless it involves the adjacent neurologic and vascular structures [10]. Cranial nerves may be involved with clinical features of cranial nerve palsies. Patients can be present with anosmia if the olfactory nerves are involved in the anterior cranial fossa at the cribriform plate [11]. It may compress the optic nerve and spread to the orbit inducing visual impairment and proptosis. From the third to the sixth cranial nerves may be involved in the cavernous sinus with diplopia, facial nevralgia and ophthalmoplegia. In the posterior cranial fossa, the disease may present with features of lower cranial nerve palsy (such as facial nerve palsy, dizziness, hearing loss, tinnitus in the ear and regurgitation on swallowing), long tract signs (like weakness of one or both upper and lower limbs) and cerebellar signs (such as dysarthria, gait disturbance and ataxia) [12].

Table 6.2 Features of malignant otitis externa [13]

Criteria to diagnose malignant otitis externa	Staging of the malignant otitis externa
– Refractory otitis externa – Severe nocturnal otalgia – Purulent otorrhoea – Presence of *Pseudomonas spp.* and granulation tissue in the external auditory canal – Diabetes or an immunocompromised state	Stage 1. Purulent otorrhoea, otalgia (out of proportion), granulation tissue on otoscopy Stage 2. Disease extends to soft tissues and skull base. Involvement of cranial nerves (XI, XII) Stage 3. Intracranial extension

Because of the unspecific nature of clinical signs with skull base osteomyelitis, a high index of suspicion must be maintained for patients with combination of fever, headache, neck pain or torticollis with or without cranial nerve palsy and without apparent septic focus.

Skull base osteomyelitis is often related to temporal bone and as previously stated in Chap. 5, two types of osteomyelitis can be recognized in skull base referring to temporal bone: one developing into the mastoid and the middle ear cleft (lateral temporal bone) and the other developing into the petrous apex, the otic capsule and the clivus (medial temporal bone). Although, lateral temporal bone osteomyelitis is principally caused by malignant external otitis [13] (Table 6.2), acute mastoiditis and suppurative otitis media, medial temporal bone is a true skull base osteomyelitis secondary to malignant external otitis and also by sphenoid sinusitis and other skull base infection. This difference becomes important because the clinical manifestation of both types of osteomyelitis differ considerably [14].

Central Skull Base Osteomyelitis

Central skull base osteomyelitis typically affects middle-aged men with underlying diabetes mellitus. For Ridder et al., the most frequent complaints are pain (80 %), conductive hearing loss (80 %) and otorrhea (30 %). Cranial nerve palsies are seen in 70 % of cases, mostly the VIIth (35 %) and Xth (20 %) cranial nerves [15]. More specifically, central skull base osteomyelitis unrelated to auricular etiology manifests with intractable headache and/or atypical facial pain in 28 % of cases followed by sinonasal symptoms (24 %). Fever is relatively uncommon, being only noted in 17 % of cases [16]. Cranial nerve palsies are seen in more than one patient out of two, most usually being the VI, IX and XI respectively [17]. In comparison to malignant otitis media which interests the facial cranial nerve in the majority of cases. This is secondary to epicenter of the infectious process which is more laterally (temporal bone) in malignant otitis media. Involvement of both VI and lower cranial nerves (IX, X and XI) are considered in the suspicion of clival pathology [18] (see Chap. 15). Ophthalmoplegia (most often VI) and paresis of XII should raise the suspicion of a malignant tumor of the nasopharynx [19, 20]. An isolated cranial nerve deficit is also being reported [21]. Additionally, several serious complications have been reported in the literature occurring from skull base osteomyelitis including numerous cranial neuropathies, cavernous sinus extension with or without thrombosis, meningitis or brain involvement [4, 6, 16, 22]. Tomovic et al. report an unusual case of a previously healthy and immunocompetent adult who developed meningitis, central skull base osteomyelitis, and occipital condylar cerebrospinal fluid rhinorrhea from sphenoid sinusitis [23].

Septic cavernous sinus thrombosis presents with fever, headache, diplopia, and retro-orbital pain. Depending on the specific cranial nerves involved, ptosis, proptosis, chemosis, hyperesthesia, and decreased corneal reflexes may be present [24, 25]. Venous engorgement of the retinal veins and papilledema are also usually present. Classic symptoms of septic transverse sinus thrombosis include headache and otitis [26]. Intracranial suppurative thrombophlebitis may also be a complication of Gradenigo's syndrome with spread of infection around the carotid sheath and surrounding venous plexus; patients with sigmoid sinus and internal jugular vein thrombosis may present with neck pain and posterior fossa syndrome [27].

Other unusual clinical manifestations have been reported with skull base osteomyelitis like Collet-Sicard syndrome (unilateral palsy of the IX–XII cranial nerves) [28, 29], lateral medullary syndrome or Wallenberg's syndrome (sensory deficits affecting the trunk and extremities on the opposite side of the lesion and sensory deficits affecting the face and cranial nerves on the same side with the lesion) [30, 31], Gradenigo's syndrome (ipsilateral facial pain, lateral abducens nerve palsy and otorrhea) [27, 32, 33], Villaret's syndrome (multiple lower cranial nerve palsies and sympathetic chain involvement) [34, 35] and bilateral Xth cranial nerve palsy [36]. Skull base osteomyelitis can also manifest as an isolated cerebrovascular accident due to occlusion of the internal carotid artery and an invasion of the vessel wall by the microorganisms [6, 26, 37].

Lateral Skull Base Osteomyelitis

Lateral temporal osteomyelitis is often related to malignant otitis externa: patient, often elderly, diabetic and immunocompromised, had slow and gradual symptoms including severe otalgia and unilateral otorrhea [38]. The presence of ear canal granulations and excessive pain in the setting of chronic otitis externa are highly suggestive. Cranial nerve palsies typically affect the facial nerve in about half of cases [13, 39]. However, spread to the petrous apex may involve the abducens, trigeminal and optic nerves [40]. Spread to the jugular foramen may affect the lower cranial nerves (15 %). More rarely, infections may extend into the orbit/eye and brain parenchyma.

Schweitzer suggested the following warning signs of temporal bone osteomyelitis: deep pain (temporal, parietal, postauricular, retroorbital), intermittent foul otorrhea and spiking fever, preauricular cellulitis, woody induration of pinna, chronic mastoid cutaneous fistula, fibrotic mastoid granulation tissue, intermittent facial twitching suggestive of facial canal dehiscence [41]. However, these variable clinical symptoms are difficult to estimate from previous case series because of frequent inclusion of patients with malignant otitis externa without confirmed skull base osteomyelitis. Sometimes, symptoms of lateral skull base osteomyelitis can be more rapid and fulminant. Some patients present with a dural sinus thrombosis, cerebral infarct, meningitis or brain abscess [42, 43].

These clinical signs and symptoms are non specific and may also been seen in other pathologies affecting ear, neck and throat areas such as abscess formation in the external auditory canal (Luc's abscess), post-auricular, retromastoid, zygomatic, sternocleidomastoid muscle (Bezold's abscess), jugulo-digastric muscle (Mouret's abscess), parapharyngeal and retropharyngeal, postanginal shock (Lemierre's syndrome) or meningitis. Also skull base malignancy may have clinical signs similar to skull base infection (see Chap. 9).

Cranial Osteomyelitis Associated with Operation or Head Injury

The clinical features of skull bone osteomyelitis occurring in association with craniotomy, head injury or traumatic scalp wound are less stereotypic than those occurring with sinusitis or ear infection. The onset of symptoms is more insidious and the clinical course more prolonged, masked, in part, by the underlying neurological illness and less pathogenic infected organisms. Indeed, patients are less likely to exhibit florid systemic signs of infection perhaps because of limiting extradural and extracranial membranes formed in response to the surgical procedures. However, attention should be paid to the possible development of any new focal neurologic deficits or worsening of pre-existing ones.

Postoperative

Early detection of a craniotomy flap infection is important by locking out for the local, regional and systemic signs of infection. Symptoms, which appear several days to weeks postoperatively, include slowly progressive headache and fever with increasing tenderness, erythema, warmth and swelling at the initial surgical site [44–50]. For Bhaskar et al., fever was significantly absent with *Propionibacterium acnes* infections [47]. Patients may develop or already have one or more cerebrospinal fluid fistulae. After some days of infection, pus formed in the bone can spread either into the cranium and cause abscess/empyema and meningitis, or spread outwards into the subgaleal or subcutaneous planes (extracranially). In this event, skin breakdown and purulent or serous discharge may follow (Fig. 6.7). More seriously, a cutaneous or deep scalp dehiscence may occur exposing the underlying skull bone (Fig. 6.8). Suspicion of skull base osteomyelitis may be more difficult clinically following mastoidectomy or facial surgery [15, 51].

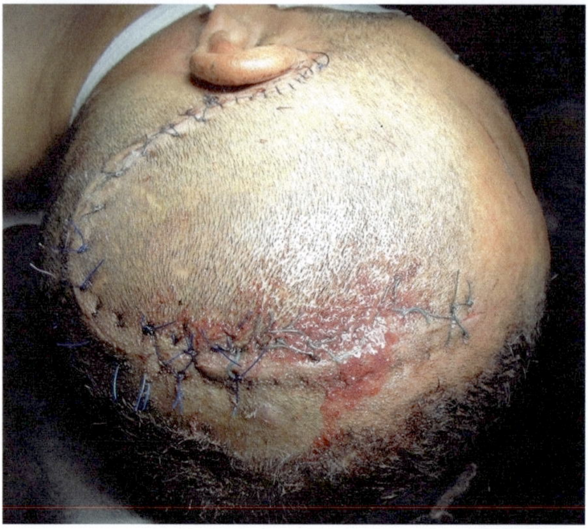

Fig. 6.7 Purulent discharge secondary to deep incisional infection occurring within the second post-operative week

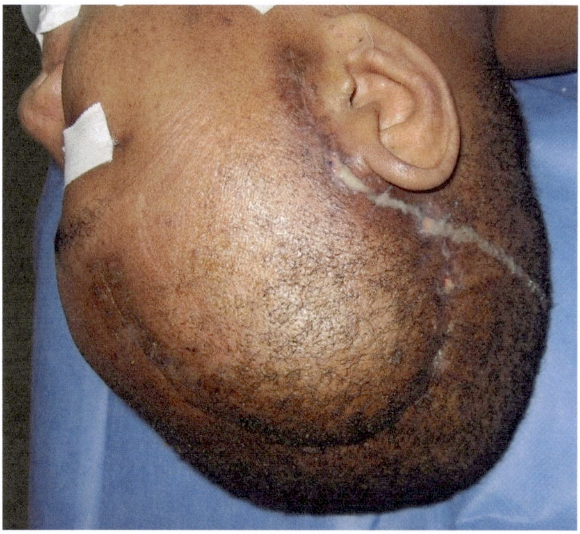

Fig. 6.8 Cutaneous and deep scalp dehiscence with purulent discharge occurring 4 weeks post-operatively

In our series of 13 patients with a postoperative osteomyelitis (four patients had a primary craniotomy at another institution), the time from the causative operation to presentation ranged from 2 weeks to 25 years. Bone flap osteomyelitis was seen alone (four cases) or in combination with extradural empyema (six cases), brain abscess (one case) or both (two cases). Clinical signs of surgical site infection were encountered in 11 patients (84 %), however 8 patients were afebrile (61 %). A wound purulent discharge was seen in four patients (30 %).

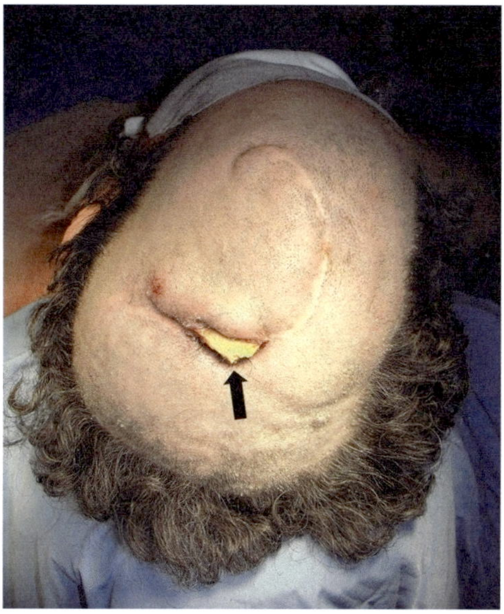

Fig. 6.9 A 47-year-old woman who had a polymethylmethacrylate cranioplasty placed 25 years previously after initial craniotomy for brain tuberculoma. The acrylic plate become infected and over time become exposed with surrounding osteomyelitis

A 47-old-woman had a frontal infected polymethylmethacrylate cranioplasty with surrounding osteomyelitis occurring 25 years after initial craniotomy for brain tuberculoma (Fig. 6.9). Another 51-old-man presented with a parietal bone flap osteomyelitis 11 years after evacuation of an acute subdural hematoma. Wilson et al. described a 40-year-old woman with no evidence of immuno-suppression in whom bone-flap osteomyelitis due to corynebacteria became clinically apparent 24 years after craniotomy [52]. The long latency period for some chronic bone flap infection should be highlighted. This may be due to indolent infection in a remaining suture or seeding of a new infection in a poorly vascularized region [53]. Some anecdotic cases may be completely asymptomatic, with the diagnosis made only on routine postoperative scanning [49].

Also, foreign devices implanted into the central nervous system or extracranially such as bone flap fixating material may serve as nidi for infection.

As mentioned above, otorhinologic, ophthalmologic, oral, dental and general systems examination should be performed to identify a particular setting or source of infection as well as a concomitant disease.

Head Injury

There have been occasional case reports of head injury causing cranial osteomyelitis. The trauma can be major or minor, depending on the mechanism of injury. In its major forms, the aggressive agent produces significant and apparent cutaneous

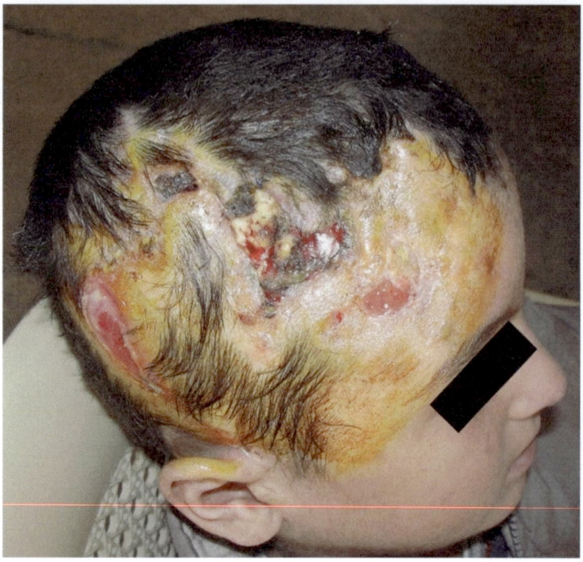

Fig. 6.10 Extensive fronto-parieto-temporal superficial wound sepsis following a severe head injury

and cranial bone lesions. However, in its minor forms, the small scalp lesions are usually ignored and misdiagnosed. If neglected, both forms may result in serious infectious complications especially cranial bone infection.

After the cranial injury, and following a longer or shorter period of time, patients may present with general and/or regional signs of infection. Headache, local pain, swelling, erythema, tenderness and edema are seen in the setting of the initial injury. The most common finding is that of superficial wound sepsis (Fig. 6.10). In the early stages, this may be manifested only by a subgaleal fluid collection that is not decreasing or by worsening of wound pain and tenderness [54]. Also, scars or local disturbance of wound healing may be noted along with local signs of suppuration (Fig. 6.11). The wound may break down with the drainage of purulent material (Fig. 6.12). Concomitant injuries should be taken into consideration. Seizures, new focal neurologic signs or deterioration of level of consciousness may appear when infection spread intracranially, often late findings [55]. According to Avasthi and colleagues, a case of recurrent pyogenic meningitis was presented. The focus for recurrent meningeal infection was frontal bone osteomyelitis secondary to a road accident which the patient sustained 10 years earlier [56]. In some patients, the primary condition or preceding trauma may previously impair the neurological situation and this will mask any new subtle modifications. The administration of antibiotics and anticonvulsants also may delay or modify disease presentation. In rare cases, the patient may be asymptomatic. Valeron-Almazan et al. reported a patient with an extensive scalp ulcer secondary to chronic osteomyelitis discovered more than 50 years after the causal trauma [57].

Some clinical conditions can sometimes be confused with cranial osteomyelitis secondary to craniotomy/craniectomy or head injury. The most important

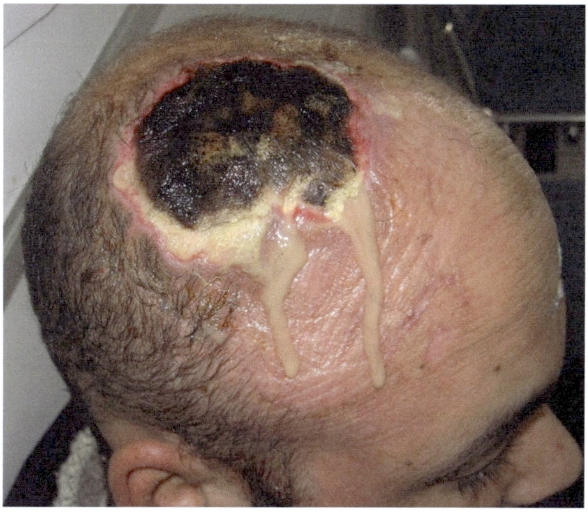

Fig. 6.11 Post-traumatic scars with local signs of suppuration on the right parietal area

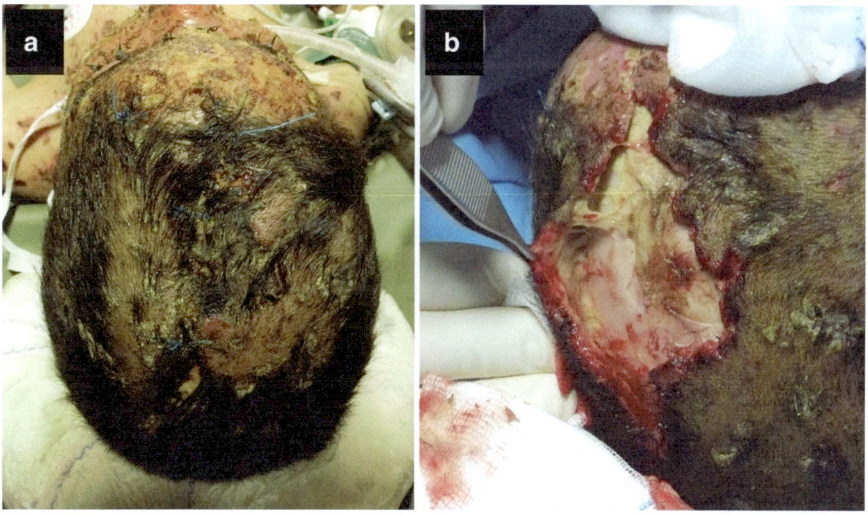

Fig. 6.12 Large traumatic scalp injury with spontaneous drainage of purulent material (**a**). Operative view showing detachment of the scalp, subgaleal suppuration, and the underlying cranial bone (**b**)

differential diagnosis is that of underlying craniocerebral injury and complicating intracranial sepsis collection or meningitis. As stated previously, these intracranial infectious complications can also be encountered late in the course of cranial bone infection (see Chap. 9).

Cranial Osteomyelitis Associated with Hematogenous Spread of Infection

Septic hematogenic metastasis is rare but possible complication in osteomyelitis of the flat and small bones [58, 59]. Because sepsis can begin in different parts of the body, it can have many different symptoms. Rapid breathing and a change in mental status, such as reduced alertness or confusion, may be the first signs to indicate that sepsis is starting [58]. Other common symptoms include: fever and shaking chills or, alternatively, a very low body temperature, decreased urination, rapid pulse, rapid breathing, nausea and vomiting and diarrhea. However, osteomyelitis usually presents with a slow insidious progression of local signs and symptoms. There have been rare case reports of hematogenous osteomyelitis of the skull, mainly secondary to specific bacteria or fungi (see Chap. 14). On the other side, many cases manifested with septicemia and meningitis especially in children with infected cephalhematoma [5, 60, 61] (see Chap. 15). However, the cause of cranial bone infection may remain cryptogenic in spite of all the investigations [62–66]. Anyway, patients should undergo meticulous general systems examination to detect probable systemic repercussion of cranial osteomyelitis, search for potential source of infection and to exclude other diseases.

Nakwan et al. reported a case of an 18-day-old neonate who was diagnosed with an infected cephalhematoma caused by *Escherichia coli* complicated with septicemia, meningitis, and skull osteomyelitis. Clinically, there was an increasing bilateral parieto-occipital swelling and fever for 7 days prior to admission [5]. More recently, Hayashi et al. described a 69-year-old woman with septicemia and recurrent meningitis complicated by skull base osteomyelitis due to *Gemella haemolysans*. A secondary septic pulmonary embolism was highly suspected. The most important neurologic manifestation was abducens nerve palsy [67]. In the same way and according to DeVries, a metastatic frontal osteomyelitis with epidural bacterial abscess was reported in a 4-year-old boy, who was treated 1 week earlier for a pulmonary empyema [58].

References

1. Marx RE. Chronic osteomyelitis of the jaws. Oral Maxillofac Surg Clin North Am. 1991;3:367.
2. Shin JW, Choi IG, Jung SN, Kwon H, Shon WI, Moon SH. Pott puffy tumor appearing with a frontocutaneous fistula. J Craniofac Surg. 2012;23(2):e158–60. doi:10.1097/SCS.0b013e31824cdcc0.
3. Davidson L, McComb JG. Epidural-cutaneous fistula in association with the Pott puffy tumor in an adolescent. Case report. J Neurosurg. 2006;105(3 Suppl):235–7.
4. Peer Mohamed B, Carr L. Neurological complications in two children with Lemierre syndrome. Dev Med Child Neurol. 2010;52(8):779–81. doi:10.1111/j.1469-8749.2010.03718.x.
5. Nakwan N, Nakwan N, Wannaro J, Dissaneevate P, Kritsaneepaiboon S, Chokephaibulkit K. Septicemia, meningitis, and skull osteomyelitis complicating infected cephalhematoma

caused by ESBL-producing Escherichia coli. Southeast Asian J Trop Med Public Health. 2011;42(1):148–51.

6. He J, Lam JC, Adlan T. Clival osteomyelitis and hypoglossal nerve palsy-rare complications of Lemierre's syndrome. BMJ Case Rep. 2015. pii: bcr2015209777. doi:10.1136/bcr-2015-209777.
7. el Alaoui Faris M, Birouk N, Slassi I, Jiddane M, Chkili T. [Thrombosis of the upper longitudinal sinus and syphilitic cranial osteitis]. Rev Neurol (Paris). 1992;148(12):783–5. French.
8. Lew DP, Waldvogel FA. Osteomyelitis. Lancet. 2004;364(9431):369–79.
9. Akhaddar A, Elasri F, Elouennass M, Mahi M, Elomari N, Elmostarchid B, Oubaaz A, Boucetta M. Orbital abscess associated with sinusitis from odontogenic origin. Intern Med. 2010;49(5):523–4.
10. Asimakopoulos P, Supriya M, Kealey S, Vernham GA. A case-based discussion on a patient with non-otogenic fungal skull base osteomyelitis: pitfalls in diagnosis. J Laryngol Otol. 2013;127(8):817–21. doi:10.1017/S002221511300145X.
11. Ducic Y. Management of osteomyelitis of the anterior skull base and craniovertebral junction. Otolaryngol Head Neck Surg. 2003;128(1):39–42.
12. Akhaddar A, El Mostarchid B, Gazzaz M, Boucetta M. Cerebellar abscess due to Lactococcus lactis. A new pathogen. Acta Neurochir (Wien). 2002;144(3):305–6.
13. Levenson MJ, Parisier SC, Dolitsky J, Bindra G. Ciprofloxacin: drug of choice in the treatment of malignant external otitis (MEO). Laryngoscope. 1991;101(8):821–4.
14. Prasad SC, Prasad KC, Kumar A, Thada ND, Rao P, Chalasani S. Osteomyelitis of the temporal bone: terminology, diagnosis, and management. J Neurol Surg B Skull Base. 2014;75(5):324–31. doi:10.1055/s-0034-1372468.
15. Ridder GJ, Breunig C, Kaminsky J, Pfeiffer J. Central skull base osteomyelitis: new insights and implications for diagnosis and treatment. Eur Arch Otorhinolaryngol. 2015;272(5):1269–76. doi:10.1007/s00405-014-3390-y.
16. Ganhewa AD, Kuthubutheen J. A diagnostic dilemma of central skull base osteomyelitis mimicking neoplasia in a diabetic patient. BMJ Case Rep. 2013. pii: bcr2012007183. doi:10.1136/bcr-2012-007183.
17. Johnson AK, Batra PS. Central skull base osteomyelitis: an emerging clinical entity. Laryngoscope. 2014;124(5):1083–7. doi:10.1002/lary.24440.
18. Kulkarni V, Rajshekhar V. Chronic non-healing ulcers of the scalp after trauma. Postgrad Med J. 2000;76(897):437, 450–1.
19. Clark MP, Pretorius PM, Byren I, Milford CA. Central or atypical skull base osteomyelitis: diagnosis and treatment. Skull Base. 2009;19(4):247–54. doi:10.1055/s-0028-1115325.
20. Keane JR. Combined VIth and XIIth cranial nerve palsies: a clival syndrome. Neurology. 2000;54(7):1540–1.
21. Patel B, Souqiyyeh A, Ali A. A case of transient, isolated cranial nerve VI palsy due to skull base osteomyelitis. Case Rep Infect Dis. 2014;2014:369867. doi:10.1155/2014/369867.
22. Bhatt YM, Pahade N, Nair B. Aspergillus petrous apicitis associated with cerebral and peritubular abscesses in an immunocompetent man. J Laryngol Otol. 2013;127(4):404–7. doi:10.1017/S0022215113000315.
23. Tomovic S, Friedel ME, Liu JK, Eloy JA. Community-acquired methicillin-resistant Staphylococcus aureus skull base osteomyelitis with occipital condylar cerebrospinal fluid leak in an immunocompetent patient. Laryngoscope. 2012;122(5):977–81. doi:10.1002/lary.23253.
24. Soga Y, Oka K, Sato M, Kabata T, Kawasaki T, Kawano H, Hayano M. Cavernous sinus thrombophlebitis caused by sphenoid sinusitis—report of autopsy case. Clin Neuropathol. 2001;20(3):101–5.
25. Assefa D, Dalitz E, Handrick W, Lietz R, Braun W, Michalski H. Septic cavernous sinus thrombosis following infection of ethmoidal and maxillary sinuses: a case report. Int J Pediatr Otorhinolaryngol. 1994;29(3):249–55.

26. Severino M, Liyanage S, Novelli V, Cheesborough B, Saunders D, Gunny R, Rossi A. Skull base osteomyelitis and potential cerebrovascular complications in children. Pediatr Radiol. 2012;42(7):867–74. doi:10.1007/s00247-011-2340-8.
27. Hehl K, Tisch M, Lampl L, Draf W, Stussak G, Frey G. [Bilateral Gradenigo syndrome—on the value of an integrated therapy concept including hyperbaric oxygenation and chronic destructive inflammation of the skull base]. HNO. 1992;40(8):318–21. German.
28. Lee SJ, Weon YC, Cha HJ, Kim SY, Seo KW, Jegal Y, Ahn JJ, Ra SW. A case of atypical skull base osteomyelitis with septic pulmonary embolism. J Korean Med Sci. 2011;26(7):962–5. doi:10.3346/jkms.2011.26.7.962.
29. Sibai TA, Ben-Galim PJ, Eicher SA, Reitman CA. Infectious Collet-Sicard syndrome in the differential diagnosis of cerebrovascular accident: a case of head-to-neck dissociation with skull-based osteomyelitis. Spine J. 2009;9(4):e6–10. doi:10.1016/j.spinee.2008.05.012.
30. Kim JS. Pure lateral medullary infarction: clinical–radiological correlation of 130 acute, consecutive patients. Brain. 2003;126(Pt 8):1864–72.
31. Ng J, Connolly DJ, Rittey CD, Mordekar SR. Skull base osteomyelitis leading to lateral medullary syndrome in a child. Eur J Paediatr Neurol. 2007;11(2):111–4.
32. Gradenigo G. [On circumscribed leptomeningitis and on abducens paralysis of post-otitic origin—Sulla leptomeningite circoscritta e sulla paralisi dell' abducente di origine otitica]. G Accad Med Torino. 1904;10:59–64. 361–7. Italian.
33. Matis GK, de A Silva DO, Chrysou OI, Karanikas MA, Birbilis TA. Giuseppe Gradenigo: much more than a syndrome! Historical vignette. Surg Neurol Int. 2012;3:122. doi:10.4103/2152-7806.102343.
34. Unnikrishnan R, Faizal BP, Pillai MGK, Paul G. Villaret's syndrome—a rare presentation of skull base osteomyelitis. Amrita J Med. 2013;9(2):32–4.
35. Huang KL, Lu CS. Skull base osteomyelitis presenting as Villaret's syndrome. Acta Neurol Taiwan. 2006;15(4):255–8.
36. Rowlands RG, Lekakis GK, Hinton AE. Masked pseudomonal skull base osteomyelitis presenting with a bilateral Xth cranial nerve palsy. J Laryngol Otol. 2002;116:556–8.
37. Wilkinson EP, Robinson RA, Trask DK. Skull base thrombotic mycosis. Ear Nose Throat J. 2007;86(3):137.
38. Rothholtz VS, Lee AD, Shamloo B, Bazargan M, Pan D, Djalilian HR. Skull base osteomyelitis: the effect of comorbid disease on hospitalization. Laryngoscope. 2008;118 (11):1917–24. doi:10.1097/MLG.0b013e31817fae0d.
39. Djalilian HR, Shamloo B, Thakkar KH, Najme-Rahim M. Treatment of culture-negative skull base osteomyelitis. Otol Neurotol. 2006;27(2):250–5.
40. Spielmann PM, Yu R, Neeff M. Skull base osteomyelitis: current microbiology and management. J Laryngol Otol. 2013;127 Suppl 1:S8–12. doi:10.1017/S0022215112002356.
41. Schweitzer VG. Hyperbaric oxygen management of chronic staphylococcal osteomyelitis of the temporal bone. Am J Otol. 1990;11(5):347–53.
42. Vourexakis Z, Kos MI, Guyot JP. Atypical presentations of malignant otitis externa. J Laryngol Otol. 2010;124(11):1205–8. doi:10.1017/S0022215110000307.
43. Sreepada GS, Kwartler JA. Skull base osteomyelitis secondary to malignant otitis externa. Curr Opin Otolaryngol Head Neck Surg. 2003;11(5):316–23.
44. Korinek AM, Golmard JL, Elcheick A, Bismuth R, van Effenterre R, Coriat P, Puybasset L. Risk factors for neurological site infections after craniotomy: a critical reappraisal of antibiotic on 4578 patients. Br J Neurosurg. 2005;19(2):155–62.
45. Lal S, McCutcheon IE. Infections after craniotomy. In: Hall WA, McCutcheon IA, editors. Infections in neurosurgery. Park Ridge, IL: American Association of Neurological Surgeons Publications; 2000.
46. Abu Hamdeh S, Lytsy B, Ronne-Engström E. Surgical site infections in standard neurosurgery procedures—a study of incidence, impact and potential risk factors. Br J Neurosurg. 2014;28 (2):270–5. doi:10.3109/02688697.2013.835376.

47. Bhaskar IP, Inglis TJ, Lee GY. Clinical, radiological, and microbiological profile of patients with autogenous cranioplasty infections. World Neurosurg. 2014;82(3–4):e531–4. doi:10.1016/j.wneu.2013.01.013.
48. Nisbet M, Briggs S, Ellis-Pegler R, Thomas M, Holland D. Propionibacterium acnes: an under-appreciated cause of post-neurosurgical infection. J Antimicrob Chemother. 2007;60(5):1097–103.
49. Levitt MR, Gabikian P, Pottinger PS, Silbergeld DL. Propionibacterium acnes osteomyelitis occurring 23 years after craniotomy: case report and review of literature. Neurosurgery. 2011;69(3):E773–9. doi:10.1227/NEU.0b013e31821964ba.
50. Uhari M, Rantala H, Herva E. Perioperative dissemination of Salmonella. Arch Dis Child. 1987;62(10):1079–80.
51. Barber AJ, Hanlon R, Rogers SN. Skull base osteomyelitis after maxillectomy: a rare complication. Br J Oral Maxillofac Surg. 2009;47(4):310–2. doi:10.1016/j.bjoms.2009.01.010.
52. Wilson IF, Candia GJ, Worthington MG, Sullivan JG. Chronic osteomyelitis due to corynebacteria in a postcraniotomy bone flap. Clin Infect Dis. 1999;28(6):1323–4.
53. Rasmussen S, Ohrström JK, Westergaard L, Kosteljanetz M. Post-operative infections of osteoplastic compared with free bone flaps. Br J Neurosurg. 1990;4(6):493–5.
54. Barry J, Fridley J, Sayama C, Lam S. Infected subgaleal hematoma following blunt head trauma in a child: case report and review of the literature. Pediatr Neurosurg. 2015;50(4):223–8. doi:10.1159/000433442.
55. Lin YT, Chen CT, Lai JP. Post-traumatic fronto-ethmoid osteomyelitis treated with free muscle transfer. J Plast Reconstr Aesthet Surg. 2010;63(6):963–9. doi:10.1016/j.bjps.2009.03.017.
56. Avasthi G, Parti A, Gupta SN, Goel R. Frontal bone osteomyelitis causing recurrent meningitis. J Assoc Physicians India. 1991;39(5):409–10.
57. Valerón-Almazán P, Gómez-Duaso AJ, Rivero P, Vilar J, Dehesa L, Santana N, Carretero G. Extensive, non-healing scalp ulcer associated with trauma-induced chronic osteomyelitis. Ann Dermatol. 2011;23 Suppl 3:S364–7. doi:10.5021/ad.2011.23.S3.S364.
58. DeVries S. Metastatic epidural bacterial abscess in a 4-year-old boy. JAMA Neurol. 2013;70(5):648–9. doi:10.1001/jamaneurol.2013.1942.
59. Radosavljević R, Zivković V, Mojsilović Z. [Chronic recurrent hematogenous osteomyelitis of the skull bones and other sites]. Med Pregl. 1984;37(1–2):47–9.
60. Blom NA, Vreede WB. Infected cephalhematomas associated with osteomyelitis, sepsis and meningitis. Pediatr Infect Dis J. 1993;12(12):1015–7.
61. Bléry M, Chagnon S, Picard A, Babin C. [Cranial osteitis: a report on four cases, including a Gradenigo-Lannois syndrome (author's transl)]. J Radiol. 1980;61(11):677–81.
62. Prasad A, Madan VS, Suri ML, Buxi TB. Cryptogenic osteomyelitis of the skull and intracerebral abscess. Childs Nerv Syst. 1992;8(3):142–3.
63. Tacon LJ, Parkinson JF, Hudson BJ, Brewer JM, Little NS, Clifton-Bligh RJ. Headache of a diagnosis: frontotemporal pain and inflammation associated with osteolysis. Med J Aust. 2008;189(10):591–2.
64. Kumar GS, Raj PM, Chacko G, Lalitha MK, Chacko AG, Rajshekhar V. Cranial melioidosis presenting as a mass lesion or osteomyelitis. J Neurosurg. 2008;108(2):243–7. doi:10.3171/JNS/2008/108/2/0243.
65. Amit A, Sudish K, Pople IK. Primary calvarial cryptococcal osteomyelitis in a patient with idiopathic lymphopenia. Acta Neurochir (Wien). 2008;150(7):713–4. doi:10.1007/s00701-008-1608-8.
66. Qiu Y, Zhang J, Liu G, Zhong X, Deng J, He Z, Jing B. Retrospective analysis of 14 cases of disseminated Penicillium marneffei infection with osteolytic lesions. BMC Infect Dis. 2015;15:47. doi:10.1186/s12879-015-0782-6.
67. Hayashi T, Uchiumi H, Yanagisawa K, Ogawa Y, Handa H, Tsukamoto N, Nojima Y. Recurrent Gemella haemolysans meningitis in a patient with osteomyelitis of the clivus. Intern Med. 2013;52(18):2145–7.

Chapter 7
Laboratory Findings

Contents

Abbreviations

AFB Acid-fast bacilli
CRP C-reactive protein
CSF Cerebrospinal fluid
ESR Erythrocyte sedimentation rate
HIV Human immunodeficiency virus
PCR Polymerase chain reaction

Biologic parameters that may be elevated in cases of osteomyelitis are blood leukocyte level, erythrocyte sedimentation rate (ESR), and C-reactive protein (CRP). However, microbiologic and histopathological examinations of bone remain the gold standard for diagnosing skull osteomyelitis. Anyway, biological findings should always be interpreted in combination with clinical and imaging data and should not be used separately.

Inflammatory Parameters

Routine laboratory studies have proven to be of little value in the diagnosis of skull osteomyelitis. The peripheral blood cell count is frequently normal (more than two third of cases) or only mildly elevated with increased polymorphonuclear leukocyte

A. Akhaddar, *Cranial Osteomyelitis*, DOI 10.1007/978-3-319-30268-3_7

counts [1–9]. In fact, white blood cell counts exceeding 20,000/mL are usually indicative of concomitant meningitis, parameningeal suppurations or some other co-existing systemic infection [10–15].

Inflammatory biomarkers were highly variable in their expression in cranial osteomyelitis. When biomarkers are elevated, they suggest osteomyelitis in the appropriate clinical setting of pain and radiological lesions. Biomarkers of inflammation may reveal an ESR and CRP [4, 16]. Although CRP level may be more useful than ESR because it reveals elevation earlier, these inflammatory parameters are nonspecific. Additionally, ESR is not constantly reliable because fever, dehydratation, and current treatment with antibiotics may cause an elevation [17]. Interpretation of the ESR or CRP level can be more problematic postoperatively because each is elevated by surgery in general, the CRP level returns to normal more quickly, but without a baseline value (often not previously obtained), a trend cannot be determined. Bhaskar et al. found only one-third (4 of 12 patients who had CRP measured) of patients with autogenous cranioplasty infection showed a significant increase in CRP (72–120 mg/L) and another third showed mild increases (10–24 mg/L) [18]. However, patients with high CRP had increased white cell counts as well. For many authors, CRP level may be more useful to follow the clinical response to therapy, mostly in the case of postoperative infection [18–23]. Skull bone infection should not be excluded in a patient with no fever, normal white blood cells count, abnormal ESR and negative blood culture [9, 24, 25]. In comparison with other types of osteomyelitis, osteomyelitis due to mycobacteria and fungi causes lower elevations in the CRP level, erythrocyte sedimentation rate, and white-cell count. Mild to moderate anemia may be seen related to inflammation [26]. Serum chemistries should also be obtained to assess for the presence of electrolyte imbalances, and the coagulation profile should be obtained in anticipation of surgical intervention. Procalcitonin levels are more specific as diagnostic tests and helpful in follow-up, but measurements of procalcitonin are more expensive and it lacks sensitivity [19, 27, 28].

The results of cerebrospinal fluid (CSF) analysis are also non-specific. There is usually a mild mononuclear pleocytosis, with white cell counts <100/mL unless there is co-existing meningitis [15, 16]. CSF protein content is slightly elevated and hypoglycorrhachia is generally absent except in the face of frank meningitis [10]. Cultures are usually sterile, especially in patients who have received antibiotics. Because lumbar puncture is potentially dangerous in the presence of intracranial suppuration and given the fact that the CSF findings are non-specific at best, lumbar puncture is contraindicated in patients with suspected intracranial empyema and/or brain abscess [29]. In a large study of 280 patients with intracranial suppurations, 33 cases (11.7 %) had a neurological deterioration following a lumbar puncture, and 3 died (1 %) [30].

Blood Cultures

It is important to obtain blood cultures in all patients with osteomyelitis, especially in those patients where hematologic spread is suspected [2, 11, 16, 31–38]. Hematogenous spread is often monomicrobial but rarely positive in the neurocranium. All the 20 patients with skull base osteomyelitis reported by Spielmann and colleagues have uniformly negative blood cultures [39].

Molecular Studies

Identification of microorganisms is crucial for the successful treatment of osteoarticular infections. Molecular methods are more sensitive than culture-dependent methods but may suffer from a lack of specificity [40]. In general, molecular studies are not needed for the etiological diagnosis in cranial osteomyelitis. However, nucleic acid amplification techniques (mainly polymerase chain reaction or PCR) and Interferon gamma enzyme linked immunosorbent assay (QuantiFERON-TB Gold testing) have recently become available with great improvements in sensitivity and specificity for the diagnosis of some difficult-to-grow organisms, such as *Mycobacterium tuberculosis* [41–43]. Levy et al. recommend the use of conventional broad-range PCR for culture-negative bone and joint specimens [40].

Additional studies to diagnose active tuberculosis should be performed—for example, sputum acid-fast bacilli (AFB) smears and cultures, urine AFB culture, and tuberculin skin testing in patients with suspected systemic tuberculosis [44, 45].

Human immunodeficiency virus (HIV) tests should be done in all patients with clinically suspected HIV infection. Luzzati et al. reported a young patient with calvarial tuberculosis as the first symptom of human immunodeficiency virus-1 positivity [46]. Also, serologic tests for syphilis should be performed when suspected [47, 48].

Selection of the appropriate specimens for the detection of causative organisms is crucial in treating infectious diseases. Whenever possible, antimicrobial therapy should be held until appropriate specimens are collected. It is also important to collect as much material as possible from fluid, purulent material and tissue specimens (deeper wound, sinus tract or abscess particularly at the time of surgical drainage). The diagnostic yield can be improved if we consider that bone or soft tissue biopsies using a strict protocol to avoid contamination are preferred over swabs. Material should then be sent for Gram stain, routine aerobic and anaerobic cultures and fungal culture with favorable transport conditions (anaerobic transport medium). The microbiological laboratory should always be informed when some difficult-to-grow organisms are suspected because the diagnosis may be missed using routine laboratory methods. This is the case for *Mycobacteria spp.*, *Brucella spp*. [49], *Actinomycosis spp*. [50], *Nocardia spp*. [1, 51] and fungi [52]. The latest can often be identified by the appearance in tissue even if the cultures are negative.

Ideally, both culture and histologic examination should be done together. In addition, histopathological analysis is useful, because the presence of leukocytes in the specimens distinguishes infection from contamination. Furthermore, the presence of granulomas suggests particular causes, such as brucellosis or tuberculosis [44, 49]. Cultures from potentially infectious sources, oral, paranasal sinus, external auditory canal, sputum and urine should be taken [3, 35]. For many of the pathogens identified in wound cultures, antimicrobial susceptibility testing is required to guide treatment and to determine whether the strain of bacteria present is likely to respond to specific antibiotics. Anyway, clinicians and biologists must work in perfect collaboration.

Microbiological Studies

As seen in Chap. 3, the skull bone and adjacent soft tissues may be infected by various microorganisms, including bacteria, fungi and parasites (Table 7.1). The causative microbiologic agents in postoperative infections are quite different from those of contiguous paranasal sinusitis or otitis. *Staphylococcus species* are a frequent cause of surgical site infections due to the patient's endogenous skin flora. While *Streptococcus species* and anaerobes are the most common bacteria related to sinogenic infections. Hematogenous spread is unusual, mostly caused by

Table 7.1 Common causative organisms in skull osteomyelitis

Cause	Pathogens
Non-specific bacteria	Aerobic Gram-positive cocci (*Staphylococcus spp.*, *Streptococcus spp.*)
	Aerobic Gram-negative bacilli (*Haemophilus influenza*, *Proteus spp.*, *E. coli*, *Pseudomonas spp.*, *Klebsiella spp.*, *Acinetobacter spp.*, *Salmonella spp.*)
	Anaerobic Gram-positive cocci (*Peptostreptococcus spp.*)
	Anaerobic Gram-negative bacilli (*Bacteroides spp.*, *Fusobacterium spp.*)
	Anaerobic Gram-positive bacilli (*Propionibacterium spp.*)
Specific bacteria	*Mycobacterium tuberculosis*
	Treponema pallidum
	Actinomyces spp.
	Nocardia spp.
Fungi	*Aspergillus spp.*
	Cryptococcus spp.
	Blastomyces spp.
	Rhizopus spp. (zygomycosis)
	Candida spp.
Parasitosis	*Echinococcus granulosis*
Virus	*Varicella-zoster virus*

specific bacteria or fungemia. In contiguous and postoperative (exogenous) osteomyelitis, infection is often polymicrobial, whereas in hematogenous (endogenous) osteomyelitis, infection is typically monobacterial. In most recent studies, hospital acquired-pathogens are increasingly resistant to multiple traditional antimicrobial drugs. Skull base osteomyelitis mostly originates from inflammations of the external auditory canal and less frequently from sinonasal infections with *Pseudomonas aeruginosa* as the most common pathologic organisms. Less often, skull base osteomyelitis is attributed to fungal agents such as *Aspergillus fumigatus*.

It's important to recognize that many osteomyelitis are polymicrobial and can even contain both anaerobic and aerobic bacteria [43, 53–55] as well as mixed fungi and bacteria [13, 56–58] (see Chap. 3). Also, culture-negative cases are not uncommon and should be taken into consideration.

Histopathologic Studies

Histopathology is a valuable aid to differential and definitive diagnosis of skull osteomyelitis especially if clinical findings, biological studies and diagnostic imaging investigations are not conclusive. Overall, acute osteomyelitis shows marrow edema, bony spicules, necrosis, and acute inflammatory cells especially granulocytic infiltration. Chronic forms demonstrate irregular fragments of devitalized bone surrounded by dense fibrous tissue heavily infiltrated by plasma cells, lymphocytes, and only a few granulocytes. Pathology has also been regarded as very helpful for identifying some "specific" osteomyelitis such as mycobacteria, fungi and parasites [44, 49, 52, 58, 59]. Please refer to Chap. 4 for more details about histopathologic results.

References

1. Nalini A, Saini J, Mahadevan A. Central nervous system nocardiosis with granulomatous pachymeningitis and osteomyelitis of skull vault. Indian J Pathol Microbiol. 2014;57(2):332–4. doi:10.4103/0377-4929.134735.
2. Prendiville S, Bielamowicz SA, Hawrych A, Deeb ZE. Isolated cryptococcal sphenoid sinusitis with septicemia, meningitis, and subsequent skull base osteomyelitis in an immunocompetent patient. Otolaryngol Head Neck Surg. 2000;123(3):277–9.
3. Akhaddar A, El Mostarchid B, Gazzaz M, Boucetta M. Cerebellar abscess due to Lactococcus lactis. A new pathogen. Acta Neurochir (Wien). 2002;144(3):305–6.
4. Ng J, Connolly DJ, Rittey CD, Mordekar SR. Skull base osteomyelitis leading to lateral medullary syndrome in a child. Eur J Paediatr Neurol. 2007;11(2):111–4.
5. Soto-Hernández JL, Morales VA, Lara Giron JC, Balderrama Bañares J. Cranial epidural empyema with osteomyelitis caused by actinomyces, CT, and MRI appearance. Clin Imaging. 1999;23(4):209–14.
6. Pincus DJ, Armstrong MB, Thaller SR. Osteomyelitis of the craniofacial skeleton. Semin Plast Surg. 2009;23(2):73–9. doi:10.1055/s-0029-1214159.

7. Baddley JW, Cobbs CS, Pappas PG. Surgical treatment of multiple skull abscesses associated with coccidioidomycosis. Mycoses. 2004;47(1–2):69–71.
8. Ketenci I, Unlü Y, Tucer B, Vural A. The Pott's puffy tumor: a dangerous sign for intracranial complications. Eur Arch Otorhinolaryngol. 2011;268(12):1755–63. doi:10.1007/s00405-011-1660-5.
9. Bullitt E, Lehman RA. Osteomyelitis of the skull. Surg Neurol. 1979;11(3):163–6.
10. Nakwan N, Nakwan N, Wannaro J, Dissaneevate P, Kritsaneepaiboon S, Chokephaibulkit K. Septicemia, meningitis, and skull osteomyelitis complicating infected cephalhematoma caused by ESBL-producing Escherichia coli. Southeast Asian J Trop Med Public Health. 2011;42(1):148–51.
11. Tattersall R, Tattersall R. Pott's puffy tumour. Lancet. 2002;359(9311):1060–3.
12. Gildener-Leapman N, Lin A. Pott's puffy tumor in a 5-year-old male and a review of the literature. Int J Pediatr Otorhinolaryngol Extra. 2012;7(2):48–51.
13. Tutela JP, Banta JC, Boyd TG, Kelishadi SS, Chowdhry S, Little JA. Scalp reconstruction: a review of the literature and a unique case of total craniectomy in an adult with osteomyelitis of the skull. Eplasty. 2014;14:e27. eCollection 2014.
14. Guillén A, Brell M, Cardona E, Claramunt E, Costa JM. Pott's puffy tumour: still not an eradicated entity. Childs Nerv Syst. 2001;17(6):359–62.
15. Blumenkopf B, Hartshorne MF, Bauman JM, Cawthon MA, Patton JA, Friedman AH. Craniotomy flap osteomyelitis: a diagnostic approach. J Neurosurg. 1987;66(1):96–101.
16. Hayashi T, Uchiumi H, Yanagisawa K, Ogawa Y, Handa H, Tsukamoto N, Nojima Y. Recurrent Gemella haemolysans meningitis in a patient with osteomyelitis of the clivus. Intern Med. 2013;52(18):2145–7.
17. Tuon FF, Russo R, Nicodemo AC. Brain abscess secondary to frontal osteomyelitis. Rev Inst Med Trop Sao Paulo. 2006;48(4):233–5.
18. Bhaskar IP, Inglis TJ, Lee GY. Clinical, radiological, and microbiological profile of patients with autogenous cranioplasty infections. World Neurosurg. 2014;82(3–4):e531–4. doi:10.1016/j.wneu.2013.01.013.
19. Michail M, Jude E, Liaskos C, Karamagiolis S, Makrilakis K, Dimitroulis D, Michail O, Tentolouris N. The performance of serum inflammatory markers for the diagnosis and follow-up of patients with osteomyelitis. Int J Low Extrem Wounds. 2013;12(2):94–9. doi:10.1177/1534734613486152.
20. Kim CW, Lee JJ, Kim HS, Won JY. Skull base osteomyelitis following a mastoidectomy. Auris Nasus Larynx. 2013;40(6):584–6. doi:10.1016/j.anl.2012.12.002.
21. Chan MS, Wong YC, Lau SP, Lau KY, Ou Y. MRI and CT findings of infected cephalhaematoma complicated by skull vault osteomyelitis, transverse venous sinus thrombosis and cerebellar haemorrhage. Pediatr Radiol. 2002;32(5):376–9.
22. Peltola H, Pääkkönen M. Acute osteomyelitis in children. N Engl J Med. 2014;370(4):352–60. doi:10.1056/NEJMra1213956.
23. Nomura M, Shin M, Ohta M, Nukui Y, Ohkusu K, Saito N. Atypical osteomyelitis of the skull base and craniovertebral junction caused by Actinomyces infection—case report. Neurol Med Chir (Tokyo). 2011;51(1):64–6.
24. Chang PC, Fischbein NJ, Holliday RA. Central skull base osteomyelitis in patients without otitis externa: imaging findings. AJNR Am J Neuroradiol. 2003;24(7):1310–6.
25. Karabatsou K, Gan YC, Christie M, Sakas D. Pott's puffy tumour: a delayed complication of surgery. Br J Neurosurg. 2001;15(5):441–2.
26. Emejulu JC, Ekweogwu OC. Complicated Pott's puffy tumour involving both frontal and parietal bones: a case report. J Infect Dis Ther. 2014;2(5):166.
27. Shen CJ, Wu MS, Lin KH, Lin WL, Chen HC, Wu JY, Lee MC, Lee CC. The use of procalcitonin in the diagnosis of bone and joint infection: a systemic review and meta-analysis. Eur J Clin Microbiol Infect Dis. 2013;32(6):807–14. doi:10.1007/s10096-012-1812-6.

28. Butbul-Aviel Y, Koren A, Halevy R, Sakran W. Procalcitonin as a diagnostic aid in osteomyelitis and septic arthritis. Pediatr Emerg Care. 2005;21:828–32.
29. Boodhoo H, Karen V. Pott's puffy tumour—the tip of an iceberg. S Afr Med J. 2006;96 (5):374–6.
30. Nadvi SS, Nathoo N, van Dellen JR. Lumbar puncture in brain abscess and subdural empyema: not an innocuous procedure. Afr J Neurol Sci. 2001;20:4–6.
31. Camargo JF, Seriburi V, Tenner M, El Khoury MY. Aspergillus osteomyelitis of the lumbar spine complicated with orbital apex syndrome: a potential role of the Batson's plexus in disease propagation. Med Mycol Case Rep. 2012;1(1):9–12. doi:10.1016/j.mmcr.2012.02.004.
32. Qiu Y, Zhang J, Liu G, Zhong X, Deng J, He Z, Jing B. Retrospective analysis of 14 cases of disseminated Penicillium marneffei infection with osteolytic lesions. BMC Infect Dis. 2015;15:47. doi:10.1186/s12879-015-0782-6.
33. Laurens MB, Becker RM, Johnson JK, Wolf JS, Kotloff KL. MRSA with progression from otitis media and sphenoid sinusitis to clival osteomyelitis, pachymeningitis and abducens nerve palsy in an immunocompetent 10-year-old patient. Int J Pediatr Otorhinolaryngol. 2008;72(7):945–51. doi:10.1016/j.ijporl.2008.02.025.
34. Senegor M, Lewis HP. Salmonella osteomyelitis of the skull base. Surg Neurol. 1991;36 (1):37–9.
35. Blyth CC, Gomes L, Sorrell TC, da Cruz M, Sud A, Chen SC. Skull-base osteomyelitis: fungal vs. bacterial infection. Clin Microbiol Infect. 2011;17(2):306–11. doi:10.1016/j.ijporl.2008.02.025.
36. Qureshi A, Quinones-Hinojosa A, Ziai W. A rare infectious presentation of a temporal bone meningioma. J Neurooncol. 2014;116(3):633–4. doi:10.1016/j.ijporl.2008.02.025.
37. Soga Y, Oka K, Sato M, Kabata T, Kawasaki T, Kawano H, Hayano M. Cavernous sinus thrombophlebitis caused by sphenoid sinusitis—report of autopsy case. Clin Neuropathol. 2001;20(3):101–5.
38. He J, Lam JC, Adlan T. Clival osteomyelitis and hypoglossal nerve palsy-rare complications of Lemierre's syndrome. BMJ Case Rep. 2015. pii: bcr2015209777. doi:10.1136/bcr-2015-209777.
39. Spielmann PM, Yu R, Neeff M. Skull base osteomyelitis: current microbiology and management. J Laryngol Otol. 2013;127 Suppl 1:S8–12. doi:10.1017/S0022215112002356.
40. Levy PY, Fournier PE, Fenollar F, Raoult D. Systematic PCR detection in culture-negative osteoarticular infections. Am J Med. 2013;126(12):1143.e25–33. doi:10.1016/j.amjmed.2013.04.027.
41. Richardus RA, Jansen JC, Steens SC, Arend SM. Two immigrants with tuberculosis of the ear, nose, and throat region with skull base and cranial nerve involvement. Case Rep Med. 2011;2011:675807. doi:10.1155/2011/675807.
42. Kostov K, Petrov I. Tuberculous spondylitis—analysis of 22 cases. Acta Neurol Belg. 2009;109(2):127–31.
43. Akhaddar A, Baallal H, Elouennass M, Elgharbaoui H, Mahi M, Boucetta M. Combined Serratia liquefaciens and Mycobacterium tuberculosis in temporal osteitis with brain extension. Surg Infect (Larchmt). 2011;12(4):329–31. doi:10.1089/sur.2010.100.
44. Morris BS, Varma R, Garg A, Awasthi M, Maheshwari M. Multifocal musculoskeletal tuberculosis in children: appearances on computed tomography. Skeletal Radiol. 2002;31 (1):1–8.
45. Ramdurg SR, Gupta DK, Suri A, Sharma BS, Mahapatra AK. Calvarial tuberculosis: uncommon manifestation of common disease—a series of 21 cases. Br J Neurosurg. 2010;24 (5):572–7. doi:10.3109/02688697.2010.495166.
46. Luzzati R, Bobicchio P, Shah D, Franchi F, Gregori M, Tacconi L. Calvarial tuberculosis as the initial presentation of AIDS. J Clin Neurosci. 2006;13(6):675–7.
47. Huang I, Leach JL, Fichtenbaum CJ, Narayan RK. Osteomyelitis of the skull in early-acquired syphilis: evaluation by MR imaging and CT. AJNR Am J Neuroradiol. 2007;28(2):307–8.

48. Kang SH, Park SW, Kwon KY, Hong WJ. A solitary skull lesion of syphilitic osteomyelitis. J Korean Neurosurg Soc. 2010;48(1):85–7. doi:10.3340/jkns.2010.48.1.85.
49. Sohn MH, Lim ST, Jeong YJ, Kim DW, Jeong HJ, Lee CS. Unusual case of occult Brucella osteomyelitis in the skull detected by bone scintigraphy. Nucl Med Mol Imaging. 2010;44(2):161–3. doi:10.1007/s13139-010-0023-2.
50. Akhaddar A, Elouennass M, Baallal H, Boucetta M. Focal intracranial infections due to Actinomyces species in immunocompetent patients: diagnostic and therapeutic challenges. World Neurosurg. 2010;74(2–3):346–50. doi:10.1016/j.wneu.2010.05.029.
51. Kostur M, Storey D. Nocardia farcinica osteomyelitis of the frontal bone five years after Nocardia brain abscess in an immunocompetent patient. J Miss State Med Assoc. 2002;43(4):111.
52. Akhaddar A, Gazzaz M, Albouzidi A, Lmimouni B, Elmostarchid B, Boucetta M. Invasive Aspergillus terreus sinusitis with orbitocranial extension: case report. Surg Neurol. 2008;69(5):490–5. doi:10.1016/j.surneu.2007.02.059.
53. Calcagno SW, Graves RM, Baum SE, Teff RJ. Polymicrobial skull osteomyelitis: a rare complication of subdural hematoma evacuation. Surg Infect (Larchmt). 2007;8(4):483–90.
54. Vitali AM. Acquired encephalocele attributable to tuberculous osteitis: case report. Neurosurgery. 2008;62(4):E976. doi:10.1227/01.neu.0000318188.18159.57.
55. Pichichero ME, Friesen HA. Polymicrobial osteomyelitis: report of three cases and review of the literature. Rev Infect Dis. 1982;4(1):86–96.
56. Ridder GJ, Breunig C, Kaminsky J, Pfeiffer J. Central skull base osteomyelitis: new insights and implications for diagnosis and treatment. Eur Arch Otorhinolaryngol. 2015;272(5):1269–76. doi:10.1007/s00405-014-3390-y.
57. Ganhewa AD, Jafri Kuthubutheen J. A diagnostic dilemma of central skull base osteomyelitis mimicking neoplasia in a diabetic patient. BMJ Case Rep. 2013:bcr2012007183. doi:10.1136/bcr-2012-007183.
58. Suchanda B, Alugolu R, Purohit A, Lakshmi V, Sundaram C. A rare concomitant tubercular and *Fonsecaea pedrosoi* fungal infection of the skull base. J Neurosci Rural Pract. 2012;3:189–91. doi:10.4103/0976-3147.98237.
59. Mukherjee KK, Kaushik R, Nada R, Khosla VK, Khandelwal N, Kak VK. Calvarial tuberculosis. Surg Neurol. 2002;57(3):195–202.

Chapter 8
Imaging Studies

Contents

Abbreviations

ADC	Apparent diffusion coefficient
CT-scan	Computed tomography scan
DWI	Diffusion-weighted imaging
FDG	Fluorodeoxyglucose
ICA	Internal carotid artery
MPR	Multiplanar reconstructions
MRI	Magnetic resonance imaging
MRS	Magnetic resonance spectroscopy
PET	Positron emission tomography
SPECT	Single-photon emission computed tomography
WI	Weighted images

The development of neuroimaging techniques, namely the computed tomography scan (CT-scan), magnetic resonance imaging (MRI) and nuclear medicine studies, had enormously improved not only initial diagnosis of this infectious disease by readily showing its location and extension, but also the monitoring of treatment results. Conventional neuroimaging can be used for detection and confirmation when the diagnosis is uncertain or to evaluate the severity of infection and extent of involvement. The choice of modality depends on the site, the clinical status and the

A. Akhaddar, *Cranial Osteomyelitis*, DOI 10.1007/978-3-319-30268-3_8

timing of the suspected infection. Because the chronic infection is, by definition, more advanced than in acute cases, radiological imaging is usually more conclusive. Detecting early infection when complete resolution is still possible is a challenge to both clinicians and radiologists. The limitations of the conventional imaging modalities necessitate utilization of functional modalities and nuclear medicine techniques are suited for these patients. Also, CT-scan and MRI are helpful for guiding fine-needle aspiration or biopsy of adjacent soft tissue in difficult access areas such as skull base osteomyelitis [1, 2].

Plain Radiographs

Skull radiographies, although useful if they show the classic findings of cranial bone destruction, may not become abnormal for 10–21 days after the onset of infection because a significant 30–50 % loss of bone density must occur before such changes become apparent [3, 4]. In addition, skull radiograph is not specific enough for diagnosing osteomyelitis in pediatric population because radiolucencies of the skull are a common finding and do not indicate local infection [5]. Conventional radiographic films may show extracranial swollen tissue, spotty areas of demineralization and variable degrees of cranial bone erosion with or without disruption of the tables. Some cases have osteolytic lesion surrounded by sclerosis and air may be seen in the diploic space (Fig. 8.1). The classic "moth-eaten" appearance (calcified necrotic bone) may not be recognized for several months following the onset of

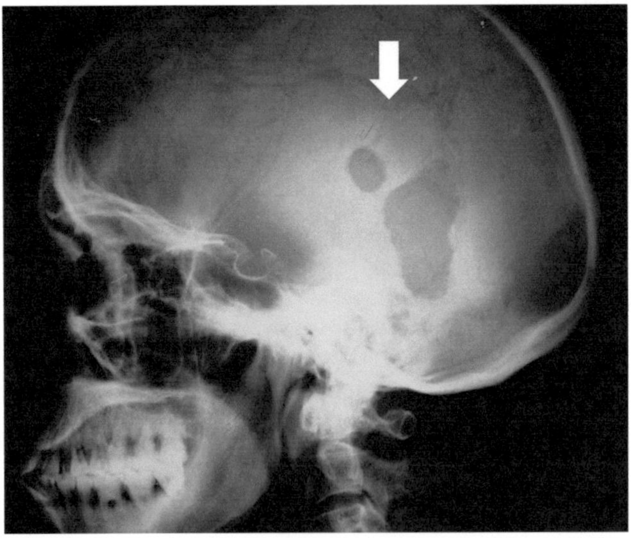

Fig. 8.1 Lateral skull plain radiography showing temporo-parietal osteolytic lesions surrounded by sclerosis

infection. On the other hand, plain radiographies have historically been used in the diagnosis of paranasal sinus and otomastoid diseases and their complications, and can offer evidence to the correct diagnosis in some conditions and in resource-limited areas [6, 7]. When postoperatively bone flap infection is suspected, plain radiography can be helpful but generally is not as sensitive in patients who have undergone a craniotomy previously (Fig. 8.2). Nevertheless, X-ray may be useful for ruling out retained foreign body (Fig. 8.3). Overall, if CT-scan and MRI are available, skull radiographies are not mandatory required.

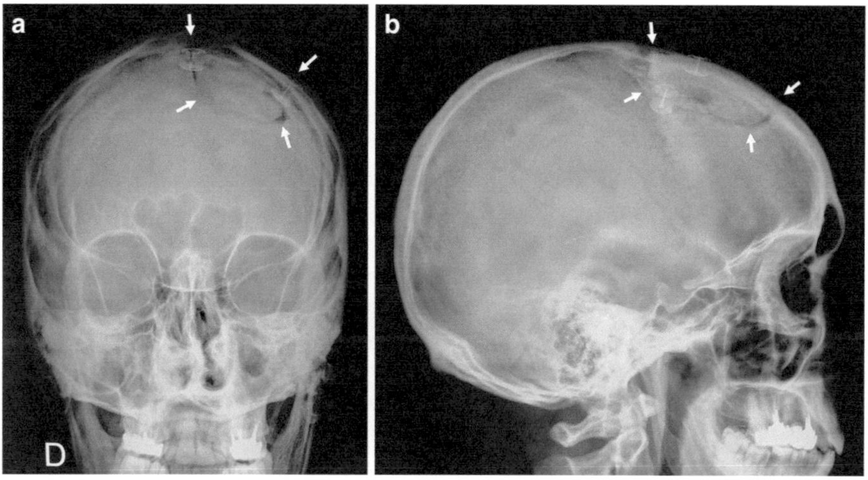

Fig. 8.2 Antero-posterior (**a**) and lateral (**b**) skull radiographies with confirmed chronic bone flap osteomyelitis

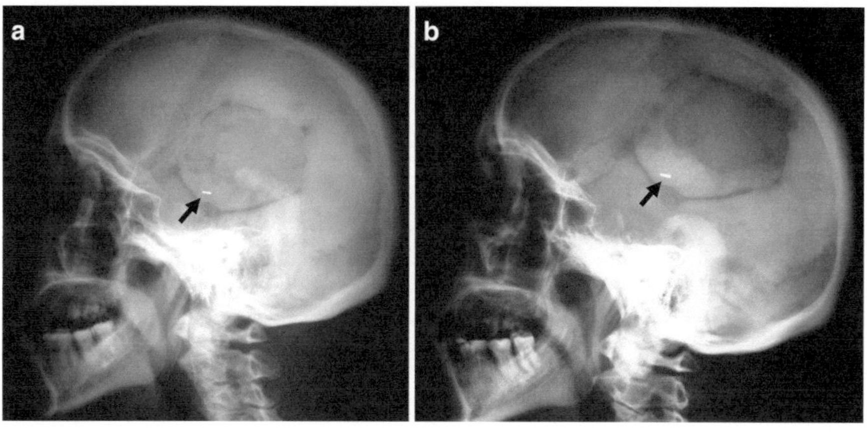

Fig. 8.3 Skull X-ray on lateral views taken 3 months (**a**) and 1 year postoperatively (**b**). Chronic osteomyelitis is identified by the presence of radiopaque sequestra which correspond to calcified necrotic bone. Note the retained metallic foreign body (*arrows*)

Computed Tomography-Scan

CT-scan is still the basic method for morphological diagnostics in cranial osteomyelitis without intracranial extension. CT-scan is also the favored technique (especially in emergency situations) because of its large availability, ease of use, and short imaging time. CT-scan is superior to MRI in assessing the bony structures and can display both osteolytic, osteosclerotic and osteogenic formations in a proper way. Technically, the cranial bones are best evaluated on CT-scan using a bone algorithm or at least when viewed using bone windows. Today, helical multidetector CT-scan allows us to make high-resolution 3D reconstructions and multiplanar reconstructions (MPR). In addition to bony changes, CT-scan is able to assess concomitant extracranial and intracranial soft tissue and dural inflammation. Intravenous injection of iodine as contrast agent is obligatory to assess alterations of the blood tissue barrier.

Compared with radiographs, the sensitivity of CT-scan is considerably higher in detecting the acute early changes of acute osteomyelitis. However, despite the availability of high-resolution CT-scan, this technique is still less sensitive than nuclear medicine imaging for the diagnosis of early osteomyelitis.

The CT-scan findings in the acute stage of osteomyelitis consist of area of rarefaction and loss of diploic bone trabeculae, demineralization/erosion/thinning of cortical bone table (Fig. 8.4), extracranial and subperiosteal abscesses (Fig. 8.5). Osteolytic defect of the table may appear secondarily (Fig. 8.6). In chronic stage, the loss of diploic bone trabeculae and the cortical bone thickening appear more evident. The most important changes are diploic bone sclerosis, cortical bone

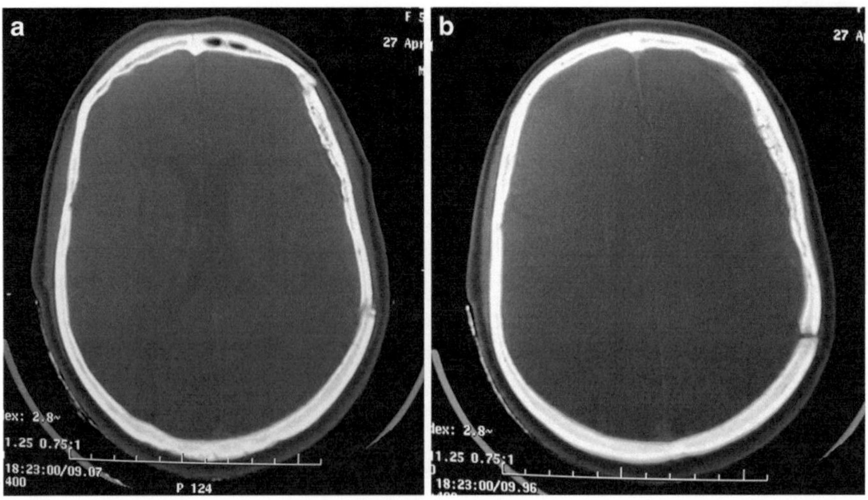

Fig. 8.4 Cranial axial CT-scan in bone windows 3 weeks postoperatively (**a** and **b**). Bone flap with loss of diploic bone trabeculae and areas of demineralization/erosion of inner table

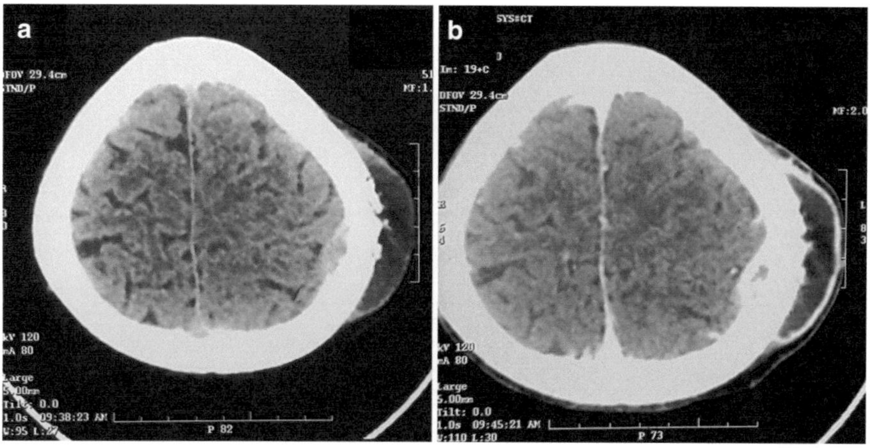

Fig. 8.5 Axial cranial CT-scan without (**a**) and with contrast injection (**b**) showing extradural and extracranial subperiosteal abscesses

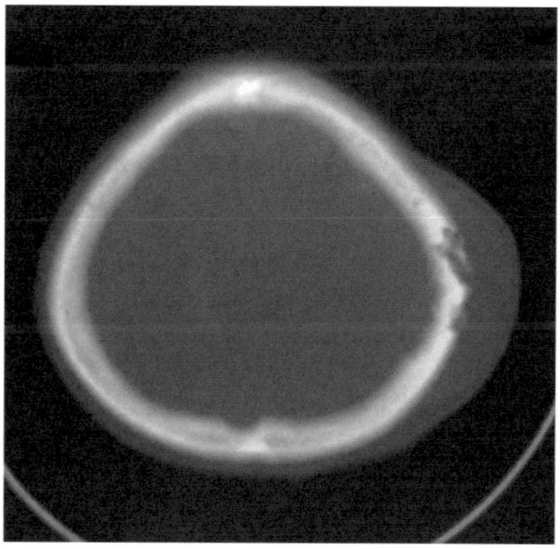

Fig. 8.6 Axial CT-scan in bone window demonstrating area of erosion and destruction of the outer table (same patient)

thickening mixed with areas of radiolucency and interruption of cortical bone (Fig. 8.7). Sequester formations are combined with more or less extensive destruction of the skull tables (Fig. 8.8).

In addition, after surgical intervention, CT-scan usually shows a scrubby subincisional space, and although strong peripheral enhancement of this cavity may denote infection (Fig. 8.9). However, false-positive results are common occurrences and accuracy is highly dependent on careful sample collection and laboratory techniques.

Additionally CT-scan is very helpful in determining if there is any intracranial component of the infection especially epidural abscess and/or subdural empyema

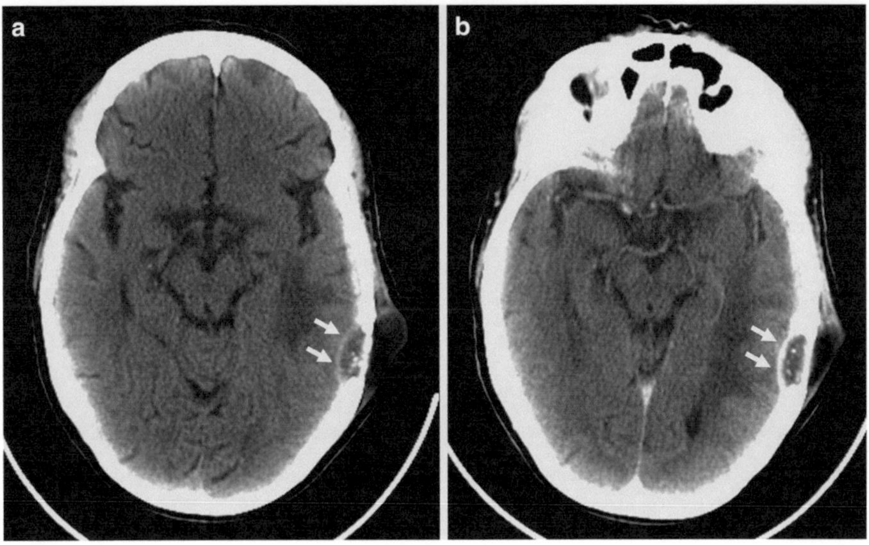

Fig. 8.7 Axial cranial CT-scan before (**a**) and after contrast injection (**b**) showing chronic osteomyelitis with temporo-parietal defect (*arrows*). Note some osseous sequestra within the osteolytic lesion

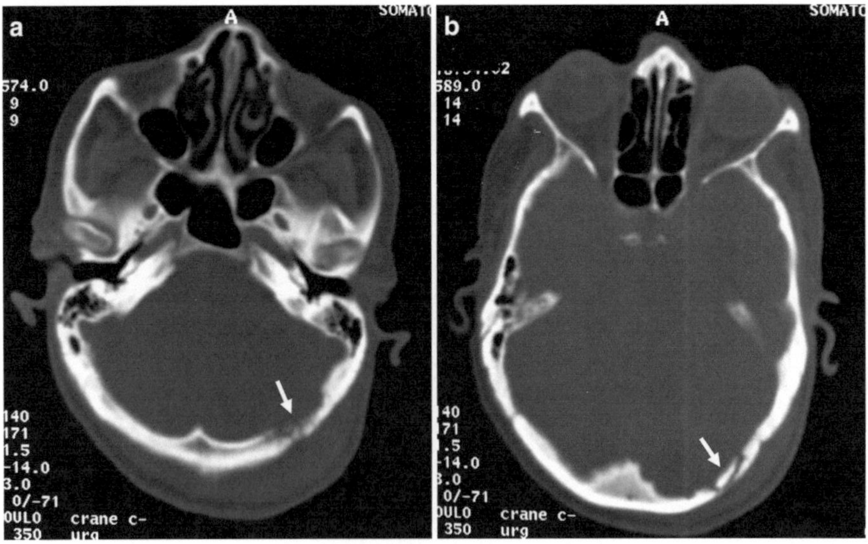

Fig. 8.8 Axial cranial CT-scan in bone windows (**a** and **b**) revealing sequester formations (*arrows*) combined with destruction of the inner skull table

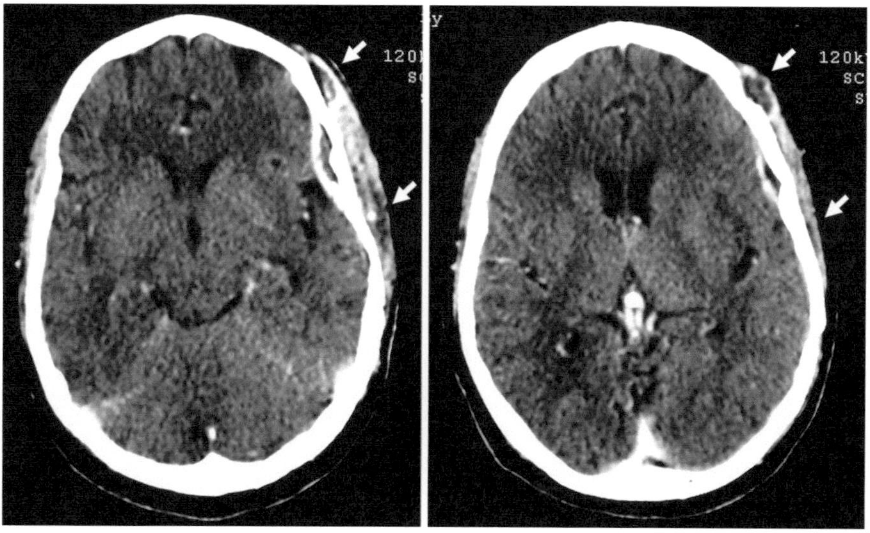

Fig. 8.9 Axial cranial CT-scan after contrast administration showing a scrubby extracranial subincisional space with strong peripheral enhancement which may denote infection (*arrows*)

[8, 9]. The appearance is that of a fluid collection with peripheral enhancement. However, the diagnosis of parameningeal infectious collection may be difficult when CT-scan is performed early in the evolution of the abscess, particularly in the posterior fossa [10, 11].

CT-scan findings for subdural empyema typically demonstrate a hypodense subdural collection over the hemisphere or along the falx with internal displacement of the gray-white junction, and effacement of the lateral ventricle, cortical sulci and basal cisterns. Mass effect is often caused more by edema than by the subdural collection itself. The peripheral margins are better delineated with the infusion of contrast material especially along the medial border of the collection at the pial surface as well as areas of underlying damage into the brain parenchyma (Fig. 8.10).

On the other hand, cranial epidural abscess appears as a poorly defined lentiform (biconvex) area of low or intermediate density. When contrast is administered, the convex inner side of the low-density lesion becomes enhanced and appears as rim enhancement caused by the inflamed dura (Fig. 8.11). CT-scan may show evidence of an intraparenchymatous mass lesion with surrounding brain edema. Peripheral rim enhancement is seen on contrast studies with a central area of hypodensity (Fig. 8.12). One of our diabetic patients presented with multiple bilateral brain abscesses associated with frontal osteomyelitis due to *Klebsiella pneumonia* (Fig. 8.13). In addition, CT-scan may study the integrity of the frontal sinus, the presence and extent of sinus or mastoid disease, and the presence of orbital involvement.

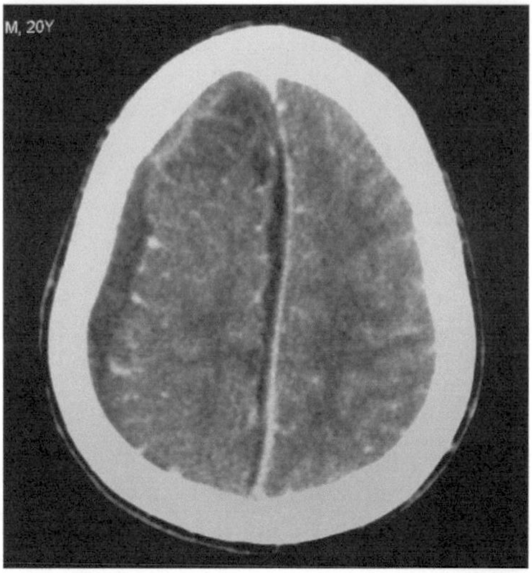

Fig. 8.10 Axial cranial CT-scan with contrast injection demonstrating interhemispheric and fronto-parietal subdural empyemas

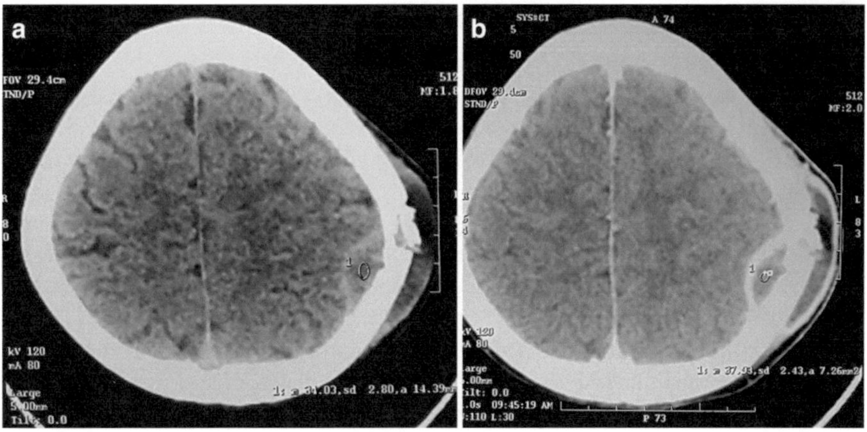

Fig. 8.11 Axial cranial CT-scan before (**a**) and after (**b**) contrast injection revealing a left parietal osteomyelitis with extracranial and epidural abscesses

In the skull base, CT-scan may be lacking initially but may later demonstrate evident bony erosion or destruction (Fig. 8.14). In some cases, no CT-scan evidence of bone erosion was seen but the diagnosis of skull base osteomyelitis was confirmed after biopsy [12, 13]. In central skull base osteomyelitis, bone erosion may involve the walls of the sphenoid sinus and the clivus. While in lateral skull base osteomyelitis erosion predominantly involves the walls of the external auditory canal, mastoid cells and occipital bone (Fig. 8.15). Diffuse nonspecific adjacent soft

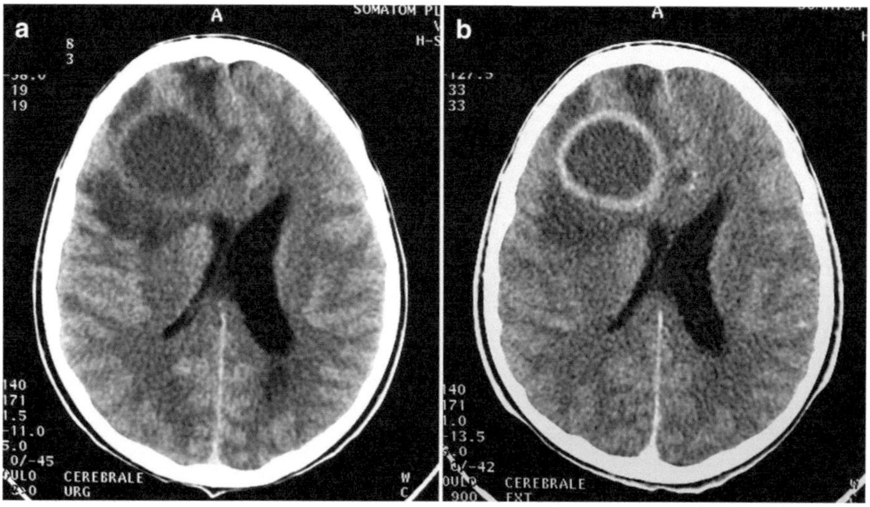

Fig. 8.12 Axial cranial CT-scan before (**a**) and after (**b**) contrast injection revealing a right frontal intraparenchymatous abscess

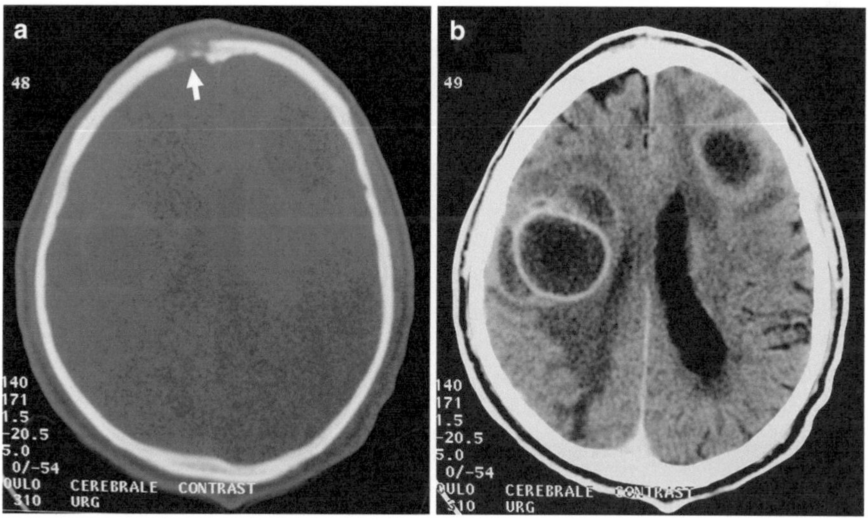

Fig. 8.13 Axial cranial CT-scan in bone (**a**) and parenchymatous (**b**) windows after contrast administration showing multiple bilateral brain abscesses associated with frontal osteomyelitis (*arrow*)

tissue swelling may be associated. Eustachian tube dysfunction may result in fluid in the mastoid and middle ear space [1, 14]. Interestingly, CT-scan may reveal bubbles of gas within the marrow spaces of the basal skull bones and within the surrounded soft tissues, meaning the existence of gas-forming micro-organisms

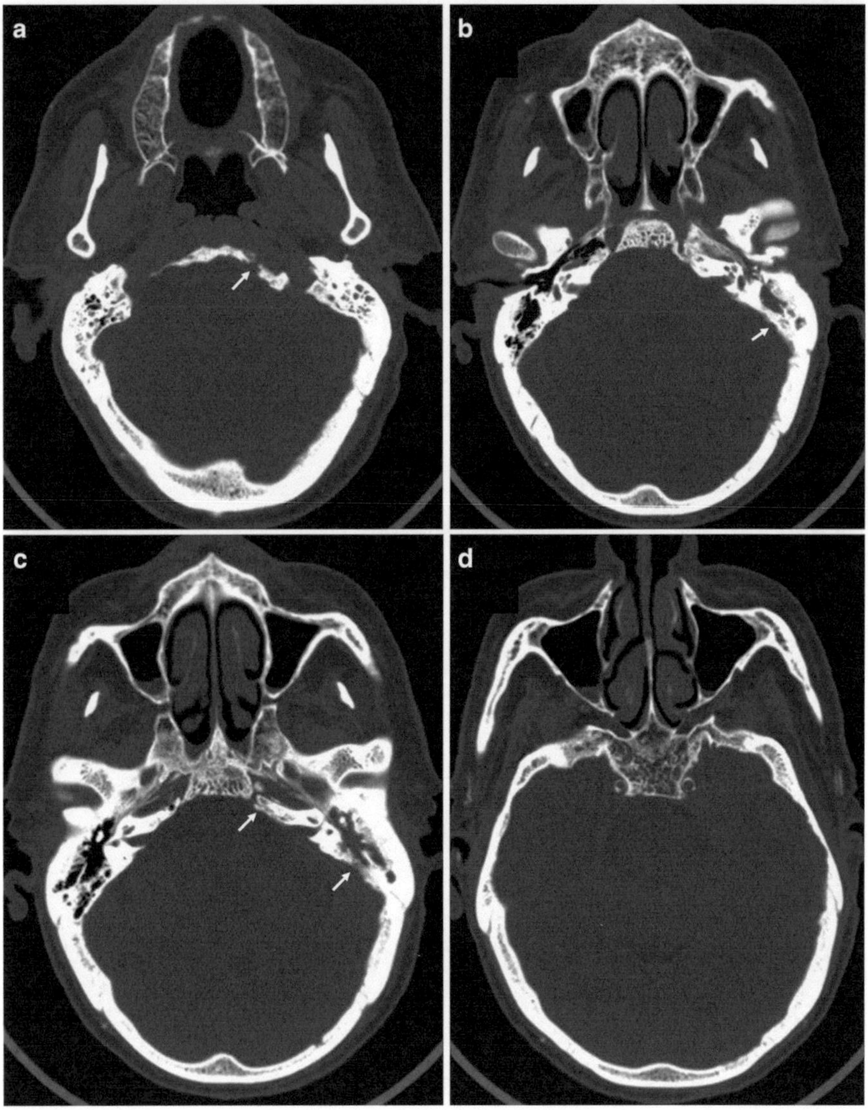

Fig. 8.14 Axial cranial CT-scan in bone windows **(a–d)** revealing chronic mastoiditis with evident clival and posterior petrous bone erosion (*arrows*) in the left side

(Fig. 8.16) [15]. After contrast administration, varying degrees of underlying dural enhancement with clear delineated abscesses may be seen, either intracranially or extracranially. Osseous lesions may fail to resolve for a long time after treatment is completed, so the use of CT-scan for monitoring of the disease course is questionable [16, 17].

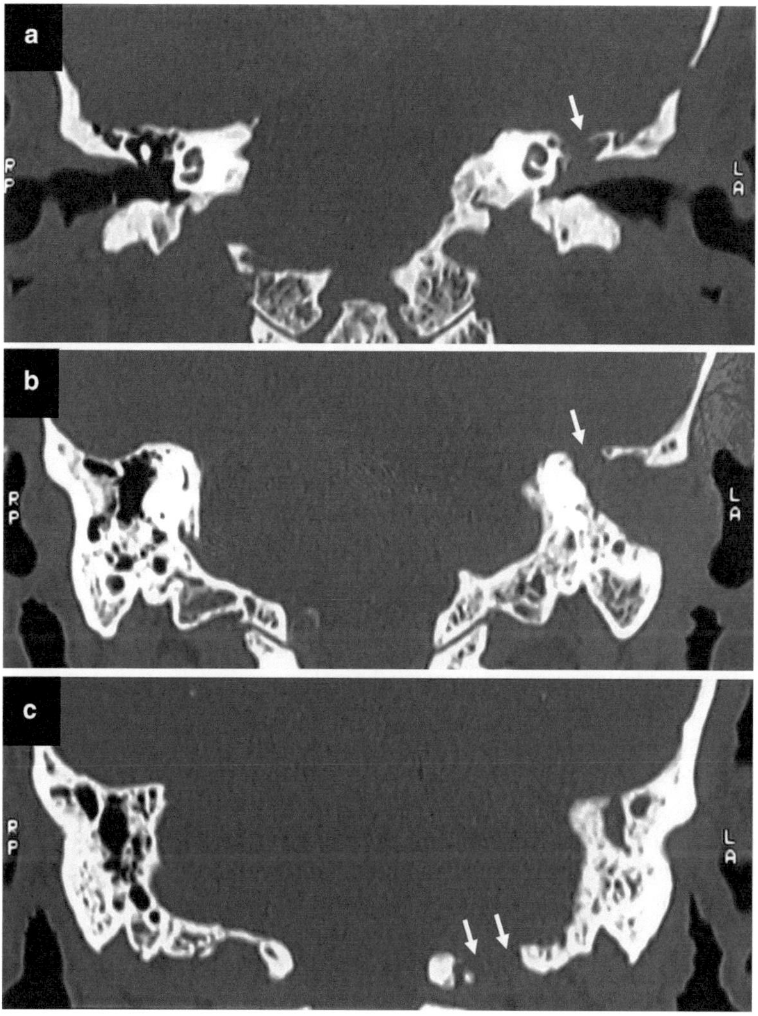

Fig. 8.15 Coronal reconstructions CT-scan in bone windows (**a–c**) showing petrous temporal skull base erosion involving the superior wall of the external auditory canal (*arrow*), mastoid cells and occipital bone (*arrows*)

Magnetic Resonance Imaging

The advantages of MRI compared to CT-scan include improvement of adjacent soft tissue contrast resolution and the extent of infection, absence of beam-hardening artifacts from bone and better interpretation of bone marrow abnormalities. MRI plays principally an increasing role in the diagnosis of the early acute stage of osteomyelitis based on the ability to detect infiltration of diploic fatty bone marrow.

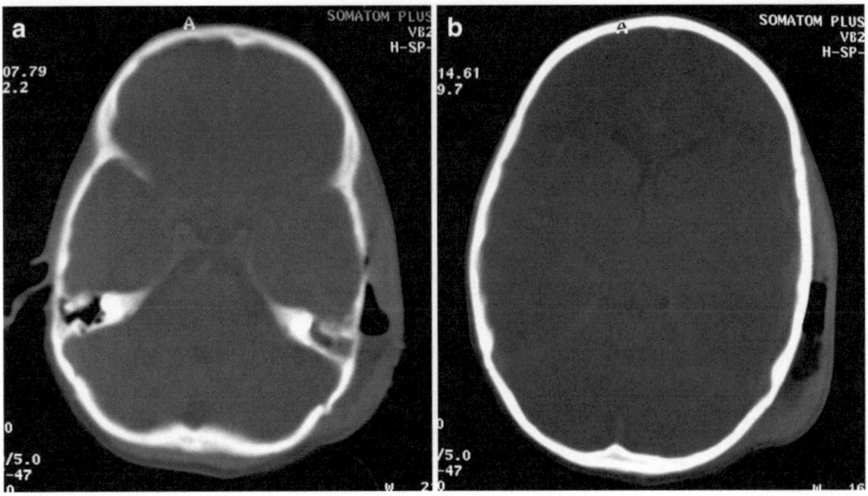

Fig. 8.16 Axial cranial CT-scan in bone windows (**a** and **b**) demonstrating opacification of left mastoid cells with large extracranial abscess formation. Note the different bubbles of gas within the collection meaning the existence of gas-forming micro-organisms

Additionally, MRI is recognized to be more sensitive for evaluating extracranial and intracranial lesions, especially parenchymal anomalies. For Hoistad and Duvall both CT-scan and MRI techniques are complementary to each other in particular for skull base study [18].

Limitations of the MRI technique include its availability and relative high cost, contraindication in patients with certain implant devices and metallic clips, and it is not tolerated by all patients because of claustrophobia or morbid obesity. In addition, young children may require sedation. In uncooperative patients, motion artifacts can impair the image quality.

On MRI, the normal cortical tables become visible as signal void on both T1-weighted images (T1-WI) and T2-weighted images (T2-WI). In adults, the marrow has high signal intensity on T1-WI due to the high fat content. In adolescents, the marrow signal is more heterogeneous because the marrow is not yet completely replaced with fat; nonetheless, the signal tends to be bilaterally symmetrical [19]. The contrast-enhanced series requires fat-suppression technique in order to facilitate recognition of pathological gadolinium enhancement within diploic bone and soft tissue. The diploë does not normally enhance with gadolinium, except for diploic veins and meninges adjacent to Pacchionian granulations [20].

The MRI findings in the acute stage of osteomyelitis consist of replacement of diploic bone fat by inflammation, enlargement of diploic (marrow) space with thinning of skull tables, T2 increase in signal intensity related to edema, T1 contrast enhancement due to blood tissue barrier disruption and extracranial and subperiosteal abscess formations.

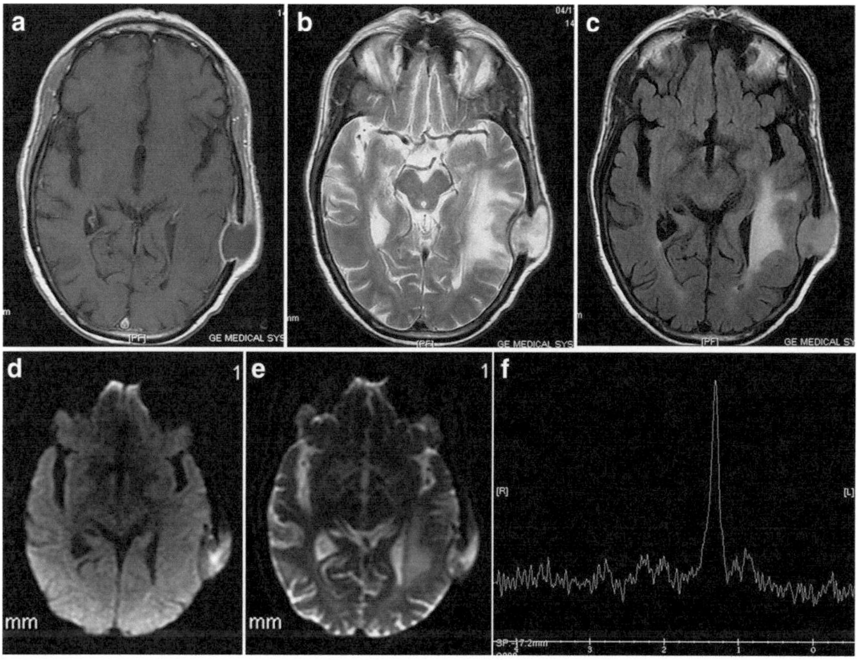

Fig. 8.17 Chronic temporo-parietal osteomyelitis. Axial cranial MRI on T1-weighted image after gadolinium administration (**a**), T2-weighted image (**b**), FLAIR sequence (**c**), diffusion weighted image (**d**), apparent diffusion coefficient map (**e**), and spectroscopy (**f**)

In chronic form, there is replacement of marrow fat by low-signal tissue with T2 increase in signal intensity related to edema, T1 gadolinium enhancement due to major inflammation, enlargement of diploic space with loss or thinning of skull tables, dissolution of cortical bone fragments leading to sequester formation and soft tissue/dural gadolinium enhancement (Fig. 8.17).

Extra-axial infectious collection (epidural abscess and subdural empyema) generally appear iso-hypointense on T1-WI with hyperintense patterns on T2-WI, they have high signal on diffusion-weighted imaging (DWI) indicating restricted diffusion (Fig. 8.18). Gadolinium enhancement helps diagnosis by showing a thickened dural surface and/or empyema wall which differentiates parameningeal suppurations from sterile collections (Fig. 8.19) [21]. Cerebral edema, cerebritis, venous infarction, mass effect and parenchymal abscess formation are also visible on MRI. DWI, apparent diffusion coefficient (ADC) images and MR spectroscopy (MRS) can confirm the diagnosis [22]. In brain abscess, subdural empyema and epidural abscess, there is restricted DWI (high signal) of the abscess cavity with corresponding low signal on ADC due to the cellularity of the cavity [23–25]. In addition, MRS may show elevated lactate (Fig. 8.17f). This finding improves the ability to differentiate other cystic structures which have low signal on DWI, from infectious collection. Orbital invasion can be resolute, in particular with fat saturation images. Overall, progressive increase in size of the collection over time is a

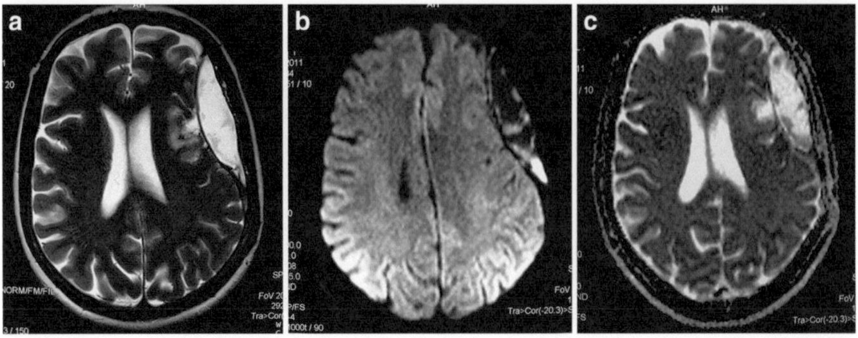

Fig. 8.18 Axial cranial MRI on T2-weighted image (**a**), diffusion-weighted image (**b**) and apparent diffusion coefficient map (**c**) showing a postoperative epidural abscess. This patient was operated 2 months previously for an adjacent cranial vault meningioma (case n°1)

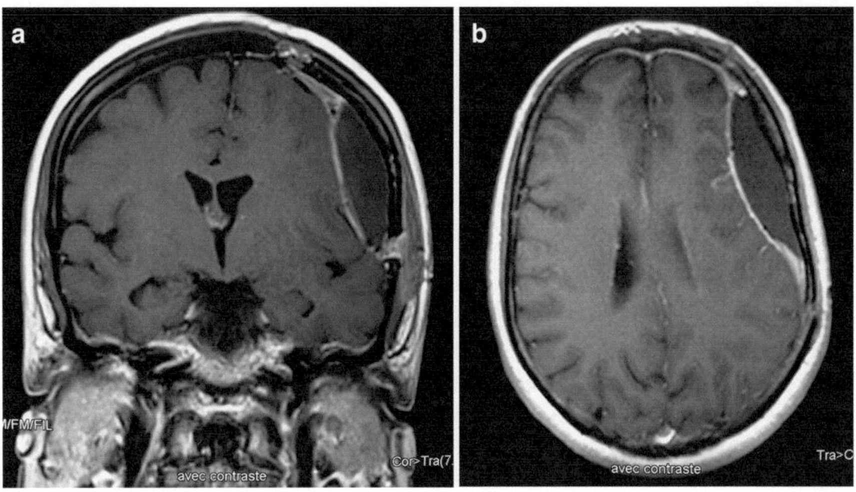

Fig. 8.19 Coronal (**a**) and axial (**b**) cranial MRI on T1-weighted images after gadolinium administration revealing a postoperative extradural abscess (case n°1)

particularly suspicious finding. In some patients, cranial osteomyelitis may be associated with a combination of multiple forms of intracranial infection such as epidural abscess, subdural empyema and brain abscess (Fig. 8.20).

In the skull base, MRI scanning is very helpful to view critical areas such as the basal foramina, cranial nerves and vascular structures [14]. For many authors, the most consistent MRI findings in central skull base osteomyelitis is focal or diffuse clival hypointensity on T1-WI relative to normal fatty marrow [26–28]. Gadolinium administration shows varying degrees of underlying dural enhancement without a clearly delineated collection (Fig. 8.21). Pre and paraclival soft tissue infiltration with obliteration of normal fat planes may be viewed, with variable extension into

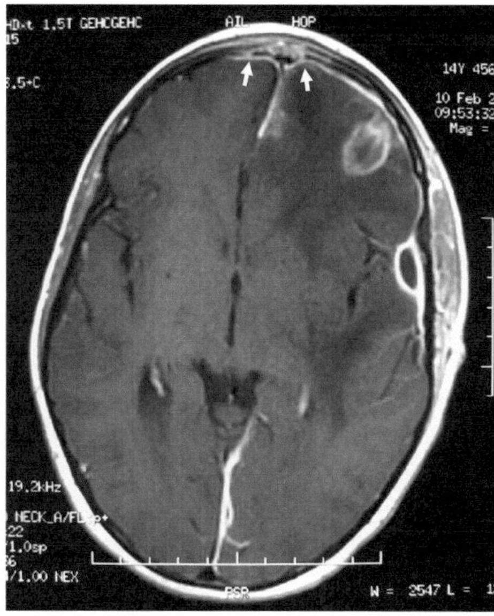

Fig. 8.20 Axial cranial MRI on T1-weighted image after gadolinium injection showing frontal bone erosions (*arrows*), thickened dural surface, left frontal brain abscess and parameningeal empyema

the cavernous sinus or the sella turcica [28–30]. If malignant otitis externa is responsible for true skull base infection, the external auditory canal and soft tissues within the subtemporal region are thickened and demonstrate reduced T1 signal. The T2-weighted sequences return isointense or slightly hyperintense signal intensity (Fig. 8.22). This is unlike the high signal that is noted in most inflammatory conditions with associated hyperemia and edema. The lower signal intensity on T2-WI is likely related to the nature of the underlying fibrotic and narcotizing pathological process [31, 32].

MRI may also be performed to differentiate an inflammatory from a neoplastic cause of an osteolytic lesion as depicted by conventional radiographs or CT-scan. Multifocal separate lesions, lack of concomitant fat involvement and substantial focal soft tissue infiltration are signs favoring a neoplasm rather than an infectious process. A retrospective study by Ozgen et al. examined the use of DWI to better distinguish skull base osteomyelitis from malignancy. This was based on the previously noted finding that diffusion-weighted sequences can help distinguish benign from malignant lymph nodes. In principle, malignant neoplasms have low ADC and benign masses have higher ADC. This study showed that ADC values of lymphomas and nasopharyngeal carcinomas were significantly lower than that of the group with skull base osteomyelitis; however the ADC values of the patients with metastatic disease overlapped with the skull base osteomyelitic group [33, 34].

Also, MRI is useful to monitor response to therapy, and the MR marrow signal intensity gradually reverted toward normal as the symptoms resolved. Other imaging techniques such as CT-scan or nuclear medicine studies are unable to follow precisely the changes occurring in the skull base bone marrow and surrounding soft tissue [1, 35].

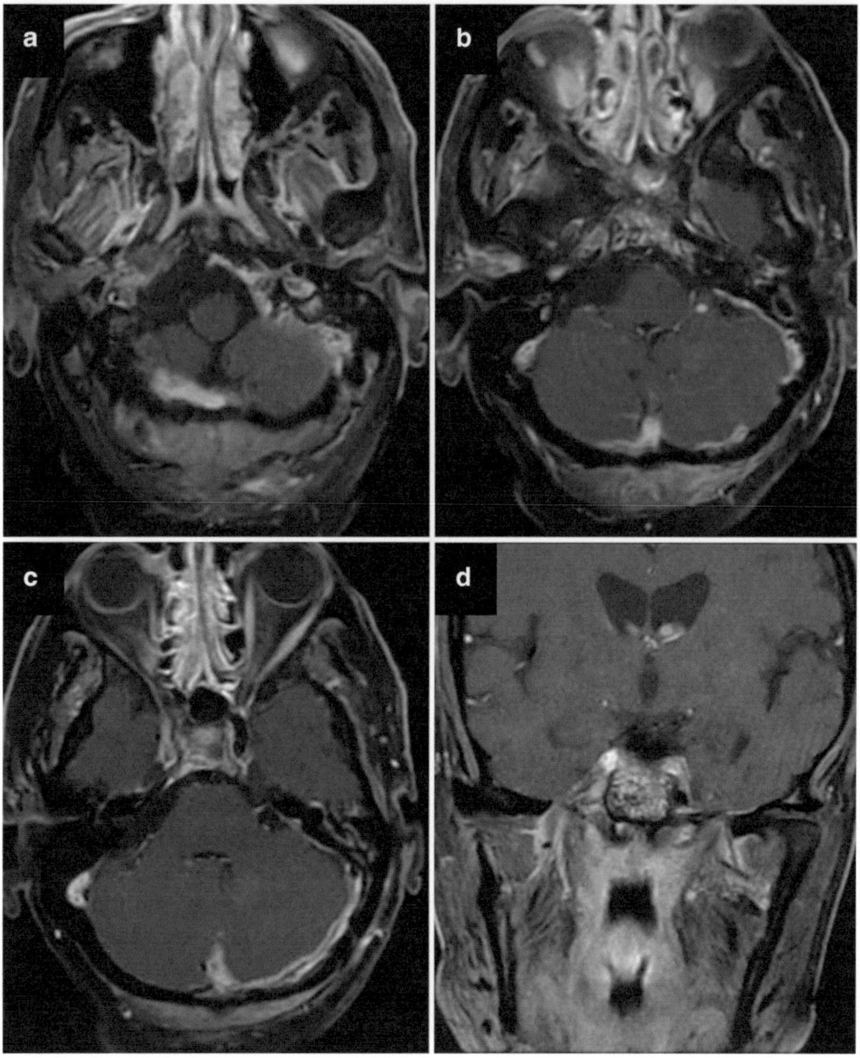

Fig. 8.21 Axial (**a–c**) and coronal (**d**) T1-weighted MRI after gadolinium injection revealing chronic central skull base osteomyelitis in the left side with adjacent dural enhancement. Note the left lateral venous sinus thrombosis (case n°2)

In patients who have undergone prior surgical intervention, MRI may not be able to distinguish between bone marrow edema or enhancement related to a reactive inflammatory phenomenon and that related to infection. Contrast CT-scan and MRI can both identify enhancing fluid collections concerning for abscess, although care must be taken not to confuse abscesses with other postoperative fluid collections, such as hematomas and seromas [36]. A plain radiography can be helpful but generally is not as sensitive as in patients who have undergone a craniotomy

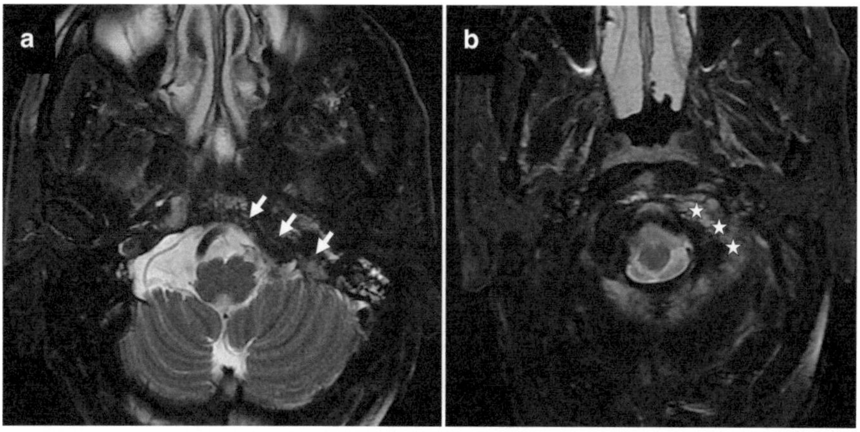

Fig. 8.22 Axial T2-weighted MRI showing left otomastoiditis with petrous bone mixed signal intensity (*arrows*) and surrounding high signal inflammatory granulomas (*stars*) (case n°2)

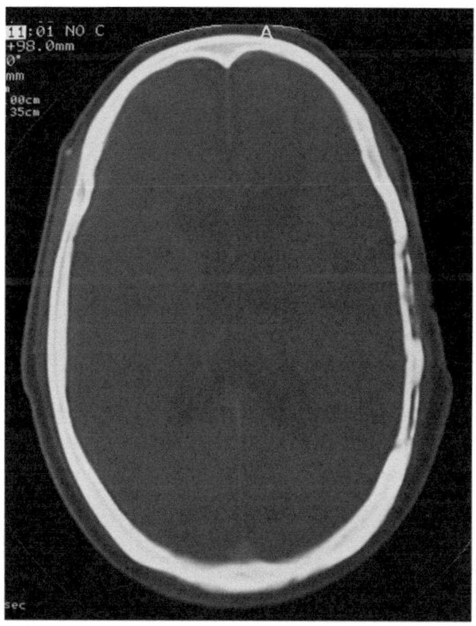

Fig. 8.23 Axial cranial CT-scan in bone window revealing chronic parietal bone flap infection with mixed areas of lucency and sclerosis. Note the erosion and destruction of the outer bone table

previously. Nevertheless, X-ray may be useful for ruling out retained foreign body. On CT-scan, bone flaps infection may either reveal areas of lucency, sclerosis (Fig. 8.23) with or without sequestrum (Fig. 8.24). Lucency and/or sclerosis appearances are not specific for osteomyelitis and can be seen in normal bone flaps. However, the existence of secondary modifications, such as overlying tracks, skin thickening, fat stranding, and adjacent fluid collections, should increase the

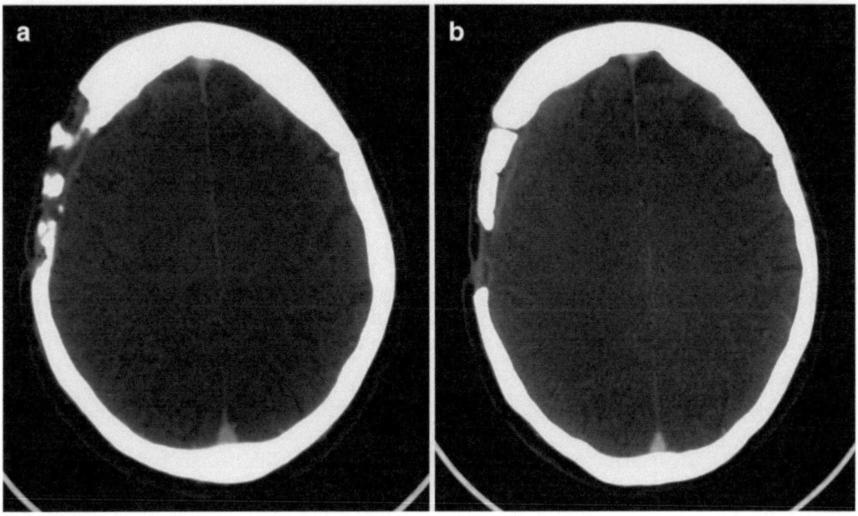

Fig. 8.24 Axial cranial CT-scan in bone windows (**a** and **b**) showing chronic frontal bone flap osteomyelitis with multiple bony sequestra

doubt of an infected bone flap. MRI can demonstrate increased T2 signal and decreased T1 signal intensity within the infected bone flap marrow. Additionally, predisposing factors include communication with paranasal sinuses, several surgeries, long intraoperative time, and surgery for preexisting intracranial infection.

Postoperative brain abscess may mimic a recurrent glioma within the previous operative cavity (Fig. 8.25). So called "pseudo-progression", with new contrast enhancing tissue due to concomitant radiation and chemotherapy, may be marked by its late time course, silent clinical presentation, and irregular form on imaging [37]. As stated previously, DWI, ADC and MRS studies are useful to aid in the differential diagnosis of a cystic or necrotic brain tumor recurrence and a postoperative abscess [38, 39]. In contrast to necrotic or cystic brain tumors that are seen as hypointense on DWI, abscesses are seen as hyperintense on DWI. This is particularly useful in the early stages of the infectious process and is a very useful modality to aid in early diagnosis and treatment of postoperative infection. Also, MRS has been applied to the examination of intracranial infectious collection. MRS of brain abscesses was found to show none of the usual detectable resonances from normal brain parenchyma or brain tumor metabolites such as N-acetyl-aspartate (NAA), phosphorylated creatine (PCr), and choline compounds (Co) [40]. Alternatively, the abscesses showed resonances from lactate, acetate, (both products of bacterial metabolism), lipids, and amino-acids. Subsequent studies have confirmed the usefulness of MRS and suggested its use in conjunction with

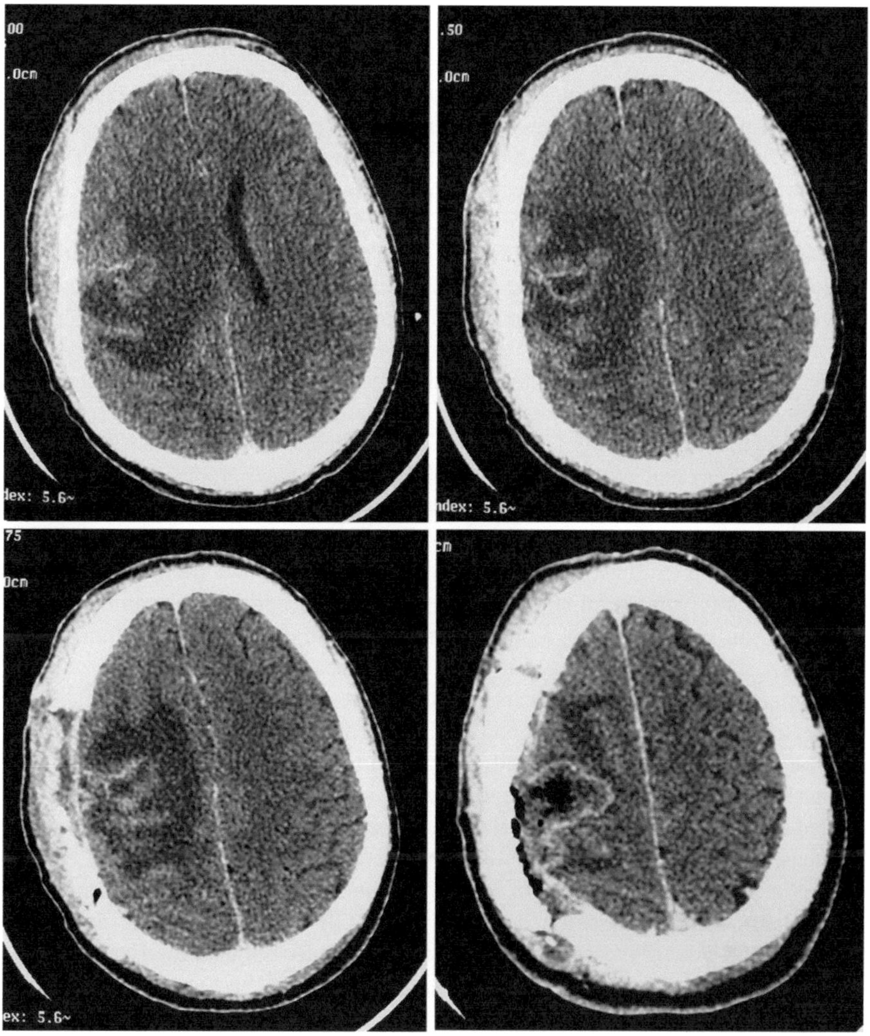

Fig. 8.25 Axial cranial CT-scan after contrast injection. Postoperative fronto-parietal brain abscess mimicking a recurrent glioma within the previous operative cavity

DWI for the differentiation of necrotic or cystic brain tumors from brain abscesses [41–43]. Additionally, nuclear scanning using labeled leukocytes which reflect migration of white blood cells into areas of inflammation can be useful in the diagnosis of osteomyelitis associated with bone surgery, trauma or prosthetic devices.

Neurovascular Explorations

Potential cerebrovascular complications may be concerned with skull base osteomyelitis especially dural venous sinus thrombosis and carotid invasions with or without ischemic infarcts [15, 44–46]. Sinovenous thrombosis is identified by contrast CT-scan or MRI/MR venography. Transverse-sigmoid sinus, cavernous sinus and internal jugular are the vascular structures more generally involved [15, 45, 47, 48]. This is due to the very close contiguity of the sigmoid sinus to the temporal bone (particularly the mastoid bone) and of the cavernous sinus to the sphenoid sinus. Clot formation is resulting in the adjacent inflammatory process that can spread to other cerebral venous sinuses with possible occlusion and distal brain parenchymal embolism [15]. On the unenhanced MRI, subacute thrombi, identified as hyperintense signals on both long and short repetition time sequences. Hemorrhagic cerebellar infarction may be associated with transverse sinus thrombosis following basal skull osteomyelitis [49]. On MR venography, a decreased or absence of flow at the dural venous sinuses may be seen [45, 50]. These findings cannot be revealed on nuclear medicine imaging [50].

Arterial complications of skull base osteomyelitis are less frequently reported [51]. Unilateral or bilateral stenosis in the internal carotid arteries can be seen in both CT-scan and MR angiography [15]. The inflammation in the cavernous sinus in central skull base osteomyelitis can easily spread on carotid siphon, causing inflammatory arteritis. Internal carotid arteries are often surrounded by inflammatory tissue; contrast involvement and wall thickening is seen [44, 52–54]. Stenosis may be seen in the petrous segment of the carotid due to petrositis [52] and in the extracranial segment due to retropharyngeal abscess [55]. In addition, internal carotid artery (ICA) stenosis can also be caused due to the mass effect or due to the spasms caused by the surrounding inflammatory tissue. ICA stenosis can be clinically asymptomatic [55]. In some patients with skull base osteomyelitis, cerebral infarcts may develop due to critical ICA stenosis or septic embolism [15, 45, 53, 54]. Flow-sensitive gradient-echo MR sequences are useful in documenting arterial thrombosis. Some patients may exhibit “watershed” infarcts due to cerebral hypoperfusion caused by bilateral ICA occlusion [56–58].

In addition to data obtained from angio-CT-scan and angio-MR evaluation may be extended to include four vessel angiography. Pseudoaneurysms may occur in the internal carotid artery or the superior cerebellar artery [46, 51, 59, 60]. Kadkhodayan et al. presented a 50-year-old woman with malignant otitis externa and bilateral temporal bone osteomyelitis presented with brisk bleeding from her left ear. She had bony dehiscence of the left carotid canal at CT-scan and extravasation from a mycotic pseudoaneurysm of the carotid petrous segment at angiography. A Pipeline embolization device was used successfully to treat this pseudoaneurysm [59].

Nuclear Medicine

The limitations of the conventional imaging modalities necessitate utilization of functional modalities and nuclear medicine techniques are suited for these patients. Nuclear medicine imaging is mostly useful in early detection of suspected osteomyelitis within 24–48 h after the onset of symptoms and consequently leads to therapy before much bone destruction occurs [4]. This imaging procedure is also valuable in identifying (asymptomatic) multifocal osseous involvement and making some differential diagnosis [61–69]. However, similar to all other imaging modalities, bone scan does not distinguish constantly inflammatory disease from an infectious or malignant process [34, 67, 70, 71]. Although radionuclide studies are sensitive, they can be time-consuming, and they have lower spatial resolution. The incidence of false-negative scans is low in neonates and in elderly patients with osteomyelitis. Additionally, it is not a good sensitive tool for assessing treatment response, as the bone scan can remain abnormal for months to years following an active osteomyelitis. Overall, nuclear medicine procedures are more sensitive than X-ray and contrasted CT-scans but less sensitive than MRI [72, 73]. Nuclear medicine imaging has been reported to be a valuable adjunct in the diagnosis of cranial osteomyelitis. However, there is poor neurosurgical literature on this subject.

A variety of nuclear medicine techniques are available for evaluation of patients with osteomyelitis such as Gallium-67 citrate, multiphase skeletal scintigraphy with Technetium-99m-methylene diphosphonate, radiolabeled leukocyte or white blood cells, single photon emission computed tomography (SPECT), positron emission tomography (PET) and labeled antibiotic imaging. However, each modality has its own strengths and weaknesses. Conventional radionuclide scintigraphy techniques are not very specific and have a low sensitivity. Gallium-67 and Technetium-99 tracers both have reasonable sensitivity [63, 69], with Gallium slightly more specific than Technetium as a tracer, but nighters have high specificity over all. Sensitivity can be raised by performing a tagged white blood cell scan [74]. The lack of anatomic detail and relatively limited spatial resolution in nuclear medicine images can be surmounted by fusion imaging. Fusion imaging consists of a combined anatomic (usually CT-scan) and a functional imaging (nuclear medicine imaging) in a single sitting in the same position [75–79]. In particular, in cases of bone infection with adjacent soft-tissue involvement, conventional CT-scan of the head fails to demonstrate any abnormality. Planar images alone of scintigraphy did not allow differentiation of soft tissue/dura from bone. However, hybrid SPECT/CT allowed better characterization of the extension of infection and provided an accurate anatomic localization of the positive focus not only in the soft tissue but also in the skull bone. This ability is of particular importance since the therapeutic approaches to soft-tissue and bone infections are different [78, 79]. In a systematic review on diagnostic accuracy and clinical value of SPECT and PET for imaging of bone and joint infections, van der Bruggen et al. concluded that SPECT/CT with Indium-111 combined with Technetium-99 seems to be the best imaging technique

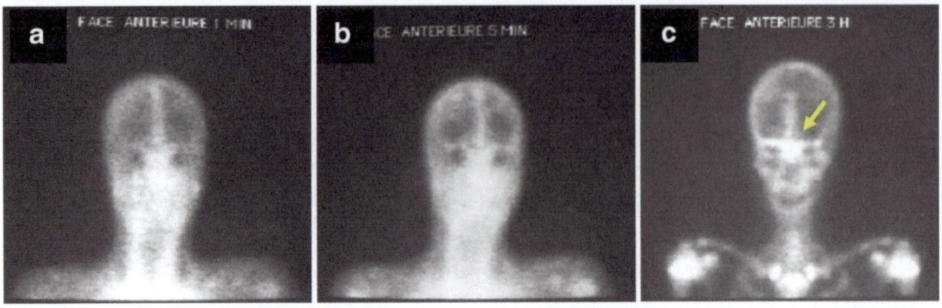

Fig. 8.26 Technetium-99m cranial bone. Anterior views at different time: 1 min (**a**), 5 min (**b**), and 3 h (**c**) showing increased radiotracer localization in the medial frontal bone near the frontal sinuses (*arrow*). This area correspond to an osteolytic lesion on CT-scan

for diagnosis of bone and joint infections. Fluorodeoxyglucose-positron emission tomography (FDG-PET) is also useful for diagnosis of osteomyelitis with improved spatial resolution over SPECT imaging, allowing more accurate localization. This localization can be further improved by adding CT-scan [79, 80].

Acute osteomyelitis is more frequently evaluated by the three phase bone scan which reveals a focal area of sequential increased perfusion, soft tissue blood pooling and late bony uptake in typical cases [81] (Fig. 8.26). In some cases bone scans show areas of decreased Technetium uptake named "cold scans" probably reflecting compromised vascular supply to the bone from thrombosis and ischemic necrosis [82]. Specificity can be improved by adding Gallium-67 imaging. The overall accuracy of combined bone/Gallium-67 imaging is about 65–80 %. However, the technique requires multiple imaging sessions over several days and difficulty in interpretation was a serious disadvantage [83]. Labeled leukocytes imaging, because of the limited spatial resolution cannot differentiate between soft tissue and bone infection. Addition of hybrid imaging techniques like SPECT/CT helps in precise anatomical localization [80, 84] (Figs. 8.27 and 8.28). Among the various conventional nuclear medicine techniques, Indium-111 labeled leukocyte is one of the most specific imaging procedures and is useful in acute infection [54, 85]. Disadvantages in imaging with Indium labeled leukocytes include need for prolonged imaging, combining with bone marrow imaging, higher radiation burden, need for handling blood and limited availability. Technetium-99m labeled leukocytes is a better alternative. A good result has been reported in a 62-year-old man with odontogenic temporal bone osteomyelitis [86]. The overall accuracy of combined leukocyte/marrow imaging for infection is approximately 90 % [83]. The role of SPECT/CT in infection imaging using Gallium-67 or Indium-111 labeled leukocytes made a better contribution to scintigraphy by improving the diagnosis, localization or definition of the extent of disease [79, 87].

In chronic and low grade osseous infections, bone/Gallium imaging and SPECT/CT are also useful [88]. For del Val Gomez et al., abnormal Gallium-67 skull uptake appears to be a sensitive (82 %) and specific (92 %) indicator of disseminated mycobacterial infection in HIV-positive patients [65]. For Horger

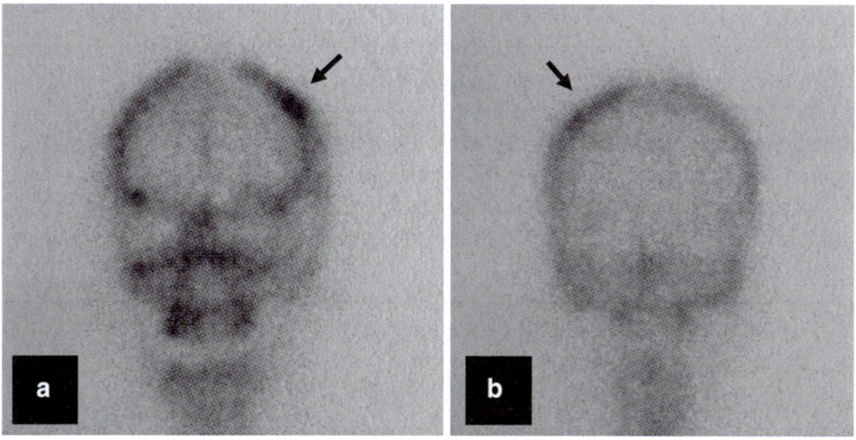

Fig. 8.27 A 52-year-old patient with left parietal chronic scalp infection and suspected adjacent cranial osteomyelitis. Cranial Tc 99m-scintigraphy shows accumulation in left side of the parietal bone on anterior (**a**) and posterior (**b**) views (case n°3)

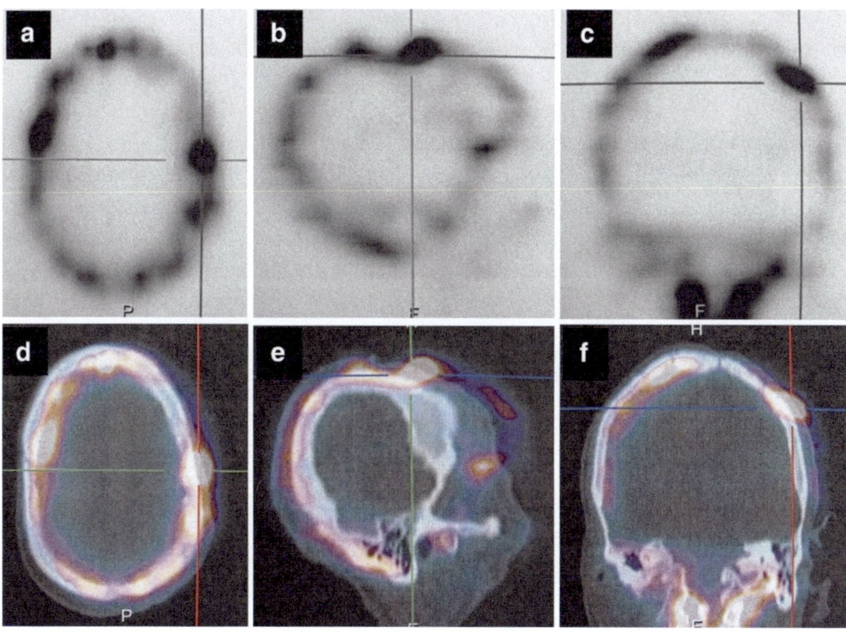

Fig. 8.28 The infected cranial bone lesion can be determined more precisely by SPECT (**a–c**) and SPECT/CT images of the head (**d–f**) (case n°3)

et al., sensitivity was identical for SPECT and SPECT/CT (100 %), whereas specificity was improved from 78 to 89 % by the use of SPECT/CT [89] (Fig. 8.28). On the other hand, the detection of osteomyelitis with 18 FDG-PET is generally excellent because the activated macrophages greedily take up FDG. A negative FDG-PET can virtually rule out osteomyelitis [90]. FDG-PET and FDG-PET/CT have many advantages over conventional nuclear medicine imaging techniques: complete image acquisition within 1 h, high sensitivity, high target-to-background contrast, and high-resolution tomographic images. PET/CT also provides exact anatomic localization of FDG uptake and increases the specificity compared with PET alone [79, 91–93]. In addition, bone scans imaging is particularly useful in some cases of chronic osteomyelitis with a predominant sclerosing radiographic appearance where bone repair mechanisms clearly mask necrosis and resorption [94].

Several authors have discussed the importance of nuclear medicine imaging in the management of skull-base osteomyelitis [34, 67, 78, 95–102]. Bone scans have been found useful as an initial screening tool, while Gallium scans have been used to follow response to therapy [95–97]. Gallium scans show areas of active inflammation and can give useful information about the involvement of soft tissue and bony structures [17]. Together, technetium and gallium scans can be used to differentiate between necrotizing otitis externa and skull-base osteomyelitis. A positive gallium scan and normal technetium scan indicate necrotizing otitis externa, while a skull-base osteomyelitis usually results in positive gallium and technetium scans [95, 96, 101]. For Sharma et al., SPECT-CT seems to be useful, but not superior to planar bone scintigraphy, SPECT, or CT, for diagnosis of skull base osteomyelitis [97].

Bruni et al. emphasize the usefulness of SPECT/CT for the Technetium99m-hexamethylpropylene amine oxime-labeled leukocyte in a patient with suspected temporal osteomyelitis [78]. The Indium-111 labeled leukocyte was used by Okpala et al. in diagnosing malignant otitis externa. In some situations, this scan was found to be negative in the presence of infection and therefore a negative scan cannot exclude malignant otitis externa. One explanation given for the poor sensitivity of the test is the difficulty in counting slow turnover radio-labeled leucocytes [103]. PET is a commonly used technique for detecting metastatic disease. This is based on the principle that many tumors preferentially take up fluorodeoxyglucose. PET may have a role in diagnostic dilemmas because the presence of disseminated metastases would make the diagnosis of malignancy more likely. However, increased uptake at the local site in the skull base can occur in the presence of infection as well as malignancy [33, 34].

Ultrasound Imaging

Ultrasonography of swelling has been used to distinguish subgaleal abscess from other soft tissue collections and masses. However, the physical properties of bone do not usually lend themselves to ultrasonographic investigation, because of the reflection of sound waves at a soft tissue-bone interface. The sonographic appearance of the scalp abscess is that of a heterogeneous hypoechoic lesion adjacent to the outer table of the cranial vault with occasionally a vascular periphery

[103, 104]. There was also disruption to the cranial vault with the mass appearing to extend intracranially via this external cortex defect [6, 104–106]. Increased vascularity of the collection may be seen in color Doppler image [105]. For Chen et al. cranial ultrasound has been useful in differentiating subdural empyema from anechoic reactive subdural effusion in pediatric population with meningitis [107]. Transfontanelar ultrasounds are used to explore the brain and the ventricles, but its use is limited to the first 18 months of life when the anterior fontanel is still open. Also, ultrasonography may be helpful in assessing the contents of the orbit.

Electroencephalography

Abnormalities on electroencephalography may be localized and can help in excluding a more generalized intracranial disease, such as encephalitis. Unilateral slow waves (delta, 1–3 per second) characterize the usual electroencephalographic findings in cases of cerebral abscess. A careful search should be made for a source of infection throughout the body. Although each of these studies has the potential to add information in the diagnosis and management of skull craniomyelitis, not all are routinely used.

Other testing should be guided by the history and findings of physical examination.

References

1. Chang PC, Fischbein NJ, Holliday RA. Central skull base osteomyelitis in patients without otitis externa: imaging findings. AJNR Am J Neuroradiol. 2003;24(7):1310–6.
2. Kacl GM, Carls FR, Moll C, Debatin JF. Interactive MR-guided biopsies of maxillary and skull-base lesions in an open-MR system: first clinical results. Eur Radiol. 1999;9:487–92.
3. Waldvogel FA, Medoff G, Swartz MN. Osteomyelitis: a review of clinical features, therapeutic considerations and unusual aspects. N Engl J Med. 1970;282(4):198–206.
4. Handmaker H, Leonards R. The bone scan in inflammatory osseous disease. Semin Nucl Med. 1976;6(1):95–105.
5. Harris VJ, Meeks W. The frequency of radiolucencies underlying cephalohematoma. Radiology. 1978;129:389–91.
6. Prasad R, Verma N, Mishra OP, Srivastava A. Osteomyelitis of skull with underlying brain abscess. Indian J Pediatr. 2011;78(8):1005–7. doi:10.1007/s12098-011-0369-1.
7. Gupta P, Varshney S, Chaterjee B, Saxena RK. Mastoid abscess caused by Nocardia in a child with visceral leishmaniasis. Trop Doct. 2005;35(1):45–6.
8. Nathoo N, Nadvi SS, van Dellen JR. Cranial extradural empyema in the era of computed tomography: a review of 82 cases. Neurosurgery. 1999;44(4):748–53.
9. Nathoo N, Nadvi SS, van Dellen JR, Gouws E. Intracranial subdural empyemas in the era of computed tomography: a review of 699 cases. Neurosurgery. 1999;44(3):529–35.
10. Rich PM, Deasy NP, Jarosz JM. Intracranial dural empyema. Br J Radiol. 2000;73 (876):1329–36.

11. van de Beek D, Campeau NG, Wijdicks EF. The clinical challenge of recognizing infratentorial empyema. Neurology. 2007;69(5):477–81.
12. Seabold JE, Simonson TM, Weber PC, Thompson BH, Harris KG, Rezai K, Madsen MT, Hoffman HT. Cranial osteomyelitis: diagnosis and follow-up with In-111 white blood cell and Tc-99m methylene diphosphonate bone SPECT, CT, and MR imaging. Radiology. 1995;196(3):779–88.
13. Rowlands RG, Lekakis GK, Hinton AE. Masked pseudomonal skull base osteomyelitis presenting with a bilateral Xth cranial nerve palsy. J Laryngol Otol. 2002;116(7):556–8.
14. Cavel O, Fliss DM, Segev Y, Zik D, Khafif A, Landsberg R. The role of the otorhinolaryngologist in the management of central skull base osteomyelitis. Am J Rhinol. 2007;21 (3):281–5.
15. Severino M, Liyanage S, Novelli V, Cheesborough B, Saunders D, Gunny R, Rossi A. Skull base osteomyelitis and potential cerebrovascular complications in children. Pediatr Radiol. 2012;42:867–74. doi:10.1007/s00247-011-2340-8.
16. Epstein JS, Ganz WI, Lizak M, Grobman L, Goodwin WJ, Dewanjee MK. Indium 111-labeled leukocyte scintigraphy in evaluating head and neck infections. Ann Otol Rhinol Laryngol. 1992;101(12):961–8.
17. Parker KM, Nicholson JK, Cezayirli RC, Biggs PJ. Aspergillosis of the sphenoid sinus: presentation as a pituitary mass and postoperative gallium-67 imaging. Surg Neurol. 1996;45 (4):354–8.
18. Hoistad DL, Duvall III AJ. Sinusitis with contiguous abscess involvement of the clivus and petrous apices. Case report. Ann Otol Rhinol Laryngol. 1999;108(5):463–6.
19. Bourekas EC, Lanzieri CF. The calvarium. Semin Ultrasound CT MRI. 1994;15(6):424–53.
20. West MS, Russell EJ, Breit R, Sze G, Kim K. Calvarial and skull based metastases: comparison of nonenhanced and Gd-DPTA enhanced MR images. Radiology. 1990;174 (1):85–91.
21. Dill SR, Cobbs CG, McDonald CK. Subdural empyema: analysis of 32 cases and review. Clin Infect Dis. 1995;20(2):372–86.
22. Tsuchiya K, Osawa A, Katase S, Fujikawa A, Hachiya J, Aoki S. Diffusion-weighted MRI of subdural and epidural empyemas. Neuroradiology. 2003;45(4):220–3.
23. Bink A, Gaa J, Franz K, Weidauer S, Yan B, Lanfermann H, Seifert V, Zanella FE. Importance of diffusion-weighted imaging in the diagnosis of cystic brain tumors and intracerebral abscesses. Zentralbl Neurochir. 2005;66(3):119–25.
24. Reiche W, Schuchardt V, Hagen T, Il'yasov KA, Billmann P, Weber J. Differential diagnosis of intracranial ring enhancing cystic mass lesions—role of diffusion-weighted imaging (DWI) and diffusion-tensor imaging (DTI). Clin Neurol Neurosurg. 2010;112(3):218–25. doi:10.1016/j.clineuro.2009.11.016.
25. Wong AM, Zimmerman RA, Simon EM, Pollock AN, Bilaniuk LT. Diffusion-weighted MR imaging of subdural empyemas in children. AJNR Am J Neuroradiol. 2004;25(6):1016–21.
26. Prabhu SP, Zinkus T, Cheng AG, Rahbar R. Clival osteomyelitis resulting from spread of infection through the fossa navicularis magna in a child. Pediatr Radiol. 2009;39(9):995–8. doi:10.1007/s00247-009-1283-9.
27. Rusconi R, Bergamaschi S, Cazzavillan A, Carnelli V. Clivus osteomyelitis secondary to Enterococcus faecium infection in a 6-year-old girl. Int J Pediatr Otorhinolaryngol. 2005;69 (9):1265–8.
28. Johnson AK, Batra PS. Central skull base osteomyelitis: an emerging clinical entity. Laryngoscope. 2014;124(5):1083–7. doi:10.1002/lary.24440.
29. Taranath A, Prelog K. Sella turcica collection due to skull base osteomyelitis. Pediatr Radiol. 2005;35(4):451.
30. Alleyne Jr CH, Vishteh AG, Spetzler RF, Detwiler PW. Long-term survival of a patient with invasive cranial base rhinocerebral mucormycosis treated with combined endovascular, surgical, and medical therapies: case report. Neurosurgery. 1999;45(6):1461–3.

31. Adams A, Offiah C. Central skull base osteomyelitis as a complication of necrotizing otitis externa: imaging findings, complications, and challenges of diagnosis. Clin Radiol. 2012;67 (10):e7–16. doi:10.1016/j.crad.2012.02.004.
32. Sando I, Harada T, Okano Y, Saito R, Caparosa RJ. Temporal bone histopathology of necrotizing external otitis. A case report. Ann Otol Rhinol Laryngol. 1981;90(2 Pt 1):109–15.
33. Ozgen B, Oguz KK, Cila A. Diffusion MR imaging features of skull base osteomyelitis compared with skull base malignancy. AJNR Am J Neuroradiol. 2011;32(1):179–84. doi:10.3174/ajnr.A2237.
34. Ganhewa AD, Kuthubutheen J. A diagnostic dilemma of central skull base osteomyelitis mimicking neoplasia in a diabetic patient. BMJ Case Rep. 2013. pii: bcr2012007183. doi: 10.1136/bcr-2012-007183.
35. Fanning NF, Laffan EE, Shroff MM. Serial diffusion-weighted MRI correlates with clinical course and treatment response in children with intracranial pus collections. Pediatr Radiol. 2006;36(1):26–37.
36. Ginat DT, Duhaime AC. Imaging the postoperative scalp and cranium. In: Ginat DT, Westesson PLA, editors. Atlas of postsurgical neuroradiology, imaging of the brain, spine, head, and neck. Berlin: Springer; 2012.
37. Nabavi A, Knerlich-Lukoschus F, Stark AM. Postoperative intracranial infections. In: Hall WA, Kim PD, editors. Neurosurgical infectious disease. Surgical and nonsurgical management. New York: Thieme Medical Publishers; 2014.
38. Guzman R, Barth A, Lövblad KO, El-Koussy M, Weis J, Schroth G, Seiler RW. Use of diffusion-weighted magnetic resonance imaging in differentiating purulent brain processes from cystic brain tumors. J Neurosurg. 2002;97(5):1101–7.
39. Mascalchi M, Filippi M, Floris R, Fonda C, Gasparotti R, Villari N. Diffusion-weighted MR of the brain: methodology and clinical application. Radiol Med. 2005;109(3):155–97.
40. Lai PH, Ho JT, Chen WL, Hsu SS, Wang JS, Pan HB, Yang CF. Brain abscess and necrotic brain tumor: discrimination with proton MR spectroscopy and diffusion-weighted imaging. AJNR Am J Neuroradiol. 2002;23(8):1369–77.
41. Lai PH, Hsu SS, Ding SW, Ko CW, Fu JH, Weng MJ, Yeh LR, Wu MT, Liang HL, Chen CK, Pan HB. Proton magnetic resonance spectroscopy and diffusion-weighted imaging in intracranial cystic mass lesions. Surg Neurol. 2007;68 Suppl 1:S25–36.
42. Muccio CF, Caranci F, D'Arco F, Cerase A, De Lipsis L, Esposito G, Tedeschi E, Andreula C. Magnetic resonance features of pyogenic brain abscesses and differential diagnosis using morphological and functional imaging studies: a pictorial essay. J Neuroradiol. 2014;41 (3):153–67. doi:10.1016/j.neurad.2014.05.004.
43. Horská A, Barker PB. Imaging of brain tumors: MR spectroscopy and metabolic imaging. Neuroimaging Clin N Am. 2010;20(3):293–310. doi:10.1016/j.nic.2010.04.003.
44. Soga Y, Oka K, Sato M, Kabata T, Kawasaki T, Kawano H, Hayano M. Cavernous sinus thrombophlebitis caused by sphenoid sinusitis—report of autopsy case. Clin Neuropathol. 2001;20(3):101–5.
45. He J, Lam JC, Adlan T. Clival osteomyelitis and hypoglossal nerve palsy-rare complications of Lemierre's syndrome. BMJ Case Rep. 2015. pii: bcr2015209777. doi: 10.1136/bcr-2015-209777.
46. Alvernia JE, Patel RN, Cai DZ, Dang N, Anderson DW, Melgar M. A successful combined endovascular and surgical treatment of a cranial base mucormycosis with an associated internal carotid artery pseudoaneurysm. Neurosurgery. 2009;65(4):733–40. doi:10.1227/01.NEU.0000351773.74034.5E.
47. Assefa D, Dalitz E, Handrick W, Lietz R, Braun W, Michalski H. Septic cavernous sinus thrombosis following infection of ethmoidal and maxillary sinuses: a case report. Int J Pediatr Otorhinolaryngol. 1994;29(3):249–55.
48. Peer Mohamed B, Carr L. Neurological complications in two children with Lemierre syndrome. Dev Med Child Neurol. 2010;52(8):779–81. doi:10.1111/j.1469-8749.2010.03718.x.

49. Chan MS, Wong YC, Lau SP, Lau KY, Ou Y. MRI and CT findings of infected cephalhaematoma complicated by skull vault osteomyelitis, transverse venous sinus thrombosis and cerebellar haemorrhage. Pediatr Radiol. 2002;32(5):376–9.
50. Lee SJ, Weon YC, Cha HJ, Kim SY, Seo KW, Jegal Y, Ahn JJ, Ra SW. A case of atypical skull base osteomyelitis with septic pulmonary embolism. J Korean Med Sci. 2011;26 (7):962–5. doi:10.3346/jkms.2011.26.7.962.
51. Blyth CC, Gomes L, Sorrell TC, da Cruz M, Sud A, Chen SC. Skull-base osteomyelitis: fungal vs. bacterial infection. Clin Microbiol Infect. 2011;17(2):306–11. doi:10.1111/j.1469-0691.2010.03231.x.
52. Visosky AM, Isaacson B, Oghalai JS. Circumferential petrosectomy for petrous apicitis and cranial base osteomyelitis. Otol Neurotol. 2006;27:1003–13.
53. Chandra S, Goyal M, Mishra NK, Gaikwad SB. Invasive aspergillosis presenting as a cavernous sinus mass in immuno competent individuals; report of 3 cases. Neuroradiology. 2000;42(2):108–11.
54. Wilkinson EP, Robinson RA, Trask DK. Skull base thrombotic mycosis. Ear Nose Throat J. 2007;86(3):137.
55. Hudgins PA, Dorey JH, Jacobs IN. Internal carotid artery narrowing in children with retropharyngeal lymphadenitis and abscess. AJNR Am J Neuroradiol. 1998;19:1841–3.
56. Ng J, Connolly DJ, Rittey CD, Mordekar SR. Skull base osteomyelitis leading to lateral medullary syndrome in a child. Eur J Paediatr Neurol. 2007;11(2):111–4.
57. Bentham JR, Pollard AJ, Milford CA, Anslow P, Pike MG. Cerebral infarct and meningitis secondary to Lemierre's syndrome. Pediatr Neurol. 2004;30:281–3.
58. Atmaca MM, Barlas NY, Çoban O. Skull base osteomyelitis presenting with facial paralysis, low cranial nerve palsies and bilateral carotid involvement: a case report. Turkish J Neurol. 2015;21(1):27–30.
59. Kadkhodayan Y, Shetty VS, Blackburn SL, Reynolds MR, Cross III DT, Moran CJ. Pipeline embolization device and subsequent vessel sacrifice for treatment of a bleeding carotid pseudoaneurysm at the skull base: a case report. J Neurointerv Surg. 2013;5(5):e31. doi:10.1136/neurintsurg-2012-010394.
60. Ong A, Blyth CC, Bency R, Vicaretti M, Harun A, Meyer W, Shingde M, Gilroy N, Chapman J, Chen SC. Fatal mycotic aneurysms due to Scedosporium and Pseudallescheria infection. J Clin Microbiol. 2011;49(5):2067–71. doi:10.1128/JCM.02615-10.
61. Coyne K, Browne R, Anagnostopoulos C, Nwokolo N. Syphilitic periostitis in a newly diagnosed HIV-positive man. Int J STD AIDS. 2006;17(6):421–3.
62. Gómez Martínez MV, Gallardo FG, Cobo Soler J, Babé Romero J, Rios Ferreiros M, Valencia Ortega E. [Osteitis in secondary syphilis]. Rev Esp Med Nucl. 2003;22(6):424–6. Spanish.
63. Sohn MH, Lim ST, Jeong YJ, Kim DW, Jeong HJ, Lee CS. Unusual case of occult Brucella osteomyelitis in the skull detected by bone scintigraphy. Nucl Med Mol Imaging. 2010;44 (2):161–3. doi:10.1007/s13139-010-0023-2.
64. Römer W, Nomayr A, Uder M, Bautz W, Kuwert T. SPECT guided CT for evaluating foci of increased bone metabolism classified as indeterminate on SPECT in cancer patients. J Nucl Med. 2006;47:1102–6.
65. del Val Gomez M, Gallardo FG, Cobo J, Castro-Beiras JM. Abnormal gallium-67 skull uptake: a sign of peripheral marrow activation in HIV-positive patients with disseminated mycobacterioses. J Nucl Med. 1995;36(12):2211–3.
66. Kurup S, Jose R, Chandy ML. Diagnostic utility of gallium 67 SPECT/CT and role of pentoxifylline-tocopherol in chronic multifocal osteomyelitis. Oral Health Dent Manag. 2014;13(3):821–5.
67. Chakraborty D, Bhattacharya A, Gupta AK, Panda NK, Das A, Mittal BR. Skull base osteomyelitis in otitis externa: the utility of triphasic and single photon emission computed tomography/computed tomography bone scintigraphy. Indian J Nucl Med. 2013;28(2):65–9. doi:10.4103/0972-3919.118222.

68. Panos GZ, Karydis I, Velakoulis SE, Falagas ME. Multi-skeletal Pneumocystis jiroveci (carinii) in an HIV-seropositive patient. Int J STD AIDS. 2007;18(2):134–7.
69. Park KH, Lee MS, Hong IK, Sung JY, Choi SH, Park SO, Shin MJ, Chung HW, Lee SH. Bone involvement in secondary syphilis: a case report and systematic review of the literature. Sex Transm Dis. 2014;41(9):532–7. doi:10.1097/OLQ.0000000000000164.
70. Giuseppe M, Varacalli S, Ciofalo A. Osteomyelitis of the skull base with atypical onset and evolution. Ann Otol Rhinol Laryngol. 2000;109:326–30.
71. Doudouh A, Oufroukhi Y, Biyi A, Belasri S. [Tuberculous osteitis of frontal bone simulating lytic metastasis of papillary thyroid carcinoma: a case report]. Med Nucl. 2012;36(11):674–7. French.
72. Weber PC, Seabold JE, Graham SM, Hoffmann HH, Simonson TM, Thompson BH. Evaluation of temporal and facial osteomyelitis by simultaneous In-WBC/Tc-99m-MDP bone SPECT scintigraphy and computed tomography scan. Otolaryngol Head Neck Surg. 1995;113(1):36–41.
73. Noyek AM, Witterick IJ, Kirsh JC. Radionuclide imaging in otolaryngology-head and neck surgery. Arch Otolaryngol Head Neck Surg. 1991;117(4):372–8.
74. Datz FL. Indium-111-labeled leukocytes for the detection of infection: current status. Semin Nucl Med. 1994;24(2):92–109.
75. Goldsmith SJ, Vallabhajosula S. Clinically proven radiopharmaceuticals for infection imaging: mechanisms and applications. Semin Nucl Med. 2009;39(1):2–10. doi:10.1053/j.semnuclmed.2008.08.002.
76. Kumar R, Basu S, Torigian D, Anand V, Zhuang H, Alavi A. Role of modern imaging techniques for diagnosis of infection in the era of 18F-fluorodeoxyglucose positron emission tomography. Clin Microbiol Rev. 2008;21(1):209–24. doi:10.1128/CMR.00025-07.
77. Gemmel F, Dumarey N, Welling M. Future diagnostic agents. Semin Nucl Med. 2009;39(1):11–26. doi:10.1053/j.semnuclmed.2008.08.005.
78. Bruni C, Padovano F, Travascio L, Schillaci O, Simonetti G. Usefulness of hybrid SPECT/CT for the 99mTc-HMPAO-labeled leukocyte scintigraphy in a case of cranial osteomyelitis. Braz J Infect Dis. 2008;12(6):558–60.
79. van der Bruggen W, Bleeker-Rovers CP, Boerman OC, Gotthardt M, Oyen WJ. PET and SPECT in osteomyelitis and prosthetic bone and joint infections: a systematic review. Semin Nucl Med. 2010;40(1):3–15. doi:10.1053/j.semnuclmed.2009.08.005.
80. Horger M, Eschmann SM, Pfannenberg C, Storek D, Vonthein R, Claussen CD, Bares R. Added value of SPECT/CT in patients suspected of having bone infection: preliminary results. Arch Orthop Trauma Surg. 2007;127(3):211–21.
81. Palestro CJ. Radionuclide imaging of osteomyelitis. Semin Nucl Med. 2015;45(1):32–46. doi:10.1053/j.semnuclmed.2014.07.005.
82. Pennington WT, Mott MP, Thometz JG, Sty JR, Metz D. Photopenic bone scan osteomyelitis: a clinical perspective. J Pediatr Orthop. 1999;19(6):695–8.
83. Palestro CJ, Torres MA. Radionuclide imaging in orthopedic infections. Semin Nucl Med. 1997;27(4):334–45.
84. Sethi RS, Mittal B, Bhattacharya A, Singh B. Tc99m MDP bone SPECT in a case of osteomyelitis of the skull. Indian J Nucl Med. 2010;25(1):25–6. doi:10.4103/0972-3919.63597.
85. Sfakianakis GN, Al-Sheikh W, Heal A, Rodman G, Zeppa R, Serafini A. Comparisons of scintigraphy with In-111 leukocytes and Ga-67 in the diagnosis of occult sepsis. J Nucl Med. 1982;23(7):618–26.
86. Kao CH, Wang SJ. Spread of infectious complications of odontogenic abscess detected by technetium-99m-HMPAO-labeled WBC scan of occult sepsis in the intensive care unit. J Nucl Med. 1992;33(2):254–5.
87. Bar-Shalom R, Yefremov N, Guralnik L, Keidar Z, Engel A, Nitecki S, Israel O. SPECT/CT using 67Ga and 111In-labeled leukocyte scintigraphy for diagnosis of infection. J Nucl Med. 2006;47(4):587–94.

88. Fortún J, Cobo J, Cañal J, Martínez-San Millán J. Post-traumatic cranial mucormycosis in an immunocompetent patient. J Oral Maxillofac Surg. 1995;53(9):1099–102.
89. Horger M, Eschmann SM, Pfannenberg C, Storek D, Dammann F, Vonthein R, Claussen CD, Bares R. The value of SPET/CT in chronic osteomyelitis. Eur J Nucl Med Mol Imaging. 2003;30(12):1665–73.
90. Termaat MF, Raijmakers PG, Scholten HJ, Bakker FC, Patka P, Haarman HJ. The accuracy of diagnostic imaging for the assessment of chronic osteomyelitis: a systematic review and meta-analysis. J Bone Joint Surg Am. 2005;87:2464–71.
91. Love C, Palestro CJ. Radionuclide imaging of infection. J Nucl Med Technol. 2004;32:47–57.
92. Nomura M, Shin M, Ohta M, Nukui Y, Ohkusu K, Saito N. Atypical osteomyelitis of the skull base and craniovertebral junction caused by Actinomyces infection—case report. Neurol Med Chir (Tokyo). 2011;51(1):64–6.
93. Kalicke T, Schmitz A, Risse JH, Arens S, Keller E, Hansis M, Schmitt O, Biersack HJ, Grünwald F. Fluorine-18 fluorodeoxyglucose PET in infectious bone diseases: results of histologically confirmed cases. Eur J Nucl Med. 2000;27:524–8.
94. Akhaddar A, Albouzidi A, Elouennas M, Elmostarchid B, Boucetta M. Nonsuppurative calvarial thickening: a new form of Garré disease? J Neurosurg. 2009;110(4):808. doi:10.3171/2008.3.17458.
95. Chandler JR, Grobman L, Quencer R, Serafini A. Osteomyelitis of the base of the skull. Laryngoscope. 1986;96(3):245–51.
96. Benecke Jr JE. Management of osteomyelitis of the skull base. Laryngoscope. 1989;99(12):1220–3.
97. Sharma P, Agarwal KK, Kumar S, Singh H, Bal C, Malhotra A, Kumar R. Utility of (99m)Tc-MDP hybrid SPECT-CT for diagnosis of skull base osteomyelitis: comparison with planar bone scintigraphy, SPECT, and CT. Jpn J Radiol. 2013;31(2):81–8. doi:10.1007/s11604-012-0148-6.
98. Malone DG, O'Boynick PL, Ziegler DK, Batnitzky S, Hubble JP, Holladay FP. Osteomyelitis of the skull base. Neurosurgery. 1992;30(3):426–31.
99. Sreepada GS, Kwartler JA. Skull base osteomyelitis secondary to malignant otitis externa. Curr Opin Otolaryngol Head Neck Surg. 2003;11(5):316–23.
100. Damle NA, Kumar R, Kumar P, Jaganathan S, Patnecha M, Bal C, Bandopadhyaya G, Malhotra A. SPECT/CT in the diagnosis of skull base osteomyelitis. Nucl Med Mol Imaging. 2011;45(3):212–6. doi:10.1007/s13139-011-0086-8.
101. Chen JC, Yeh CF, Shiao AS, Tu TY. Temporal bone osteomyelitis: the relationship with malignant otitis externa, the diagnostic dilemma, and changing trends. ScientificWorldJournal. 2014;2014:591714. doi:10.1155/2014/591714.
102. Trück J, Thompson A, Dwivedi R, Segal S, Anand G, Kelly DF. Nonotogenic skull base osteomyelitis in children: two cases and a review of the literature. Pediatr Infect Dis J. 2015;34(9):1025–7. doi:10.1097/INF.0000000000000782.
103. Okpala NCE, Nilssen E. Radiological and radionuclide investigation of malignant otitis externa. J Laryngol Otol. 2005;119:71–5.
104. Weinberg B, Gupta S, Thomas MJ, Stern H. Pott's puffy tumor: sonographic diagnosis. J Clin Ultrasound. 2005;33(6):305–7.
105. Grant RL, Piotto L. Ultrasound detection of a subperiosteal abscess secondary to coalescent otomastoiditis. Australas Radiol. 2005;49(4):312–4.
106. Secko M, Aherne A. Diagnosis of Bezold abscess using bedside ultrasound. J Emerg Med. 2013;44(3):670–2. doi:10.1016/j.jemermed.2012.07.066.
107. Chen CY, Huang CC, Chang YC, Chow NH, Chio CC, Zimmerman RA. Subdural empyema in 10 infants: US characteristics and clinical correlates. Radiology. 1998;207(3):609–17.

Chapter 9
Differential Diagnoses: Clinical and Imaging

Contents

Diagnosis of cranial osteomyelitis can be challenging due to the variable clinical presentation of the disease and potentially subtle radiological appearances. For that reason a high index of suspicion needs to be kept in mind, mainly in patients with immunodepression, a past history of otic, dental or nasosinusal pathologies, bacteremic conditions or surgical or traumatic antecedents. In addition to medical history, clinical information and biologic data are essential for the radiologist to achieve an appropriate diagnosis and to narrow the list of differential diagnoses. At other times, histological examination is necessary.

A. Akhaddar, *Cranial Osteomyelitis*, DOI 10.1007/978-3-319-30268-3_9

Scalp and skull lesions have a wide variety of different etiologies, ranging from normal variants to congenital, traumatic, inflammatory and neoplastic lesions. Some of them are incidental findings in imaging studies, while many others manifest as palpable masses, with or without local cardinal signs of inflammation. To mention all of them is beyond the scope of this book. A summary of the most frequent imaging differential diagnoses of cranial vault and skull base osteomyelitis is given according to anatomic origin and pathogenesis of the lesions. Only the most common diagnoses are briefly addressed in this chapter.

Mimicking Clinical Presentations

The most presenting complaint of various scalp and skull lesions is a visible swelling or palpable mass with or without signs of inflammation, regardless of the primary pathology and the age of patients. Congenital lesions may be noticed at birth and may obscure a cephalhematoma. Some lesions are painful or tender to palpation. Many lesions that can affect the skin may involve the scalp. Superficial lesions confined to the dermis are usually treated by dermatologists, general surgeons and plastic surgeons, it is not until subgaleal or cranial involvement is apparent than imaging exploration and neurosurgical consultation are obtained. The history, local findings of induration/inflammation and skull tenderness will usually give a good clinical indication of the underlying cranial bone infection.

Scalp Neoplasms and Nodules

- **Malignant neoplasms** may be primary or secondary (metastasis). The most common malignant tumors of the scalp are squamous and basal cell carcinomas which predominate in adult men (Fig. 9.1). A significant proportion of these tumors can secondarily invade the cranial vault because the subgaleal plane offers little resistance [1].
- **Neurofibroma** of the scalp may accompany neurofibromatosis. It is a benign tumor that progress along the nerve of origin, sometimes into the intracranial space. In a patient with known neurofibromatosis, the discovery of painless, subcutaneous nodules of the scalp does not usually present a diagnostic problem. On magnetic resonance imaging (MRI), the lesion is heterogeneous and has low signal intensity on T1-weighted images. There is often more homogeneous marked contrast enhancement compared with other lesions that are seen within the scalp or skull. Malignant degeneration should be considered when the tumor has rapidly enlarged [2].
- **Necrobiotic granulomas** of the scalp or pseudo-rheumatoid nodules are multiple painless subcutaneous nodules of the scalp in children resulting from an inflammatory process of unknown origin known as “necrobiosis”. These granulomas

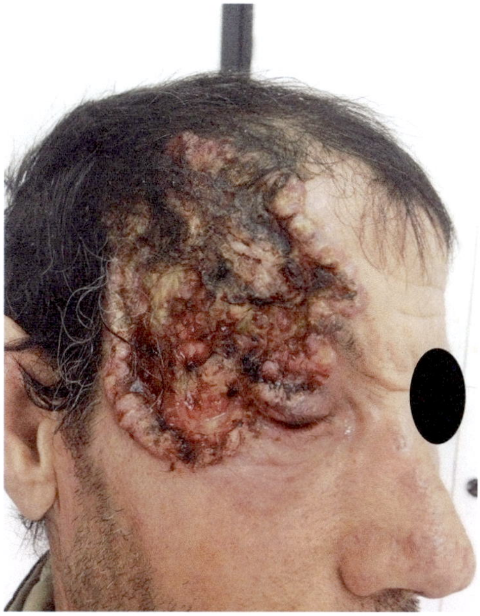

Fig. 9.1 Extensive basal cell carcinoma of frontal scalp with orbital and temporal involvement

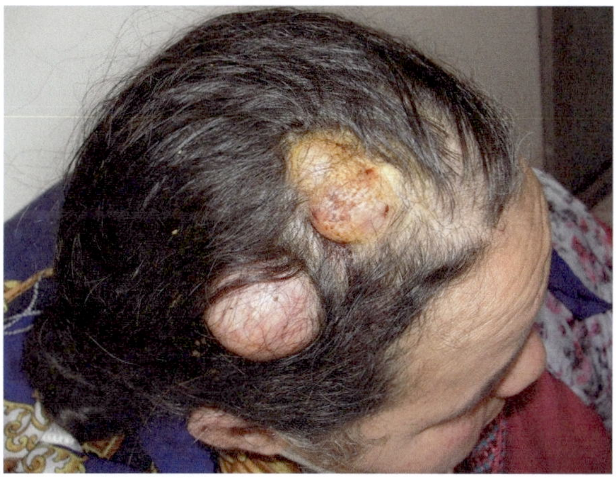

Fig. 9.2 Multiple epidermoid (sebaceous) cysts of the scalp

involve the occipital and frontal scalp, pre-tibial subcutaneous tissue and are not found near the joints. These nodules usually resolve spontaneously [3].

- **Myofibroma** is a benign mesenchymal tumor that occurs in infancy and may result in masses involving the scalp, and occasionally, the skull [4].
- **Epidermoid** and **dermoid cysts**. Both epidermoid and dermoid lesions are congenital unilocular ectodermal inclusion cysts lined by an epithelium. Epidermoid cysts, also previously known as sebaceous cyst (Fig. 9.2) are filled with debris of keratin and cholesterol from the desquamation of their thin squamous epithelial lining. Dermoid cysts are lined by a thicker epithelium and filled with

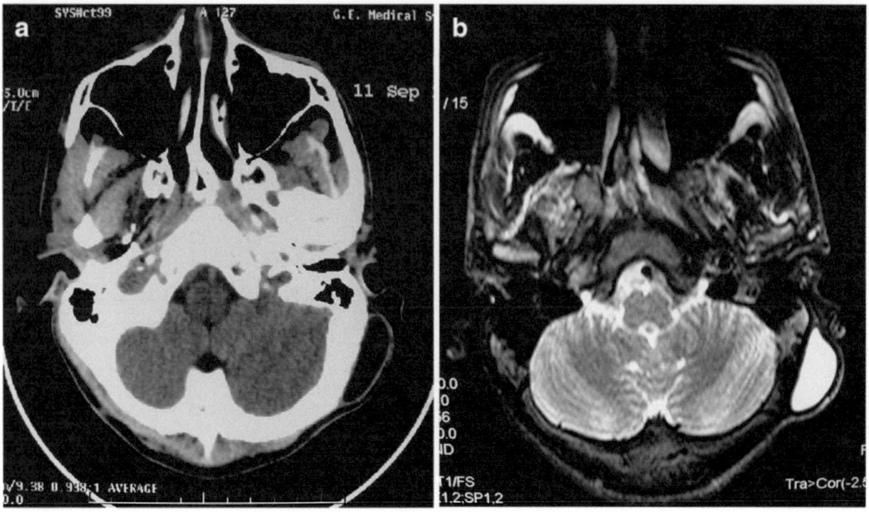

Fig. 9.3 Subgaleal retroauricular left-sided lipoma. Axial CT-scan (**a**) and MRI on T2-weighted images (**b**)

sebaceous, sweat and apocrine glands, hair and less commonly, teeth. They may be associated with dermal sinus tracts. Epidermoids tend to present more laterally while dermoids usually present closer to the midline. Both cysts may erode and expand the calvaria. Epidermoid and dermoid cysts are usually slow-growing and painless, painful if infected [5].

- **Lipoma** of the forehead is a soft, rounded or lobulated fatty tumor, usually painless, nontender, movable against the overlying skin, several centimeters in size and includes subcutaneous and subgaleal lipomas (Fig. 9.3). The growth is insidious consisting of an initial growth phase and after the quiescence phase.

Congenital Scalp Defects

Failure of closure of the cranial neural tube results in a variety of anomalies, ranging from massive encephaloceles to small skull defects through which the cranial meninges herniated without underlying cerebral abnormality.

- **Cephaloceles** are herniations of brain parenchyma due to congenital fusion defects. They are usually seen in the midline occipital area in pediatric population. They are classified as meningoencephalocele, meningocele, atretic cephalocele and gliocele, based on the neural elements they consist of. The lesion is soft, compressible, and may increase in size with Valsalva maneuvers. The overlying skin is frequently thin and discolored and neural elements may be present within the cavity with variable connection to the underlying brain parenchyma. Computed tomography-scan (CT-scan) is essential in

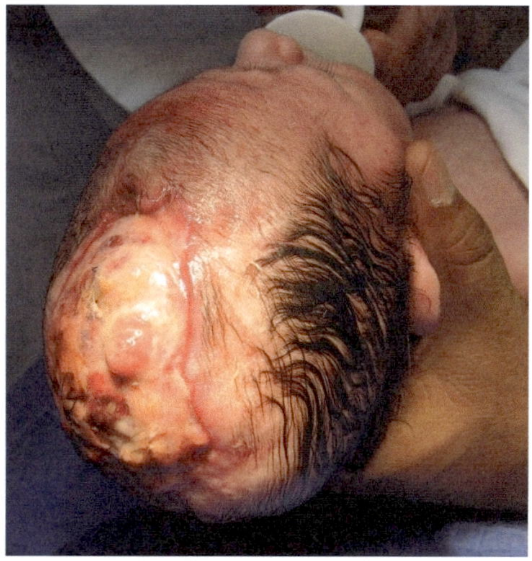

Fig. 9.4 Large scalp defect over the vertex in a new born (aplasia cutis congenital)

demonstrating the cranial bone defect and MRI is necessary in showing the sac contents and potential cerebral anomalies [6]. Vitali presented an interesting report of calvarial tuberculosis causing a cranial defect and venous sinus thrombosis and resulting in an acquired encephalocele in a 10-year-old boy. CT-scan and MRI demonstrated evidence of left occipital encephalocele with left mastoiditis, extradural granulations, bone destruction, and complete occlusion of the left sigmoid sinus [7].

– **Aplasia cutis congenita** is a full-thickness skin defect of variable size that frequently involves the scalp in the midline vertex. Less frequently, there is also a defect of the underlying skull and the dura. An irregular border of erythematous, hairless, dystrophic skin of variable width surrounds the defect, in which the raw surface of the underlying tissue appears [8]. Rarely, a small superficial skin defect may be covered by a thin, translucent, epithelial membrane that gives it the appearance of a "bulla" (Fig. 9.4).

Vascular Lesions

– "**Port wine stains**" represent dermal areas containing irregular blood vessels, usually capillaries and venules within the superficial vascular plexus. These lesions appear to result from progressive ectasia of the involved vessels rather than vessel proliferation. In the scalp, port wine stains may be markers of underlying brain involvement. About 5 % of patients with port wine stains have Sturge-Weber syndrome with abnormal pial vasculature of the ipsilateral cerebral cortex, seizures and varying degrees of cognitive impairment [2, 9].
– **Arteriovenous malformations** of the scalp also called "cirsoid aneurysms" of the scalp appear as a pulsatile, compressible mass with marked venous dilatation

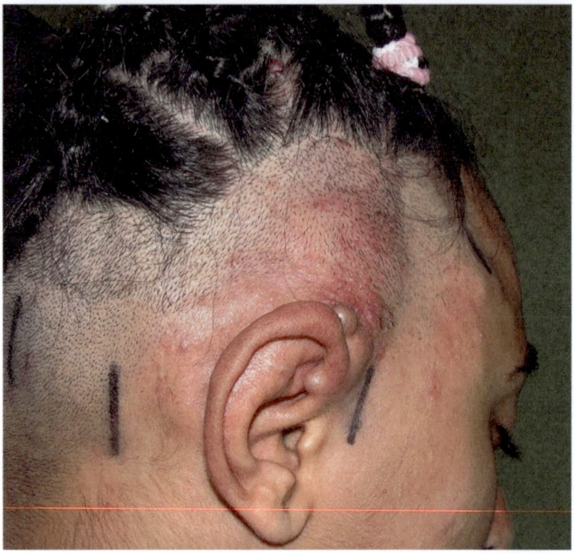

Fig. 9.5 Temporo-auricular non-traumatic arteriovenous malformation of the scalp (cirsoid aneurysm)

through the scalp and face (Fig. 9.5). In children, this vascular malformation may enlarge, with potential high-output heart failure. Most lesions are congenital, especially in infants; however some cases following head injury were reported. Conventional angiography is necessary for the diagnosis [10].

- **Sinus Pericranii** is a slow-flow anastomosis between extracranial and intracranial veins, usually involving the superior sagittal sinus. This congenital vascular lesion appears as painless swelling of the scalp, less than 1.5 cm in diameter and usually in the midline. The lesion is compressible, deflates with head elevation, and refills with Valsalva maneuver or with the head in a dependant position. On CT-scan, this vascular lesion presents as numerous small localized defects, discrete area of bone loss or complete absence of cranial bone. On MRI, there is a mixed intensity lesion with flow voids present. Communication with a vascular sinus may be demonstrated [11].
- **Pseudoaneurysm** arising from the superficial temporal artery is a potentially critical cause of palpable mass. This rare vascular lesion typically presents after a short delay following blunt trauma.

Soft Tissue Infections

The scalp is a common site of infection. However, spontaneous scalp infections are unusual, produced by almost any type of microorganisms. Access of pathogens to the subgaleal space may permit spread of infection and may mimic cranial vault osteomyelitis.

- **Chronic scalp lesions** as non-healing wound, ulcer, chronic sinus tracts, kerion or other chronic wounds can be infected with local and/or regional signs of inflammation/infection [12] (Fig. 9.6). Some forms of alopecia and/or scalp thickening may also precede scalp infection.
- **Infected scalp lesions** may mimic cranial vault osteomyelitis as erysipelas, nonnecrotizing cellulitis, impetigo, furuncles, carbuncles, folliculitis and scalp abscess (Fig. 9.7). These local infectious lesions may be extended inducing more

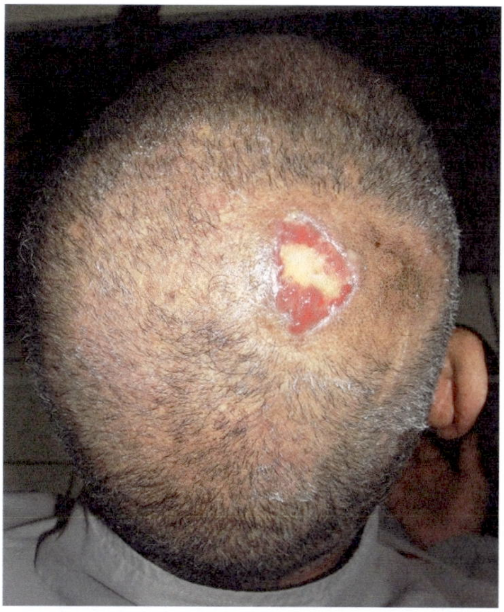

Fig. 9.6 Chronic non-healing ulcer of the scalp (right parietal region)

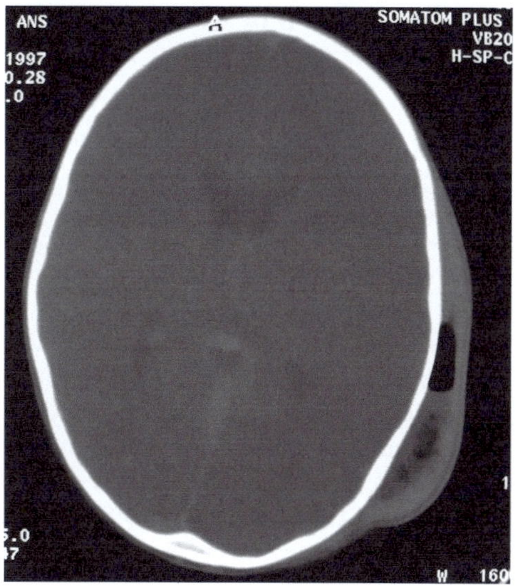

Fig. 9.7 Extensive subgaleal scalp abscess on bone windows cranial CT-scan. Note the air or gas within the suppurative collection

serious complications as staphylococcal bacteremic skin lesions, necrotizing fasciitis and more deeply cranial osteomyelitis. Then, the clinical picture can be more serious [13].

In general, tenderness out of proportion to soft-tissue findings suggests osteomyelitis rather than soft-tissue infection or cellulitis. Combined use of Indium-111 white blood cell and Tc-99m methylene di-phosphonate (MDP) bone single-photon emission computed tomography (SPECT) scans has been shown to be useful in differentiating osteomyelitis from adjacent soft tissue infection [14].

Traumatic Lesions

- **Subgaleal hematomas** are relatively common occurrences whereas cephalhematomas (effusion of blood under the pericranium) are unusual mostly occur in newborns due to pressure or injury during labour. Both hematomas usually resolve spontaneously and completely. During resolution, the hematoma liquefies producing a soft "squishy" scalp that may alarm the parents [2]. Subgaleal and subperiosteal hematomas may be infected inducing a scalp abscess with infectious signs and symptoms [15].
- **Calcified hematomas** may sometimes be relatively large and prominent, requiring surgical correction for an unacceptable cosmetic appearance [16].
- **Post-traumatic scalp nodules** are very firm nodules found fixed to the skull after trauma in children, with or without skull fracture. These periosteal reactions often resolve spontaneously.

Imaging Pattern of Cranial Vault Lesions

Focal lesions of the cranial vault may originate primarily from bony structures, or they may be secondary to invasion of the skin or intracranial lesions into bony structures. Well-defined borders and sclerotic margins are attributing to benign lesions. Slow growing tumors lead to thinning in the adjacent calvarium, whereas aggressive tumors lead to severe destruction. Also, some iatrogenic, congenital, inflammatory or normal anatomical variants can mimic cranial osteomyelitis and should be taken into consideration.

In general population, seven diagnosis include 85 % of all causes (by decreasing order) Langerhans histiocytosis, osteoma, epidermoid/dermoid cysts, metastasis, meningioma, hemangioma and fibrous dysplasia [17]. In adults, tumoral causes are predominant, particularly metastasis and myeloma; whereas in children, besides congenital defects, dermoid cysts and eosinophilic granuloma are the most frequent diagnosis [17, 18]. Small and Schaefer [19] use the mnemonic acronym **HELP ME** to remember the most frequent lesion of the calvaria (Table 9.1)

Table 9.1 The acronym mnemonic HELP ME denoting the most frequent lesion in the cranial vault [19]

Alphabetic initial	Cranial vault lesion
H	Hemangioma
E	Epidermoid/dermoid
L	Leptomeningeal cyst, leukemia/lymphoma
P	Paget's disease, postsurgical
M	Metastases, multiple myeloma
E	Eosinophilic granuloma, encephalocele

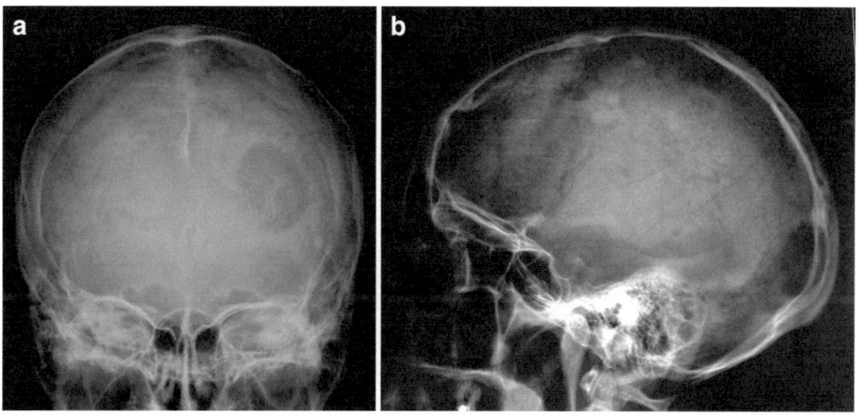

Fig. 9.8 Antero-posterior (**a**) and lateral (**b**) cranial plain radiographs demonstrating an oval-shaped osteolytic defect on the occipital bone (eosinophilic granuloma)

Eosinophilic Granuloma

Eosinophilic granuloma is the localized form of Langerhan's cell histiocytosis and occurs in children and young adults. Patient may be asymptomatic or have a palpable soft tissue mass frequently located in the parietal area. The lesions are oval or round that begin in the diploe and involve the full thickness of the cranial vault (Fig. 9.8). Peripheral sclerosis is not seen unless the lesion is in the healing period. Residual bone tissue or sequestrum may be seen into the lesion (Fig. 9.9). Multiple lesions may expand and coalesce, making the form of a "geographic map". On MRI, they appear as a soft tissue mass located in the diploe, appearing hypointense on T1-weighted images (WI), hyperintense on T2-WI, and enhancing homogeneously after gadolinium administration but without surrounding edema. Decreased signal intensity on T2-WI has been related to healing lesions with centripetal bone formation. Dural invasion is uncommon and when occurs local enhancement may be seen [17, 20, 21].

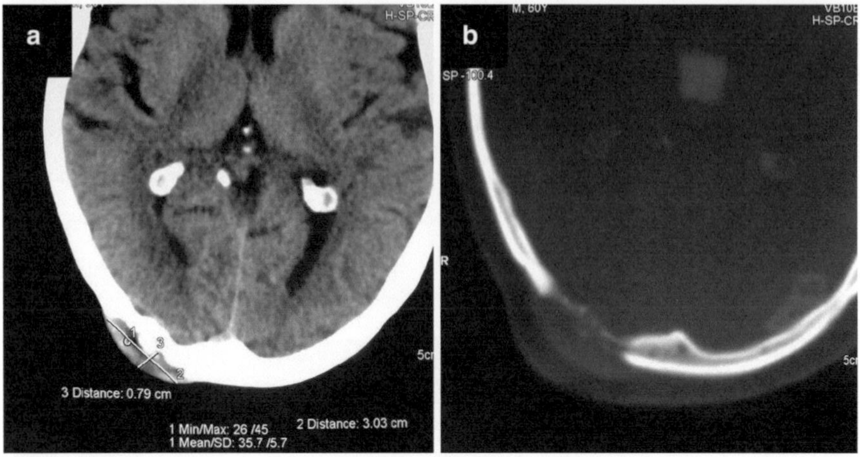

Fig. 9.9 Occipital cranial vault eosinophilic granuloma (same patient). Axial cranial CT-scan with parenchymatous (**a**) and bone windows (**b**)

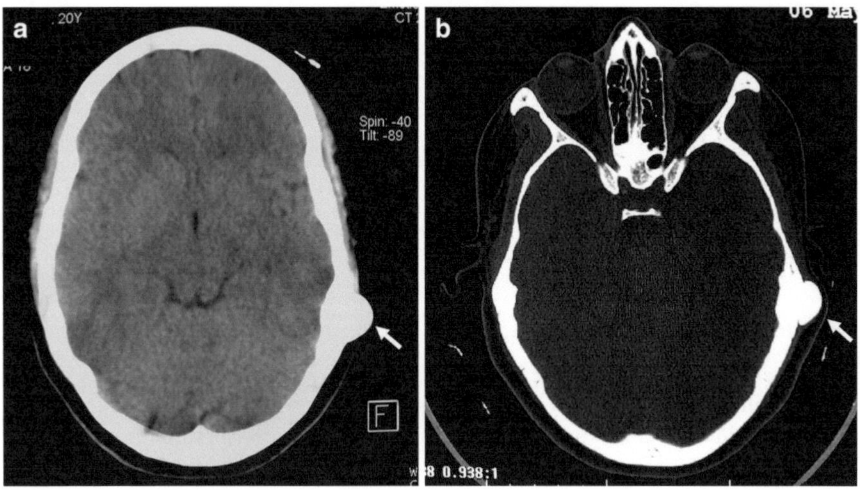

Fig. 9.10 Temporal retroauricular cranial vault osteoma arising from the outer table (*arrow*). Axial cranial CT-scan with parenchymatous (**a**) and bone windows (**b**)

Osteoma

Osteoma is a solid nodular tumor comprising mature bone. The lesion is very hard, painless and fixed on palpation without inflammatory signs. It appears most commonly in adult men between the fourth and fifth decades of life [22]. The most common location is the paranasal sinuses and near the suture lines. It may be sessile or pedunculated. On CT-scan, osteoma is dense, smooth, well-demarcated tumor that usually arises from the outer table (Fig. 9.10). Inner table osteomas may be confused with ossified meningiomas. On MRI, osteomas show signal void and an absence of soft-tissue component on all sequences. Osteoma does not enhance after contrast administration [17].

Meningioma

Meningioma represents the most common benign intracranial tumor. This neoplasm arises from the meningothelial cells and usually forms a unilobular mass with a broad-based dural attachment. Adjacent bony changes can occur in 25 % of meningiomas. Osseous formation or "hyperostosis" is the most common bony change, but bone destruction may also occur with extracranial extension [23]. Intraosseous meningioma is a rare subtype of meningioma (Fig. 9.11). It originates ectopically within the diploe and is most often located near the coronal suture. Their expansion in bones and "ground-glass" appearance may be difficult to distinct from those of fibrous dysplasia. However, meningioma usually presents in middle-aged or advanced-aged women and lead to irregularity in the inner table. The homogeneous enhancement and "dural tail" sign following contrast injection on CT-scan and MRI is highly suggestive of meningioma [24].

Osteosarcoma

An osteosarcoma is mainly a primary tumor in children, while it is secondary to Paget's disease, fibrous dysplasia and radiotherapy in adults. The osteoblastic type is the most frequent (osteogenic sarcoma). At the time of diagnosis, intracranial extension is frequent. On CT-scan, the tumor has focal sclerosis with poorly defined margins. Mineralization and a soft tissue mass in the tumor matrix may be seen. It may demonstrate a "sunburst" appearance with infiltration of the surrounding soft-tissue (Fig. 9.12). On MRI, the lesion is heterogeneous and has mixed signal on both T1 and T2-WI. After gadolinium administration, the tumor enhances heterogeneously. This tumor is highly vascular and angio-MR or conventional angiography may be valuable in preoperative planning, including consideration of arterial embolization [25].

Lipoma

Lipoma consists of mature fat cells developing in the diploe. This slow-growing expansile lytic lesion has well-defined margins. Lipoma may have sclerotic borders and, due to fatty necrosis in the lesion, central calcifications can be seen. The lesion appears as fat density on CT-scan and show a typical fat signal on MRI [26].

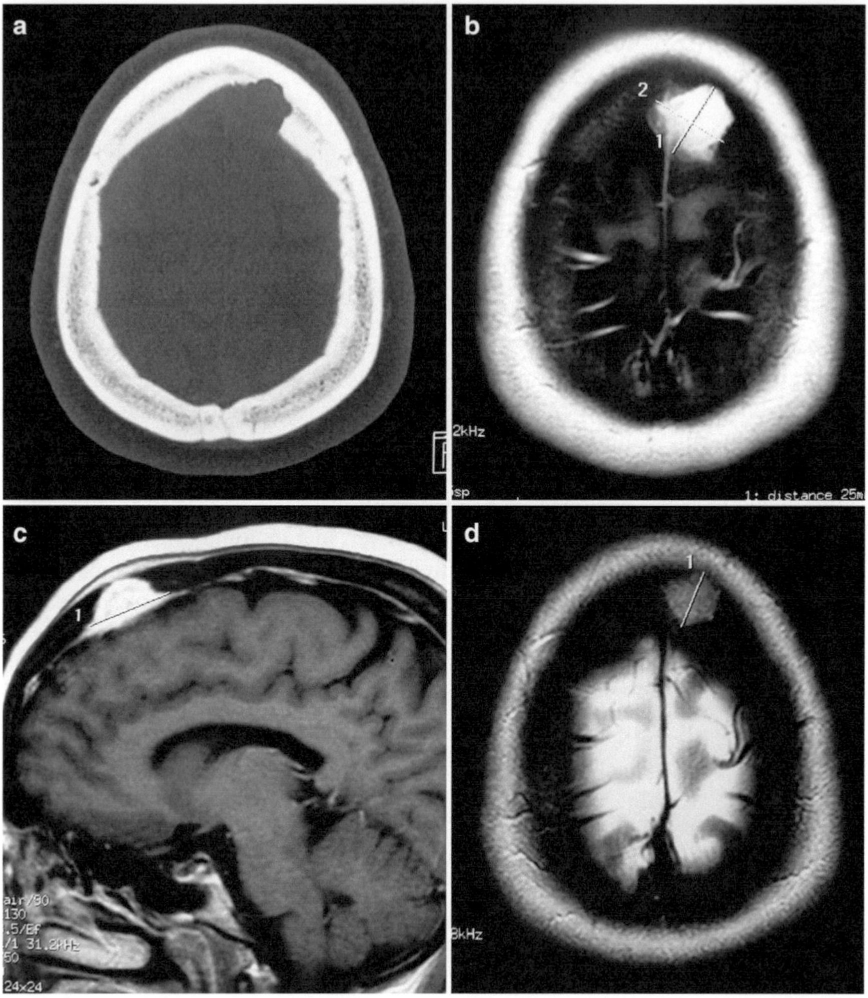

Fig. 9.11 Frontal cranial vault meningioma. Axial cranial CT-scan with bone windows (**a**). Axial (**b**) and sagittal (**c**) T1-weighted MRI following gadolinium injection. Axial T2-weighted MRI (**d**)

Fibrous Dysplasia

Fibrous dysplasia is a genetically based sporadic disorder characterized by the replacement of normal cancellous bone with abnormal fibrous tissue containing immature woven bone. This benign lesion occurs in adolescents and young adults and may involve a single bone (monostic) or multiple contiguous bones (polyostotic). In cranial vault, fibrous dysplasia usually affects the frontal and temporal bones. The presenting symptoms are related to bony expansion and frequent complaints are local swelling, proptosis, visual loss, headache and cranial

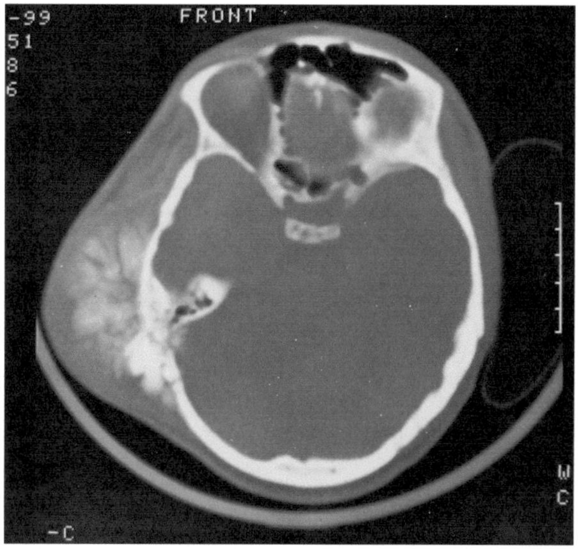

Fig. 9.12 Temporo-parietal osteosarcoma in bone window axial CT-scan

nerve palsies. On CT-scan fibrous dysplasia appears as a "ground-glass" matrix appearance (Fig. 9.13). Rarely, there may be a dense homogeneous or cystic pattern. Intra-lesional calcifications can be seen. On MRI, signal intensity varies with regard to the amount of fibrous tissue and bony matrix in the lesion. The most common type is hypointense on both T1 and T2-WI with gadolinium enhancement (Fig. 9.13). MRI is also useful to evaluate intracranial extension. Malignant degeneration is possible [27–29].

Hemangioma

Calvarial hemangioma is a solitary lesion seen generally in middle-aged women as palpable mass or can be incidentally detected. The most frequent type is cavernous, meaning that it is composed of dilated blood vessels containing within the bony trabeculae. This osteolytic lesion affects mainly the outer table with sclerotic borders. The bony striations radiating centrally to the periphery of the lesion have a characteristic "sunburst" or "honeycomb" appearance. On MRI, the lesion appears isointense within the diploic space on T1-WI with scattered hypo and hyperintensities corresponding to iron storage complexes and fatty tissue, respectively (Fig. 9.14). Focal areas of diminished signal intensity represent bony trabeculation. After gadolinium injection, the enhancement is initially focal and then diffuses [29]. T2-WI reveals a hyperintense lesion [30, 31]. Aggressive presentation with soft-tissue extension is possible [29].

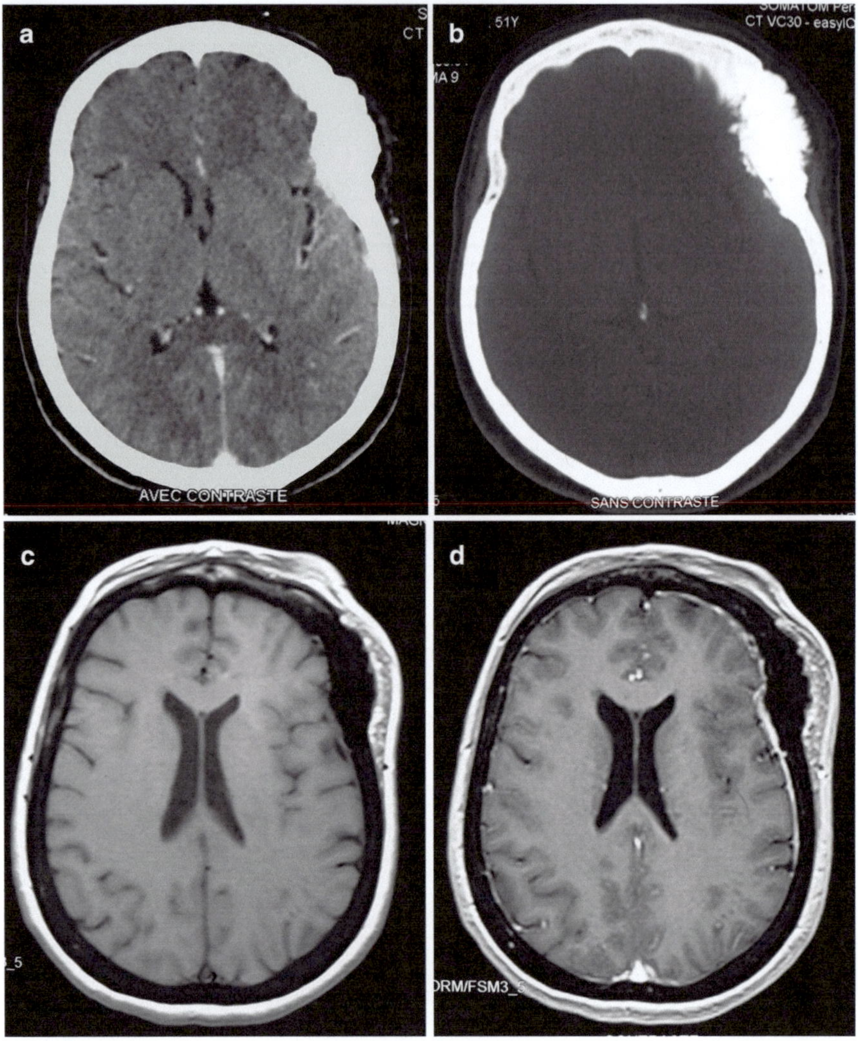

Fig. 9.13 Frontal cranial vault fibrous dysplasia. Axial cranial CT-scan with parenchymatous (**a**) and bone windows (**b**). Axial T1-weighted MRI before (**c**) and after (**d**) gadolinium injection

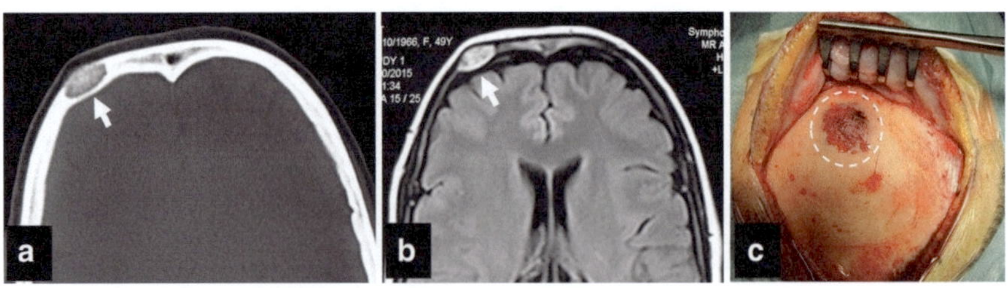

Fig. 9.14 Frontal cranial vault hemangioma (*arrow*). Axial cranial CT-scan with bone windows (**a**), axial T2-weighted MRI (FLAIR) (**b**), and operative view (**c**)

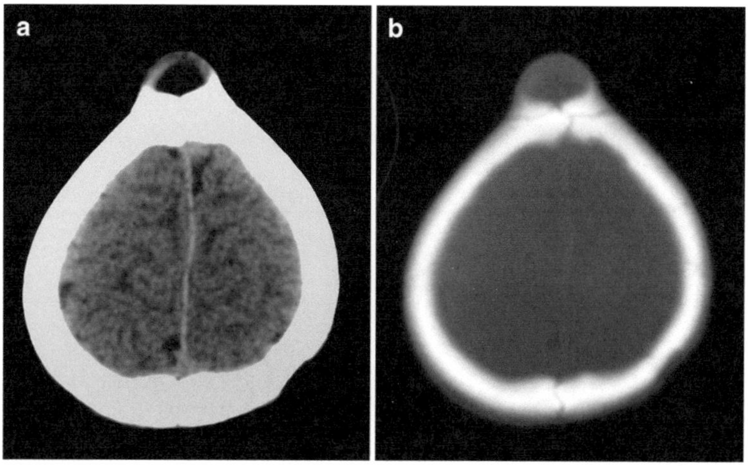

Fig. 9.15 Frontal cranial medial dermoid cyst. Axial cranial CT-scan with parenchymatous (**a**) and bone windows (**b**)

Epidermoid and Dermoid Cysts

As seen above, these congenital cysts (rarely posttraumatic) contain elements of epidermal and/or dermal origin and may erode and expand the calvaria. Pressure erosion causes remodeling and expansion of the outer and inner tables. The lesions are typically lytic and oval-shaped with a clearly sclerotic margin. Epidermoid cysts predominantly occur laterally, while dermoid cysts frequently involve the midline near the anterior fontanel (Fig. 9.15). On CT-scan, epidermoids are more homogeneous than dermoids. The latter may display calcification along their wall or internally. On MRI, epidermoids are hyperintense on T2-WI and variable intensity on T1-WI. In contrast, dermoids usually show high signal intensity on T1 and T2 WI due to their oily sebaceous secretions. However, signal intensity varies depending on the lipid content or hemorrhagic products. There is no enhancement following contrast administration in epidermoids, while the wall (capsule) of dermoids may enhance because it is often somewhat vascularized [28, 32, 33].

Metastases

Most multiple abnormal radiolucencies in the cranial vault after 50 years of age are carcinoma metastases (mostly secondary to lung and breast cancers). When the lesions are solitary and expanded, metastasis of thyroid or renal neoplasias might be suspected [22, 25] (Fig. 9.16). Metastases are usually diagnosed in the context of a

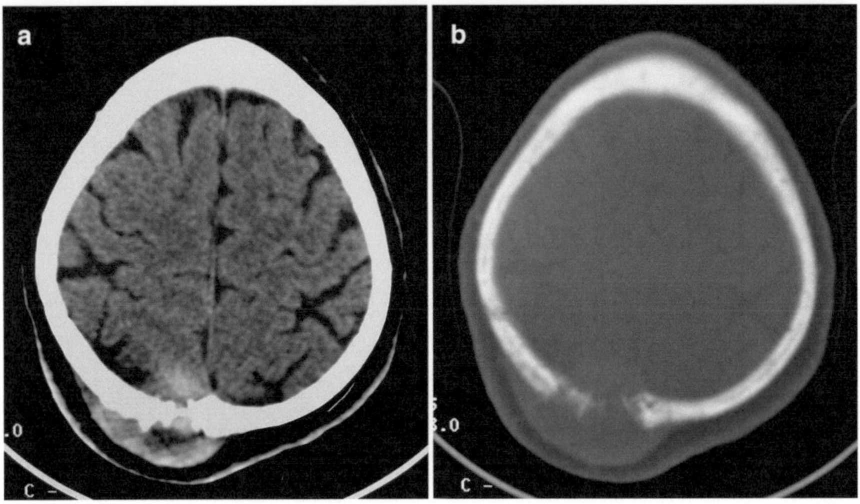

Fig. 9.16 Solitary parietal cranial bone metastasis with intra and extracranial extension. Axial cranial CT-scan with parenchymatous (**a**) and bone windows (**b**)

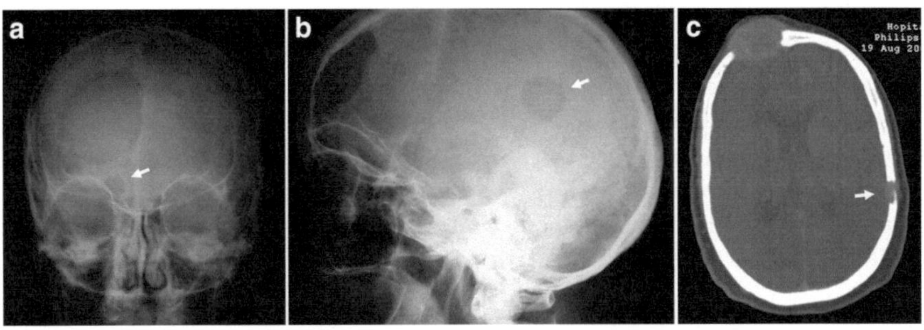

Fig. 9.17 Multiple cranial bone metastases. Antero-posterior (**a**) and lateral (**b**) cranial plain radiographs. Axial CT-scan in bone window (**c**)

known primary tumor. They are commonly asymptomatic or may be revealed by a painful swelling [29, 34]. In children, calvarial metastases due to neuroblastomas and sarcomas are the most frequent. For neuroblastoma, four patterns of calvarial involvement have been described: sutural diastasis secondary to dural involvement, sunburst appearance or linear periosteal reaction, lytic defects, and thickened bone [35]. Generally, metastases are almost exclusively osteolytic with ragged margins or permeative destruction (Fig. 9.17). Prostate and thyroid cancer metastases are usually sclerotic or mixed types. On T1-WI, hypointense areas are seen in fatty bone marrow with marked enhancement following gadolinium administration. On T2-WI, the metastases are visualized as areas of hyperintensity replacing the normal diploic space and cortical bone (Fig. 9.18). Multiple radiolucencies with well-defined borders but without reactive sclerosis are characteristic of multiple

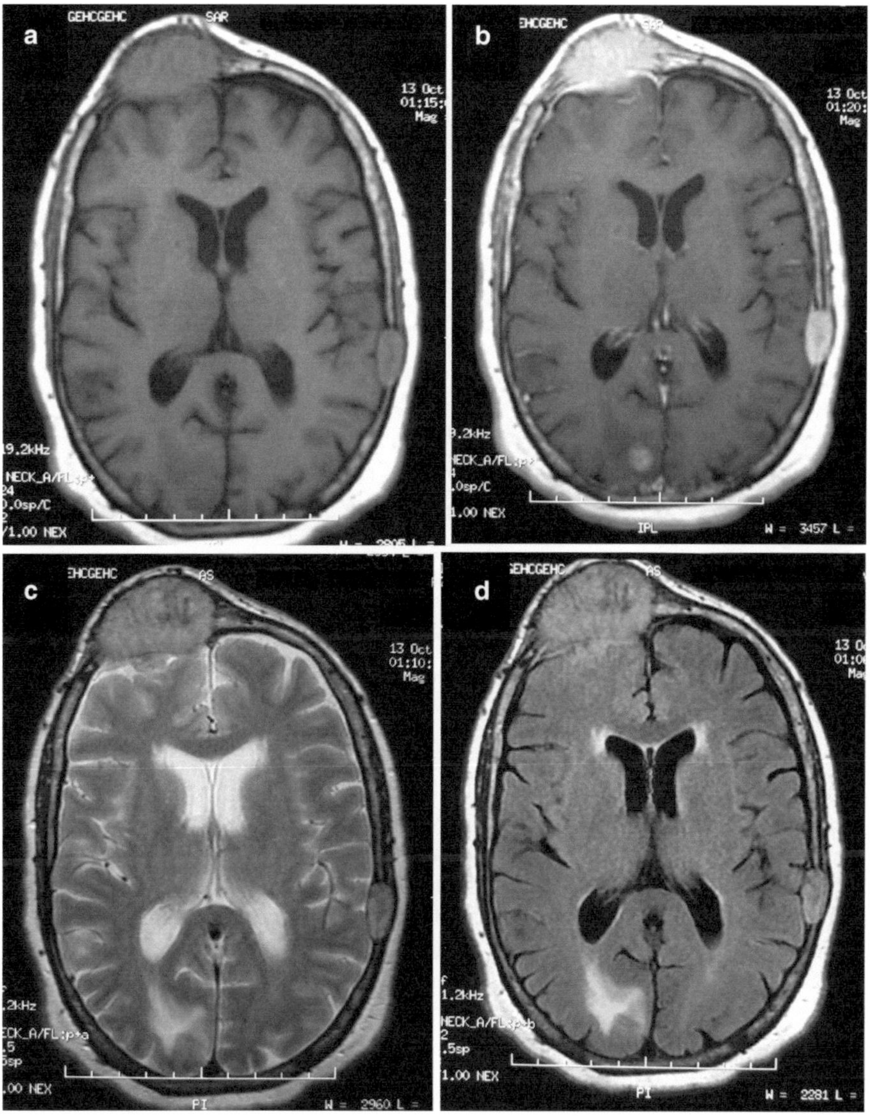

Fig. 9.18 Multiple cranial bone metastases (same patient). Axial MRI on T1 (before (**a**) and after (**b**) gadolinium injection), T2-weighted images (**c**), and FLAIR (fluid attenuated inversion recovery) sequence (**d**)

myeloma (the classic "punched-out" lesions). They may coalesce into larger osteolytic segments [29]. On MRI, a "salt-and-pepper" appearance or diffuse bone marrow replacement may be seen [28]. The diagnostic of multiple myeloma should be suspected when other skeletal lesions are seen. Rarely a focal lesion may be due to solitary plasmocytoma [25].

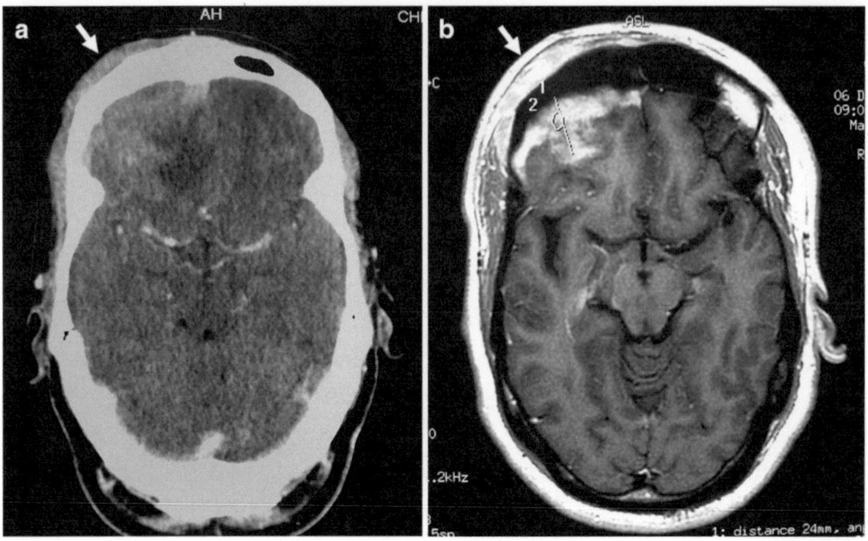

Fig. 9.19 Frontal cranial vault lymphoma with intra and extracranial extension (*arrow*). Cranial axial CT-scan after contrast administration (**a**) and T1-weighted image after gadolinium injection (**b**)

Leukemias and Lymphomas

Many of the various leukemias and lymphomas involve the cranial vault bones via bone marrow invasion. These lesions may present with pain or nasal congestion or the common clinical picture of infection with fever and anemia. Leukemias and lymphomas are rarely excised surgically because the tumor is usually responsive to current chemotherapy regimens depending on clinical stage. Surgery may be indicated for biopsy, or suspected recurrent disease or resection of apparently solitary disease [36] (Fig. 9.19).

Aneurysmal Bone Cyst

An aneurysmal bone cyst is a rapidly-growing expansive mass composed of several blood-filled spaces of variable size separated by connective tissue. It is a benign tumor mainly seen in child and young adult. This osteolytic vascular lesion had well-defined borders with multiple loculations. On MRI, aneurysmal bone cyst has mixed low and high signal areas because of blood elements in different stages. Fluid/fluid levels within the cysts themselves demonstrate a "soap-bubble" appearance. Although it may expand intracranially, the dura is rarely invaded [37].

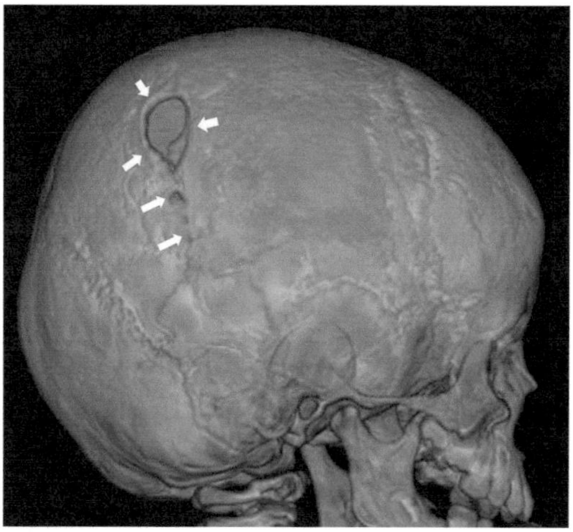

Fig. 9.20 Parietal growing skull fracture (*arrows*) on three-dimensional CT-scan reconstruction (reformatted volume-rendered)

Leptomeningeal Cyst

Leptomeningeal cysts or "Growing skull fractures" are a late complication of head traumas that occur before the age of 3 years. Skull fractures with an underlying dural laceration are the essential substrate of these lesions. The growing brain or perhaps the normal pulsation of the brain, result in herniation of the brain parenchyma or the cerebrospinal fluid into the subcutaneous tissue. A growing skull fracture is a widening of the fracture line more than 4 mm and involves both the inner and outer tables (Fig. 9.20). Growing skull fractures present as a soft, pulsatile mass beneath the scalp, with seizures, or with a progressive neurologic deficit [38]. Diagnosis is made in patients with a history of head injury, bone fracture, presence of gliosis in adjacent brain parenchyma and the presence of cystic CSF lesions [39, 40].

Pseudomeningocele

Pseudomeningoceles are the herniation of CSF or brain parenchyma into the subcutaneous tissue of the scalp due to a postoperative cranial bone defect [41] (Fig. 9.21).

Paget's Disease

Paget's disease or osteitis deformans is an incompletely understood, most likely genetically based process that cause abnormal and excessive bone remodeling [42]. It is usually asymptomatic or discovered incidentally in adults over the fifth

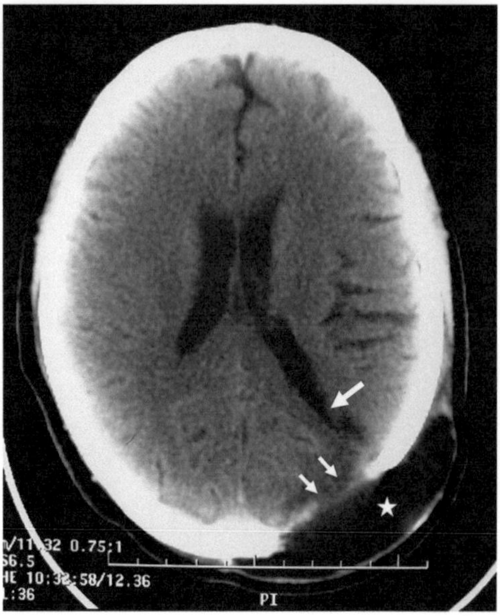

Fig. 9.21 Left parietal pseudomeningocele (*star*) on axial CT-scan. Note the direct communication of the extracranial cyst with the ipsilateral ventricle (*arrows*)

decades of age. In the skull, the entire thickness of the bone is affected, especially the frontal and occipital bones [22]. The disease progresses through three phases: an osteolytic phase, followed by a mixed phase and finally an osteosclerotic phase. In the osteolytic stage, there are lytic lesions that erode the outer table which are known as "osteoporosis circumscripta". In the osteosclerotic stage, differentiation between the inner and outer tables is lost and the diploe widens. In mixed stage, irregular regions of sclerosis demonstrate a cotton-wool shaped image. MRI demonstrate widening of the diploe and heterogeneous signal intensity depending on the stage of the disease. Complications mainly include stenosis of nerve foramina, platybasia or basilar impression. Sarcomatous transformation of Paget's disease is a rare complication that occurs later in the course of the disease [28, 43].

Further lesions in the cranial vault are given in Table 9.2 such as congenital skull defect (Fig. 9.22) and frontal sinus mucocele (Fig. 9.23).

Imaging Pattern of Skull Base Lesions

The skull base is a more complex anatomical structure than the cranial vault, therefore anatomical site of the skull base lesion further helps to narrow the very large variations of differential diagnosis (especially tumoral) (Tables 9.3 and 9.4).

Table 9.2 Differential diagnosis of cranial vault osteomyelitis according to pathogenesis of the lesions

Pathogenesis	Lesions
A. Congenital lesions	– Dermoid and epidermoid cysts
	– Dermal sinus tract
	– Encephalocele/meningocele
	– Sinus pericranii
	– Intradiploic arachnoid cyst
	– Cranium bifidum
	– Craniosynostosis
	– Congenital skull defect
B. Inflammatory lesions	– Eosinophilic granuloma
	– Sarcoidosis
	– Chronic recurrent multifocal osteomyelitis [44–46]
C. Traumatic/iatrogenic lesions	– Skull fracture
	– Surgical defect (burr hole, craniotomy and craniectomy)
	– Bone flap resorption
	– Suture diastasis
	– Intraosseous hematoma
	– Leptomeningeal cyst and growing skull fracture
	– Pseudomeningocele
D. Benign neoplastic lesions	– Lipoma
	– Hemangiopericytoma
	– Aneurysmal bone cyst
	– Osteoma
	– Osteoblastoma
	– Hemangioma
	– Meningioma
	– Neurofibroma
E. Malign neoplastic lesions	– Chondrosarcoma
	– Hemangiosarcoma
	– Multiple myeloma
	– Squamous and basal cell carcinoma
	– Osteosarcoma
	– Ewing's sarcoma
	– Leukemia and lymphoma
	– Metastases
	– Fibrosarcoma
	– Angiosarcoma
F. Metabolic	– Hyperparathyroidism
	– Osteoporosis
	– Osteogenesis imperfecta
	– Rickets
	– Renal osteodystrophy

(continued)

Table 9.2 (continued)

Pathogenesis	Lesions
G. Normal variations	– Enlarged parietal foramina
	– Parietal thinning and normal ageing calvarium
	– Pacchionian granulations or arachnoid granulations
	– Transcalvarial venous lakes and vascular channels (emissary veins)
	– Anterior and posterior fontanelle
H. Others	– Paget's disease
	– Fibrous dysplasia
	– Neurofibroma
	– Frontal sinus mucocele
	– Hemoglobinopathies
	– Hyperostosis frontalis interna
	– Radiation osteonecrosis
	– Avascular osteonecrosis

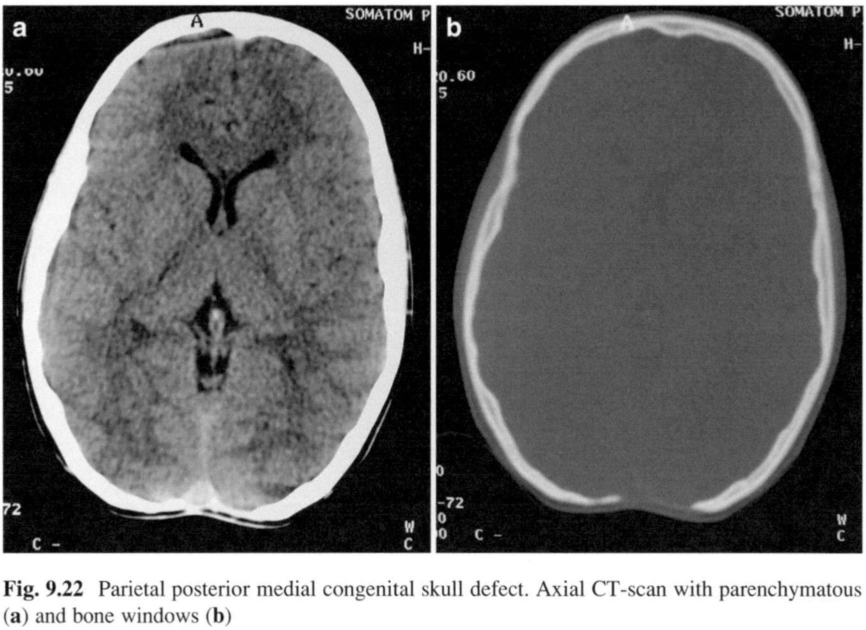

Fig. 9.22 Parietal posterior medial congenital skull defect. Axial CT-scan with parenchymatous (**a**) and bone windows (**b**)

Tumoral Lesions

Usually, tumoral lesions with skull base extension would generally result in a more focal destructive mass, rather than the diffuse infiltrative pattern observed in skull base osteomyelitis (Fig. 9.24). However, some cases were diagnosed only at

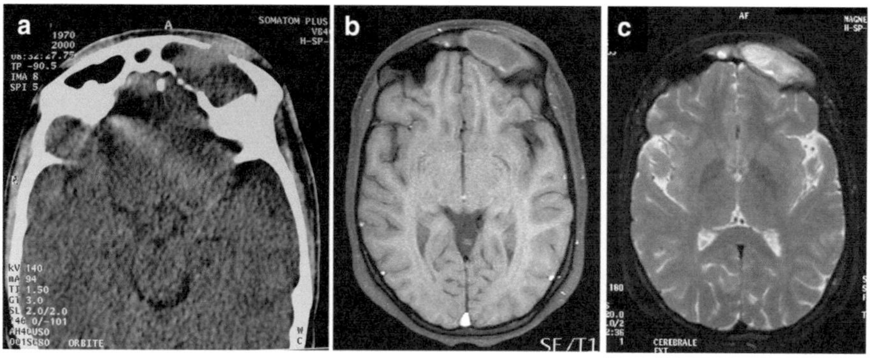

Fig. 9.23 Large left frontal mucocele. Both anterior and posterior walls of the left frontal sinus are eroded. Axial CT-scan (**a**), axial T1-weighted (**b**) and T2-weighted (**c**) images

autopsy study [60]. For Lesser et al., CT-scans of central skull base osteomyelitis show much less bony destruction relative to the MRI changes, whereas malignancy cases were associated with similar bony destruction on CT-scan and MRI [59]. In addition, the rapidity of progression of skull base infections is generally more important than in skull base malignancies. But sometimes, the diagnosis remains uncertain or completely unidentified and in these cases laboratory findings can be very helpful in limiting the differential diagnosis. Anyway, a biopsy must be achieved when the lesion is accessible [49, 55] (Fig. 9.25). In 2011, Ozgen et al. examined the use of diffusion-weighted MRI to better distinguish skull base osteomyelitis from malignancy. This was based on the previously noted finding that diffusion-weighted sequences can help distinguish benign from malignant lymph nodes. In principle, malignant neoplasms have low apparent diffusion coefficients (ADC) and benign masses have higher ADC. This study showed that ADC values of lymphomas and nasopharyngeal carcinomas were significantly lower than that of the group with skull base osteomyelitis; however the ADC values of the patients with metastatic disease overlapped with the skull base osteomyelitis group [54].

Pseudo-tumoral Lesions

Many "pseudotumors" can mimic tumoral lesions and osteomyelitis and can involve the skull base and eventually have intracranial extension such as mucocele, inflammatory pseudotumor, Wegener's granulomatosis and other granulomatous diseases involving the sinuses as well as polyposis nasi and inverted papilloma [51, 52, 56]. Obliteration of the carotid artery is often a sign indicating that a central skull base lesion is more often inflammatory and not tumoral. Once an inflammatory lesion crosses the bony wall of the skull base and comes in contact with carotid artery, the latter will get an inflamed wall and the artery will occlude rapidly. On the contrary, the lumen can be narrowed but remains open even in very advanced

Table 9.3 Differential diagnosis of skull base osteomyelitis according to the three classic anatomic divisions [47–60]

Anatomic division	Lesions
Anterior skull base	Squamous cell carcinoma
	Adenocarcinoma
	Lymphoma
	Plasmocytoma
	Melanoma
	Rhabdomyosarcoma
	Esthesioneuroblastoma
	Olfactory schwannoma
	Meningioma
	Fibrous dysplasia
	Mucocele
Central skull base	Meningioma
	Lymphoma
	Squamous cell carcinoma
	Adenocarcinoma
	Adenoid cystic carcinoma
	Juvenile angiofibroma
	Nasopharyngeal tumor
	Carotid aneurysm
	Schwannoma
	Pituitary adenoma
	Chordoma
	Chondrosarcoma
	Metastases
	Osteosarcoma
	Paget's disease
	Fibrous dysplasia
	Inflammatory pseudotumor
	Rosai-Dorfman disease
	Sarcoidosis
Posterior skull base	Paraganglioma
	Schwannoma
	Metastasis
	Meningioma
	Nasopharynx carcinoma
	Myeloma
	Chondrosarcoma

Table 9.4 Differential diagnosis of skull base osteomyelitis according to anatomic origin and pathogenesis of the lesions [47–60]

Anatomic origin	Pathogenesis	Lesions
Middle/external ear mass	Inflammatory	Acquired cholesteatoma
		Acute otitis media
		Malignant otitis externa
		Cholesterol granuloma
		Serous otitis media
		Middle ear effusion
		Tympanosclerosis
	Tumor	Glomus tympanicum
		Glomus jugular
		Facial nerve schwannoma
		Temporal bone mass
	Vascular	Aberrant internal carotid artery
		Dehiscent jugular bulb
Temporal bone mass	Tumoral	Glomus tumor
		Meningioma
		Metastasis
		Myeloma
		Lymphoma
		Nasopharyngeal carcinoma
		Rhabdomyosarcoma
		Parotid carcinoma
		Chordoma
		Chondroma/chondrosarcoma
		External auditory canal carcinoma
		Meningioma
	Non tumoral	Cholesteatoma
		Cholesterol granuloma
		Apical petrositis
		Aneurysm of petrous carotid
		Eosinophilic granuloma
	Others	Otosclerosis
		Paget's disease
		Fibrous dysplasia
		Osteopetrosis
		Renal osteodystrophy
		Hemoglobinopathy

(continued)

Table 9.4 (continued)

Anatomic origin	Pathogenesis	Lesions
Jugular foramen mass	Tumoral	Glomus jugular
		Schwannoma
		Metastasis
		Meningioma
		Chondrosarcoma
		Eosinophilic granuloma
		Lymphoma
	Non-tumoral	Enlarged jugular bulb
		Venous thrombosis

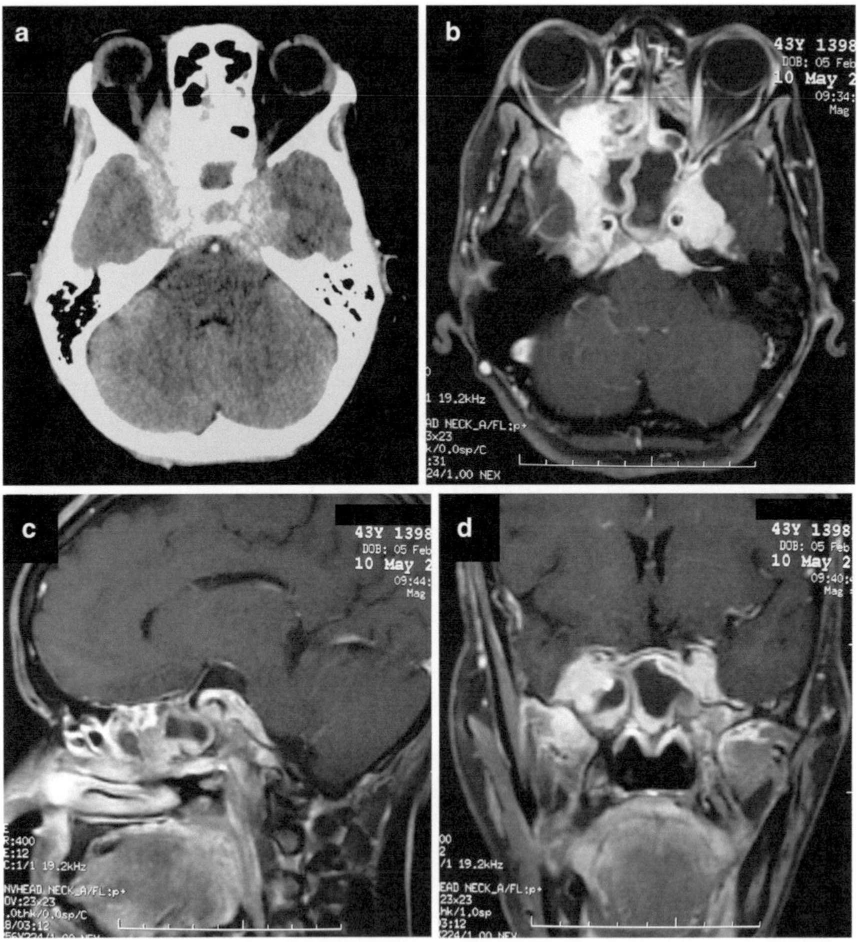

Fig. 9.24 Central skull base undifferentiated carcinoma of the nasopharyngeal type (UCNT). Note the multidirectional extension of the tumor. Axial CT-scan after contrast injection (**a**). T1-weighted MRI following gadolinium administration on axial (**b**), sagittal (**c**), and coronal (**d**) views

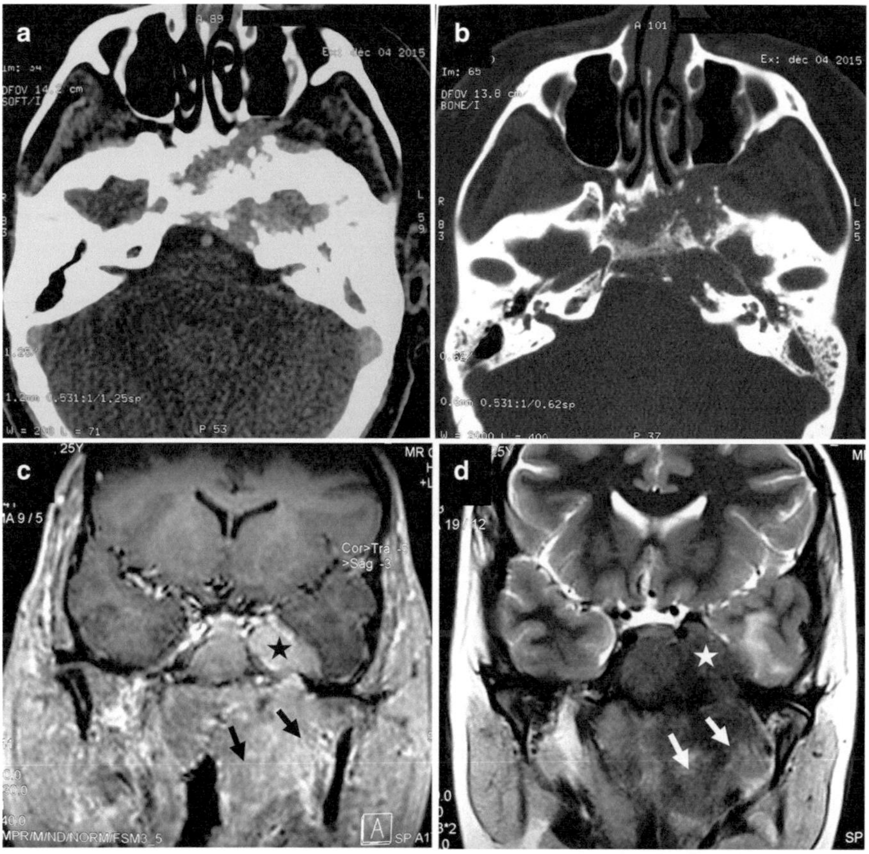

Fig. 9.25 Central skull base lymphoma with sphenoidal and clival osteolysis (diagnosed after nasopharyngeal biopsy). The tumor has an intracranial (cavernous sinus and temporal lobe) (*star*) and extracranial (infratemporal and nasopharyngeal) (*arrows*) extensions. Axial cranial CT-scan after contrast administration in parenchymatous (**a**) and bone windows (**b**). Coronal brain MRI on T1-weighted image with gadolinium enhancement (**c**) and on T2-weighted image (**d**)

tumoral lesions [47]. For Casselman, another sign to differentiate inflammatory "pseudotumor" from true tumor is the discordance between the CT-scan and the MRI findings. With an inflammatory pseudotumor, the lesion if often more hardly visible on CT-scan but is more easily seen and larger on MRI [47]. Sarcoidosis can also affect bone and soft tissue, but in osteomyelitis, the diffuse marrow abnormality and contiguous non-nodal soft tissue abnormality are more important [57, 58]. Fibrous dysplasia and Paget disease can result in abnormal marrow signal intensity on MRI, but they have a typical CT-scan appearance, cause bone expansion rather than erosion, and would not be expected to have an associated soft tissue abnormality as in osteomyelitis [53]. On Paget disease, bone resorption may be associated with high signal intensity on T2-WI and strong enhancement after gadolinium administration. Later, bone develops bone marrow containing hypointense thickened trabeculae and surrounded by thick hypointense tables. Complications mainly include stenosis of nerve foramina, platybasia, basilar impression, and sarcomatous degeneration [22, 29].

References

1. Soma PF, Chibbaro S, Makiese O, Marsella M, Diemidio P, Fricia M, Passanisi M, Catania V, Siragò P, Ventura F. Aggressive scalp carcinoma with intracranial extension: a multidisciplinary experience of 25 patients with long-term follow-up. J Clin Neurosci. 2008;15 (9):988–92. doi:10.1016/j.jocn.2007.09.014.
2. Swift DM, Sacco DJ. Scalp and skull neoplasms. In: Albright AL, Pollack IF, Adelson PD, editors. Principles and practice of pediatric neurosurgery. 2nd ed. New York: Thieme Medical Publishers; 2008.
3. Jankowski PP, Krishna PH, Rutledge JC, Waldhausen J, Avellino AM. Surgical management and outcome of scalp subcutaneous granuloma annulare in children: case report. Neurosurgery. 2008;63(5):E1002. doi:10.1227/01.NEU.0000333264.11514.FE.
4. Molés-Poveda P, Noguera L, Torrelo A. Spontaneous regression of an infantile scalp tumor. Infantile myofibromatosis. Infantile myofibromatosis. JAMA Dermatol. 2015;151(6):663–4. doi:10.1001/jamadermatol.2014.4985.
5. Smirniotopoulos JG, Chiechi MV. Teratomas, dermoids, and epidermoids of the head and neck. Radiographics. 1995;15(6):1437–55.
6. Fukuyama M, Tanese K, Yasuda F, Hayashi Y, Tanikawa A. Two cases of atretic cephalocele, and histological evaluation of skin appendages in the surrounding skin. Clin Exp Dermatol. 2015. doi:10.1111/ced.12687.
7. Vitali AM. Acquired encephalocele attributable to tuberculous osteitis: case report. Neurosurgery. 2008;62(4):E976. doi:10.1227/01.neu.0000318188.18159.57.
8. Piatt Jr JH. Congenital defects of the scalp and skull. In: Albright AL, Pollack IF, Adelson PD, editors. Principles and practice of pediatric neurosurgery. 2nd ed. New York: Thieme Medical Publishers; 2008.
9. Renfro L, Geronemus RG. Anatomical differences of port-wine stains in response to treatment with the pulsed dye laser. Arch Dermatol. 1993;129(2):182–8.
10. Kumar R, Sharma G, Sharma BS. Management of scalp arterio-venous malformation: case series and review of literature. Br J Neurosurg. 2012;26(3):371–7. doi:10.3109/02688697.2012.654838.
11. Pavanello M, Melloni I, Antichi E, Severino M, Ravegnani M, Piatelli G, Cama A, Rossi A, Gandolfo C. Sinus pericranii: diagnosis and management in 21 pediatric patients. J Neurosurg Pediatr. 2015;15(1):60–70. doi:10.3171/2014.9.PEDS13641.
12. Annabel M, Hubert L, Jacques C, Fabienne L, Emmanuelle L, Gérard L. Treatment of 2 cases of kerions with griseofulvin and oral steroids. Arch Pediatr. 2009;16(11):1464–6. doi:10.1016/j.arcped.2009.07.023.French.
13. Yuen JC, Puri SK, Feng Z. Scalp necrotizing fasciitis with osteomyelitis of the skull from Aspergillus. J Craniofac Surg. 2002;13(6):762–4.
14. Epstein JS, Ganz WI, Lizak M, Grobman L, Goodwin WJ, Dewanjee MK. Indium 111-labeled leukocyte scintigraphy in evaluating head and neck infections. Ann Otol Rhinol Laryngol. 1992;101(12):961–8.
15. Barry J, Fridley J, Sayama C, Lam S. Infected subgaleal hematoma following blunt head trauma in a child: case report and review of the literature. Pediatr Neurosurg. 2015;50 (4):223–8. doi:10.1159/000433442.
16. Kaufman HH, Hochberg J, Anderson RP, Schochet Jr SS, Simmons Jr GM. Treatment of calcified cephalohematoma. Neurosurgery. 1993;32(6):1037–9.

17. Arana E, Martí-Bonmatí L. CT and MR imaging of focal calvarial lesions. AJR Am J Roentgenol. 1999;172(6):1683–8.
18. Gibson SE, Prayson RA. Primary skull lesions in the pediatric population: a 25-year experience. Arch Pathol Lab Med. 2007;131(5):761–6.
19. Small JE, Schaefer PW, editors. Neuroradiology key differential diagnoses and clinical questions. Philadelphia: Elsevier Saunders; 2013.
20. Okamoto K, Ito J, Furusawa T, Sakai K, Tokiguchi S. Imaging of calvarial eosinophil granuloma. Neuroradiology. 1999;41(10):723–8.
21. Azouz EM, Saigal G, Rodriguez MM, Podda A. Langerhans' cell histiocytosis: pathology, imaging and treatment of skeletal involvement. Pediatr Radiol. 2005;35(2):103–15.
22. Amaral L, Chiurciu M, Almeida JR, Ferreira NF, Mendonça R, Lima SS. MR imaging for evaluation of lesions of the cranial vault: a pictorial essay. Arq Neuropsiquiatr. 2003;61 (3A):521–32.
23. Ginsberg LE. Radiology of meningiomas. J Neurooncol. 1996;29(3):229–38.
24. Akhaddar A, Ennouali H. Intraosseous extradural meningioma of the frontal bone. Pan Afr Med J. 2014;17:69. doi:10.11604/pamj.2014.17.69.3844.
25. Yalçin O, Yildirim T, Kizilkiliç O, Hürcan CE, Koç Z, Aydin V, Sen O, Kayaselçuk F. CT and MRI findings in calvarial non-infectious lesions. Diagn Interv Radiol. 2007;13(2):68–74.
26. Sutherland JE, Dahdaleh NS, Greenlee JD, Kirby PA, Sargent MD. Large osteolytic skull tumor presenting as a small subcutaneous scalp lesion. J Am Board Fam Med. 2011;24 (6):763–7. doi:10.3122/jabfm.2011.06.100308.
27. Yoon SH, Park SH. A study of 77 cases of surgically excised scalp and skull masses in pediatric patients. Childs Nerv Syst. 2008;24(4):459–65.
28. Garfinkle J, Melançon D, Cortes M, Tampieri D. Imaging pattern of calvarial lesions in adults. Skeletal Radiol. 2011;40(10):1261–73. doi:10.1007/s00256-010-0971-8.
29. Colas L, Caron S, Cotten A. Skull vault lesions: a review. AJR Am J Roentgenol. 2015;205 (4):840–7. doi:10.2214/AJR.14.13415.
30. Akhaddar A, Laaguili J. Post-traumatic cavernous hemangioma of the frontal cranial vault. Pan Afr Med J. 2014;17:90. doi:10.11604/pamj.2014.17.90.3904.
31. Naama O, Gazzaz M, Akhaddar A, Belhachmi A, Asri A, Elmostarchid B, Elbouzidi A, Kadiri B, Boucetta M. Cavernous hemangioma of the skull: 3 case reports. Surg Neurol. 2008;70(6):654–9. doi:10.1016/j.surneu.2007.05.052.
32. Ajja A, Akhaddar A, Naama O, Guazzaz M, Belhachmi A, Asri Abad C, Elmoustarchid B, Boucetta M. [Intradiploic epidermoid cyst of the occipital bone]. Neurochirurgie. 2007;53 (5):367–70. French.
33. Akhaddar A, Jiddane M, Chakir N, El Hassani R, Moustarchid B, Bellakhdar F. Cerebellar abscesses secondary to occipital dermoid cyst with dermal sinus: case report. Surg Neurol. 2002;58(3–4):266–70.
34. Cherif El Asri A, El Mostarchid B, Akhaddar A, Boucetta M. Chronic subdural hematoma revealing skull metastasis. Intern Med. 2011;50(7):791.
35. Egelhoff JC, Zalles C. Unusual CNS presentation of neuroblastoma. Pediatr Radiol. 1996;26 (1):51–4.
36. El Asri AC, Akhaddar A, Baallal H, Boulahroud O, Mandour C, Chahdi H, Mikdame M, Gazzaz M, El Mostarchid B, Boucetta M. Primary lymphoma of the cranial vault: case report and a systematic review of the literature. Acta Neurochir (Wien). 2012;154(2):257–65. doi:10.1007/s00701-011-1124-0.
37. Guida F, Rapanà A, Conti C, Cagliari E, Civelli F, Trincia G. Cranial aneurysmal bone cyst: a diagnostic problem. With a review of the literature. Childs Nerv Syst. 2001;17(4–5):297–301.
38. Akhaddar A, Mercier P, Diabira S, Fournier D, Menei P. Growing skull fracture combined with schizencephaly. Pan Arab J Neurosurg. 2011;15(2):87–9.
39. Sanford RA. Prevention of growing skull fractures: report of 2 cases. J Neurosurg Pediatr. 2010;5(2):213–8. doi:10.3171/2009.9.PEDS09180.

40. Prasad GL, Gupta DK, Mahapatra AK, Borkar SA, Sharma BS. Surgical results of growing skull fractures in children: a single centre study of 43 cases. Childs Nerv Syst. 2015;31 (2):269–77. doi:10.1007/s00381-014-2529-x.
41. Ginat DT, Duhaime AC. Imaging the postoperative scalp and cranium. In: Ginat DT, Westesson PLA, editors. Atlas of postsurgical neuroradiology, imaging of the brain, spine, head, and neck. Berlin: Springer; 2012.
42. Ralston SH, Langston AL, Reid IR. Pathogenesis and management of Paget's disease of bone. Lancet. 2008;372(9633):155–63. doi:10.1016/S0140-6736(08)61035-1.
43. Brouard R, Wybier M, Miquel A, Laredo JD. The lucent rim: a radiographic and computed tomography sign of Paget's disease of the skull. Eur Radiol. 2006;16(6):1308–11.
44. Wedman J, van Weissenbruch R. Chronic recurrent multifocal osteomyelitis. Ann Otol Rhinol Laryngol. 2005;114(1 Pt 1):65–8.
45. Watanabe T, Ono H, Morimoto Y, Otsuki Y, Shirai M, Endoh A, Naito M, Inoue Y, Hongo T. Skull involvement in a pediatric case of chronic recurrent multifocal osteomyelitis. Nagoya J Med Sci. 2015;77(3):493–500.
46. Kurup S, Jose R, Chandy ML. Diagnostic utility of galium 67 SPECT/CT and role of pentoxifylline-tocopherol in chronic multifocal osteomyelitis. Oral Health Dent Manag. 2014;13(3):821–5.
47. Casselman JW. The skull base: tumoral lesions. Eur Radiol. 2005;15(3):534–42.
48. Naama O, Ajja A, Gazzaz M, Albouzidi A, Belhachmi A, Asri A, Akhaddar A, El Moustarchid B, Kadiri B, Labraimi A, Boucetta M. Primary Ewing sarcoma of the skull base with cerebral extension. A case report. J Neuroradiol. 2007;34(1):68–9.
49. Ganhewa AD, Jafri Kuthubutheen J. A diagnostic dilemma of central skull base osteomyelitis mimicking neoplasia in a diabetic patient. BMJ Case Rep. 2013;2013:bcr2012007183. doi:10.1136/bcr-2012-007183.
50. Subburaman N, Chaurasia MK. Skull base osteomyelitis interpreted as malignancy. J Laryngol Otol. 1999;113(8):775–8.
51. Yokoyama T, Inoue S, Imamura J, Nagamitsu T, Jimi Y, Katoh S, Kameda H, Abiko S. Sphenoethmoidal mucoceles with intracranial extension—three case reports. Neurol Med Chir (Tokyo). 1996;36(11):822–8.
52. Sharma A, Deshmukh S, Shaikh A, Dabholkar J. Wegener's granulomatosis mimicking skull base osteomyelitis. J Laryngol Otol. 2012;126(2):203–6. doi:10.1017/S0022215111002064.
53. Chang PC, Fischbein NJ, Holliday RA. Central skull base osteomyelitis in patients without otitis externa: imaging findings. AJNR Am J Neuroradiol. 2003;24(7):1310–6.
54. Ozgen B, Oguz KK, Cila A. Diffusion MR imaging features of skull base osteomyelitis compared with skull base malignancy. AJNR Am J Neuroradiol. 2011;32(1):179–84. doi:10.3174/ajnr.A2237.
55. Clark MP, Pretorius PM, Byren I, Milford CA. Central or atypical skull base osteomyelitis: diagnosis and treatment. Skull Base. 2009;19(4):247–54. doi:10.1055/s-0028-1115325.
56. Alyono JC, Shi Y, Berry GJ, Recht LD, Harsh IV GR, Jackler RK, Corrales CE. Inflammatory pseudotumors of the skull base: meta-analysis. Otol Neurotol. 2015;36(8):1432–8. doi:10.1097/MAO.0000000000000818.
57. Carlson ML, White Jr JR, Espahbodi M, Haynes DS, Driscoll CL, Aksamit AJ, Pawate S, Lane JI, Link MJ. Cranial base manifestations of neurosarcoidosis: a review of 305 patients. Otol Neurotol. 2015;36(1):156–66. doi:10.1097/MAO.0000000000000501.
58. Akhaddar A, Elguendouz F, Elmoustarchid B, Boucetta M. Intrasellar neurosarcoidosis with suprasellar extension. Intern Med. 2011;50(8):945.
59. Lesser FD, Derbyshire SG, Lewis-Jones H. Can computed tomography and magnetic resonance imaging differentiate between malignant pathology and osteomyelitis in the central skull base? J Laryngol Otol. 2015;129(9):852–9. doi:10.1017/S0022215115001991.
60. Wilkinson EP, Robinson RA, Trask DK. Skull base thrombotic mycosis. Ear Nose Throat J. 2007;86(3):137.

Part IV
Management of Cranial Osteomyelitis

Chapter 10
General Considerations and Surgical Therapy

Contents

Abbreviations

CSF Cerebrospinal fluid
HBOT Hyperbaric oxygen therapy

General Considerations

Prior to any successful treatment, initial diagnosis of cranial osteomyelitis should be suspected and confirmed early. The adequate diagnosis can generally be recognized based on the patient's comorbidities, the neurologic status, the duration of disease before diagnosis was established, the potential primary source of infection, biologic and imaging results, and more relevant the causative pathogen and its susceptibility patterns. Treatment of cranial bone infections is not standardized due

A. Akhaddar, *Cranial Osteomyelitis*, DOI 10.1007/978-3-319-30268-3_10

to the variable clinical presentations, locations, severities, etiologies and the lack of data from randomized controlled trials. However, it is necessary to develop a management plan and a final treatment strategy for each patient in close collaboration with otolaryngologist, microbiologist, radiologist, infectious disease specialist and plastic surgeon among others medical practitioners.

The spectrum of treatment goes from antibiotic therapy alone to combination with simple incision and drainage to invasive surgery. However, most diagnoses are delayed needing combination of surgical debridement, correction of the primary source of infection and long term use of antimicrobial agents. Hyperbaric oxygen therapy (HBOT) has also been added to the therapeutic armamentarium; but, the role of hyperbaric oxygen in the treatment of cranial osteomyelitis has not been well defined (see Chap. 12).

Commonly, therapy of acute and chronic osteomyelitis of the skull is more or less the same, since etiology and pathogenesis are somewhat identical in both. However, and based on pathophysiological data, the disease is generally more advanced in cases of chronic osteomyelitis than in acute ones.

The aims of therapy for osteomyelitis in any location in the body are: elimination of infection and removal of potential primary infectious focus, analgesia as a part of symptom control, limitation of additional spreading of the disease, preservation of anatomic structures when possible, prevention of relapse of disease and/or chronification of the infection and re-establishment of anatomy and function. To the best of our knowledge, there is no comprehensive universally accepted guideline on the management of patients with osteomyelitic cranial bone to date. Some authors believe that immediate neurosurgical intervention is necessary, whilst others insist that a more conservative approach with/without neurosurgical intervention carries similar results. As reported in the literature since 1925 [1], it appears that most case reports are still managed on an individual decision basis. Anyway, founded on our experience and that of others, we believe that principles of management of cranial osteomyelitis need to be tailored to the appropriate clinical picture, diagnosis, and treatment objective and some items should always be taken into consideration (Table 10.1).

In addition, comorbidities and underlying medical conditions should be actively addressed to improve the possibility of adequate healing. Consultation with the appropriate medical specialist will be helpful in resolving many of these underlying problems. Empirical antibiotic therapy without diagnostic work-up should never be considered. In acute infection with sepsis syndrome, blood cultures must be obtained before starting rational empiric antimicrobial treatment. When infectious material has been obtained for microbiologic and histopathologic studies, empirical antibiotic therapy should be initiated on the basis of the patient's predisposing conditions and the presumed pathogenesis of skull osteomyelitis. Generally, treatment is started with intravenous antibiotics. If the infecting agent is susceptible to drugs with excellent bioavailability, oral treatment can be started after a few days. The duration has not been tested in comparative studies. In general, a 6-week course is proposed. In case of more serious intracranial complications, which are not completely removed by surgery, a longer treatment may be required (see

Table 10.1 The 12 principles for treatment of cranial osteomyelitis

Principles	Details
Establishing adequate diagnosis	Based on history, clinical evaluation, biologic and imaging studies
Performing biopsy	In ambiguous cases to exclude others pathologies
Determining exact extension of cranial bone infection	Using imaging explorations
Evaluation and correction of any comorbidities	When possible
Control and elimination of primary source of infection	Especially sinogenic, otogenic, and odontogenic
Drainage of purulent collections and surgical bone debridement	If necessary
Collection of specimens for microbiologic and histopathologic studies	Identification of the causative agents
Starting with empiric broad-spectrum antibiotic therapy	With possible adjustment to antimicrobial susceptibility patterns
Protection of vital intracranial structures and control of cerebrospinal fluid leaks	Preventing complications
Possibility of complementary hyperbaric oxygen therapy	When available
Clinical and paraclinical Follow-up	Reevaluation if there is evidence of clinical or paraclinical worsening
Restoration of durable scalp and/or cranial bone coverage	Using scalp and/or cranial bone reconstructions

Chap. 11). Management of specific cases with unusual pathogens and those with special clinical situations are discussed in Chaps. 14 and 15 respectively.

Response to the treatment is usually based on empiric judgment and is guided clinically, biologically and occasionally with follow-up imaging studies. In cases of persistent infection despite an adequate therapy, adjuvant HBOT and potential further surgical debridement should be evaluated.

Patients with cranial osteomyelitis may be subject to many hospitalizations, surgical procedures, and long term antimicrobial regimens. Physicians should provide a clear explanation of the disease, its causes, the suggested treatment and follow-up plan to the patient. The health care team must support the patient and discuss with him his doubts, questions and concerns [2].

Neurosurgical Procedures

Extracranial Infection with Mild Osteomyelitis

Superficial soft tissue site infection with mild cranial osteomyelitis can be treated with antibiotics alone but they should be followed carefully and reevaluated if there is evidence of clinical/paraclinical worsening. Sometimes, simple percutaneous

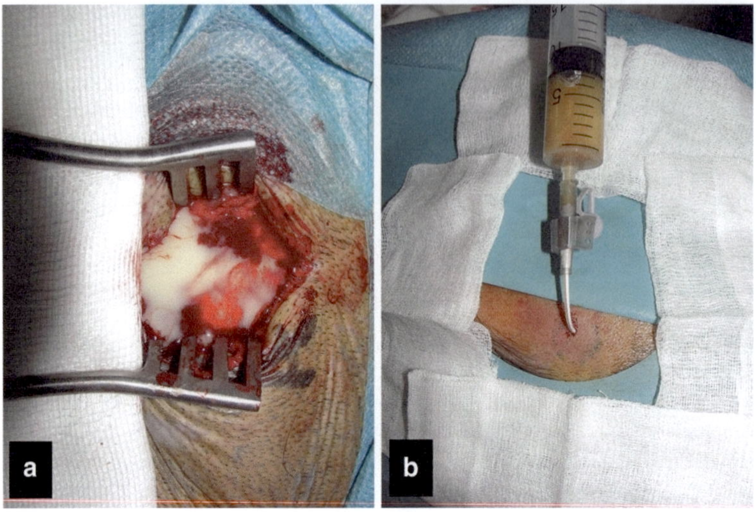

Fig. 10.1 Operative views. Limited scalp incision with drainage of small extracranial purulent fluid (**a**). Simple percutaneous collection of extracranial abscess formation (**b**)

drainage or limited scalp incision are sufficient to drain small superficial abscess and to collect specimens (avoiding skin contamination) for microbiologic and histopathologic studies (Fig. 10.1).

Cranial Vault Osteomyelitis

As soon as cranial vault osteomyelitis is suspected (clinically, biologically and on neuroimaging study) and particularly if purulent material extrudes from drained sinus tract, neurosurgical procedure is indicated. The quality and integrity of extracranial soft tissue must be evaluated for postoperative wound closure and the necessity of flap coverage. Infiltration of local anesthetic and vasoconstrictor solutions should be avoided when possible. This procedure has the danger of spreading infection in the scalp and altering the healing inflammatory response. The skin incision was centered over the osteomyelitic lesions and the sinus tract. Bleeding from the scalp can be limited by opening the wound in stages and securing hemostasis at each step. It is important to collect as much material as possible from fluid, purulent material and tissue specimens. The principles for harvesting specimens are described extensively in Chap. 3. All purulent material (soft-tissues, granulations, abscesses and bone) should be removed (Fig. 10.2). Then a careful debridement of the cranial bone should be performed. Surgical debridement remains critical to eliminate areas of necrosis and sequester, and to reduce local hypoxia and bacterial contamination (Fig. 10.3). This allowed macrophages and

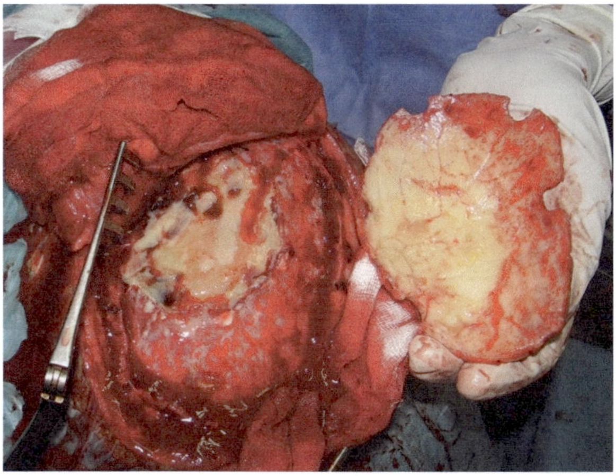

Fig. 10.2 Operative view. The wound was reopened. When the bone flap was elevated, an abundant purulent collection was observed. Yellowish pus was adherent to a Gore-tex dural plastia implanted in the previous operation for cranial vault meningioma (case number one)

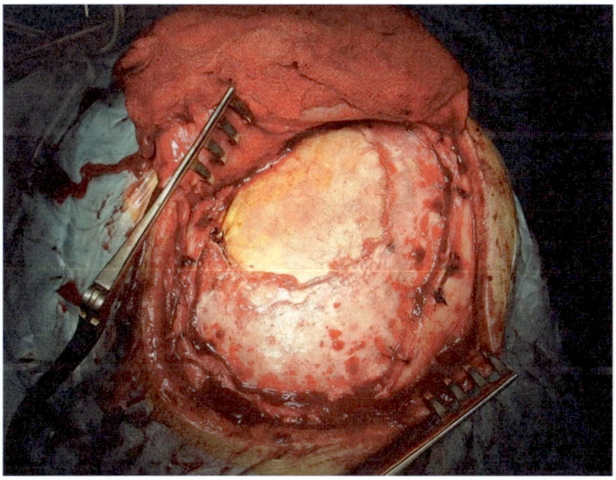

Fig. 10.3 Operative view after careful extradural drainage, debridement (soft-tissues, granulations, abscesses and bone) and washing surgical site with antiseptic products (case number one)

leukocytes from the vascular network to come in contact with the wound bed bacteria promoting phagocytosis [3]. To ensure clearance of osseous infection, a 1 cm margin of macroscopically healthy bone should be done. Greenberg emphasizes the need to bite off infected bone with rongeurs until "a normal snapping sound replaces the more muted sound made by rongeuring infected bone" [4]. All bony irregularities may be corrected with a high-speed drill, creating a shallow cavity with no overhanging bony edges. Tissue adherent to the dura should not be removed too vigorously because breaching the dura may allow the infected material to be introduced into the subarachnoid space, resulting in meningitis or deeper suppuration [5]. If needed, frontal sinus may be cranialized. Bone flaps that include part of the frontal sinus wall are especially susceptible to developing bone flap infection (Figs. 10.4, 10.5, and 10.6). Secondary extracranial lesions like sinus tracts (purulent fistula) should also be excised. Once the solid material has been

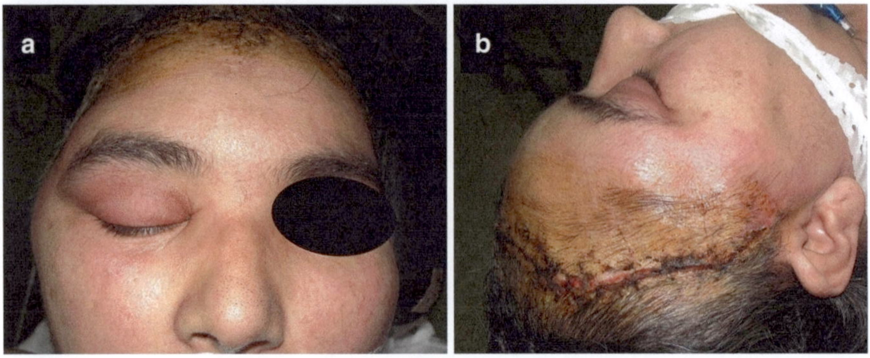

Fig. 10.4 Right fronto-temporal swelling with periorbital cellulitis (**a**). Note the wound inflammation secondary to deep incisional infection (**b**) occurring 2 weeks postoperatively (pterional approach) (case number two)

removed from the extradural space, irrigation with antibiotic solutions may be performed. An extradural closed drainage system can be used to minimize any hematoma collection, which can also become infected. Drain is left in place for no more than a few days. The wound should be closed without additional tension.

Antibiotics are continued intravenously for several days, and conversion to oral administration takes place when and if sensitivities allow. The total duration of antibiotic therapy depends on the severity of the infection but should be more than 6 weeks duration. Classically, after healing of the infection, the bone defect is closed by neurosurgeon and/or plastic surgeon (see below).

Skull Base Osteomyelitis

Further treatment difficulties arise when the cranial bone infection is largely in the skull base. The base of skull is almost inaccessible especially the central skull base area. The danger of incontrollable hemorrhage and injury to important cranial nerves is very great.

Aggressive surgical debridement of bone infection was previously considered first line-therapy for central skull base osteomyelitis. However, development of recent antimicrobial therapies allowed a less radical approach in these patients [6]. In the literature review performed by Johnson and Batra, only 43 % of patients with central skull base osteomyelitis underwent surgery for therapeutic intention. Unexpectedly, patients who were treated surgically were more likely to relapse and require supplementary courses of treatment. However, it is possible that these patients have a more advanced clinical presentation or cranial extension. The available database was unable to confirm the triumph of surgery as an action to decrease overall duration of antimicrobial treatment [7, 8]. For many authors,

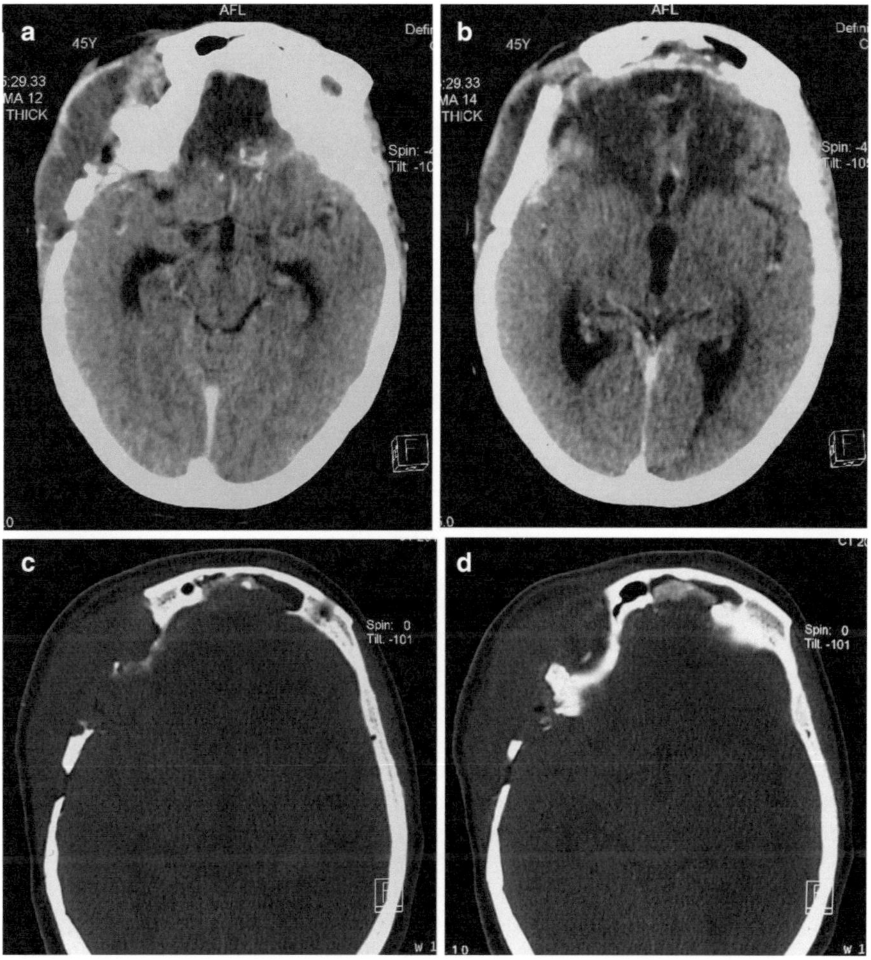

Fig. 10.5 Axial cranial CT-scan after contrast injection (**a** and **b**) and with bone windows (**c** and **d**) showing the extracranial abscess formation. Note the incomplete right frontal sinus cranialisation (case number two)

extension of the operation may be counterproductive because it may expose healthy bone to the infection [9, 10].

As stated previously for cranial vault osteomyelitis, no therapeutic criterion is available for the duration of antimicrobial therapy against skull base infection. Numerous reports have addressed this question, but opinions differ regarding the endpoint of treatment (see Chap. 11). An earlier study suggested that gallium scanning could be helpful in the evaluation of the response to therapy or disease recurrence in skull base osteomyelitis [11].

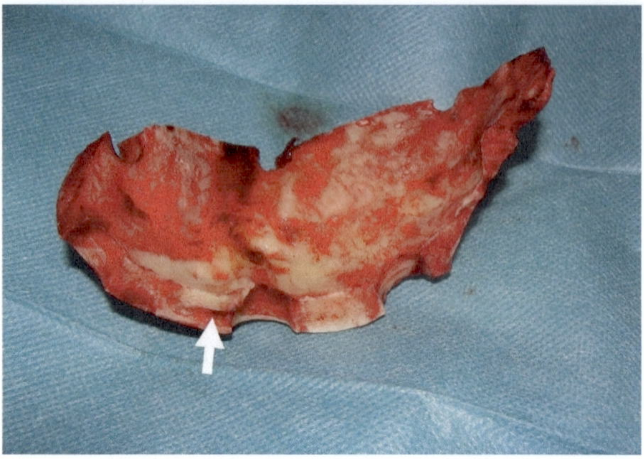

Fig. 10.6 Infected bone flap with left frontal sinus (*arrow*) (case number two)

Intracranial Suppurations

There is no consensus regarding the optimal surgical approach for intracranial purulent collections. Surgical management is indicated in almost all cases of subdural empyema for cerebral decompression, drainage of purulent material, and identification of the causative micro-organisms. Interventions include burr hole drainage, stereotactic drainage for deep-seated parafalcine or tentorial empyemas (Figs. 10.7 and 10.8), and craniotomy for irrigation, debridement, and drainage. The dura may be difficult to open because of its friability and thickness (Fig. 10.9). When visible, the pus is softly aspirated by gentle suction. Subdural collections under the craniotomy edge can be drained by passing a flat dissector into the subdural space and gently depressing the brain surface by a few millimeters. The dura should be closed after draining the empyema to avoid a cerebrospinal fluid leak. If a dural defect exists, it should be closed by using pericranial graft. For McCall et al., resorbable collagen dural substitutes can be used safely in the presence of cranial infection [12]. Purulent material tends to be in a fluid state early in the disease process and may become loculated with time. Repeat surgical procedures may be required [13].

Burr hole craniotomy for decompression with irrigation, debridement and drainage is warranted in a majority of cases of epidural abscess. However, in some cases with more solid organized granulomatous collection, a large bone flap is considered necessary (Fig. 10.10). A delay in surgical intervention has been associated with higher morbidity and mortality rates. Repeat surgical procedures may be needed in cases of persistent or recurrent suppurative infection [14–16].

All intraparenchymatous brain abscesses larger than 2 cm should be aspired (Fig. 10.11). If any abscess enlarges after 2 weeks of antibiotic therapy or fails to shrink after 4 weeks of therapy, repetition of stereotactic aspiration is suggested; however, craniotomy and excision are less commonly required [17].

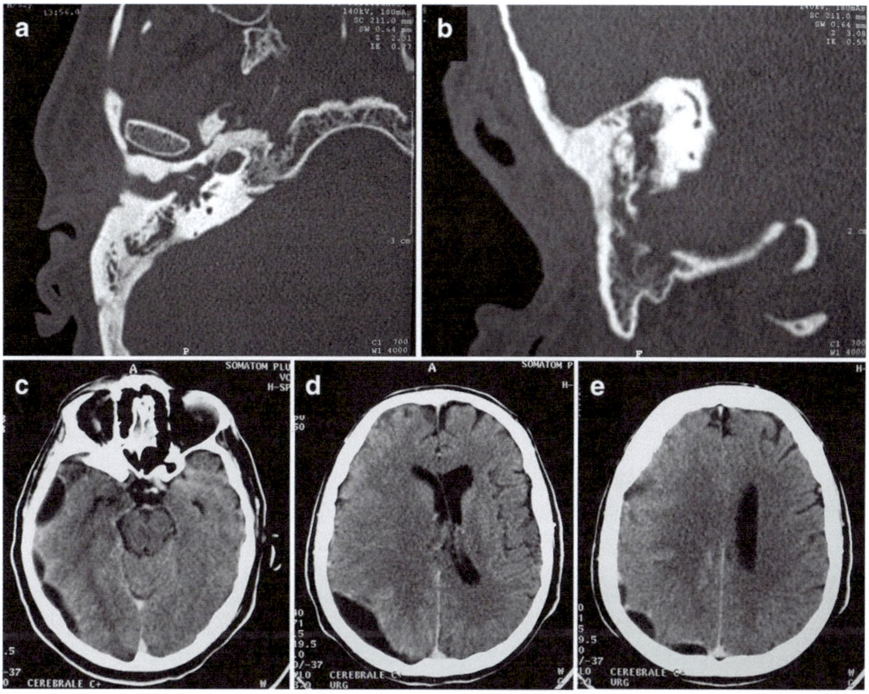

Fig. 10.7 Axial (**a**) and coronal reconstruction (**b**) CT-scan in bone windows revealing right chronic oto-mastoiditis. Axial CT-scan after contrast administration showing multiple subdural empyemas with mass effect (**c**–**e**) (case number three)

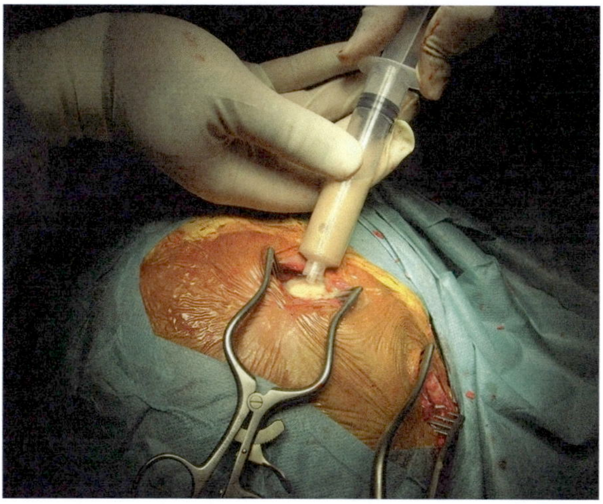

Fig. 10.8 Operative view. A thick yellowish green pus drained from the subdural space through two burr hole craniotomies (case number three)

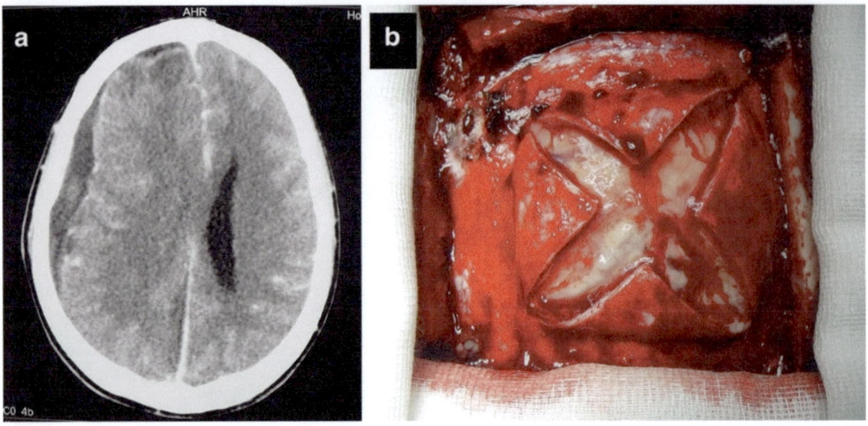

Fig. 10.9 Axial cranial CT-scan after contrast injection revealing a large right hemispheric subdural empyema (**a**). Operative view (**b**). The dura may be difficult to open because of its friability and thickness

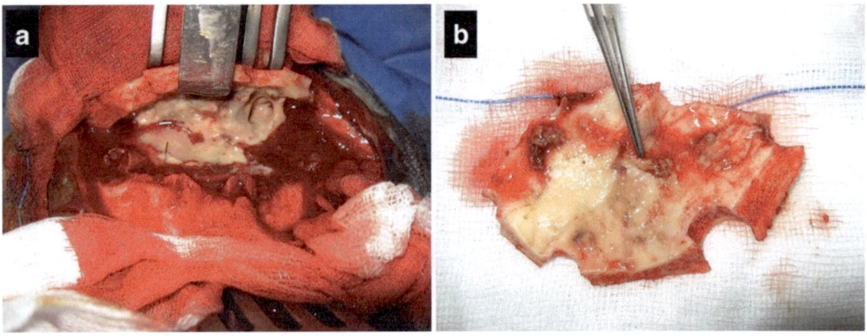

Fig. 10.10 Operative views. Craniotomy for a large epidural abscess (**a**). Note the infected cranial bone (**b**)

Other Unusual Measures

It is remarkable to note that prior to the wide availability and use of antibiotics, Baer in 1931 had underlined the beneficial effects of maggots (blow fly larvae) in soft tissue wounds infections and osteomyelitis [18]. One of the major advantages of Maggot debridement therapy is that the maggots separate the necrotic tissue from the living tissue, making a surgical debridement easier. While the concept relevance is well known in osteomyelitis, they have never gained widespread use. As mentioned by recent studies, the method remains simple and inexpensive, and appears effective [19–22]. However, to the best of our knowledge, Maggot debridement therapy was never used to treat osteomyelitis of the skull.

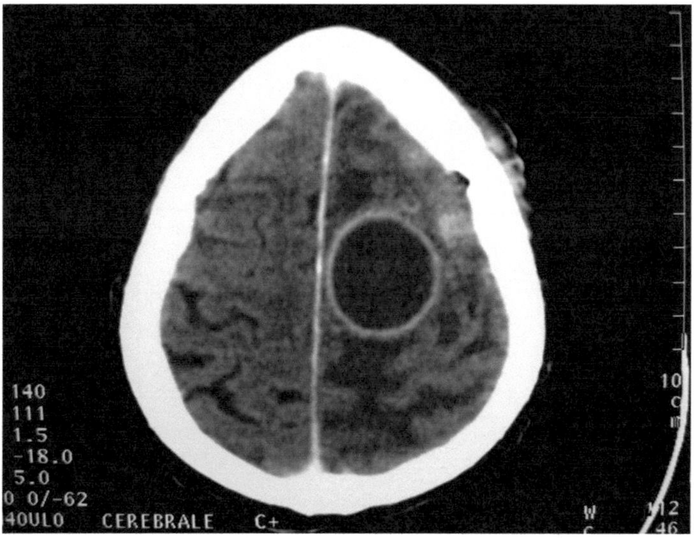

Fig. 10.11 Axial cranial CT-scan after contrast injection showing a left frontal intraparenchymatous abscess with surrounding edema

Along the same lines, honey has been applied for medicinal purposes since ancient times especially for wounds, burns and ulcers. Its antibacterial effects have been established during the past few decades [23]. Many modern medical practitioners support the use of honey in infected wounds and some suggest the prophylactic use of honey on the wounds of patients susceptible to Methicillin-resistant *Staphylococcus aureus* (MRSA) and other antibiotic-resistant bacteria [23–27] (Figs. 10.12 and 10.13). These results support the proposition that there are clinical benefits of using honey in wound care, but further research is needed [26, 28].

Surgery for Concomitant Paranasal Sinus and Ear Infection

When cranial osteomyelitis is secondary to rhinosinusitis, orodental infection or otomastoiditis, a multidisciplinary approach (neurosurgical, otorhinolaryngological and dental) is needed for many patients to eliminate the primary source of infection. Concomitant antibiotic treatment of sinusitis or otomastoiditis needs to be continued if present [29]. Aggressive surgical treatment against the source of the infection must be sought as soon as possible, regardless of the need for cranial and/or intracranial surgical intervention [30, 31]. However, when needed, it is better to plan and perform sinogenic and/or otogenic surgical procedures under the same anesthetic if deemed necessary by the neurosurgeon.

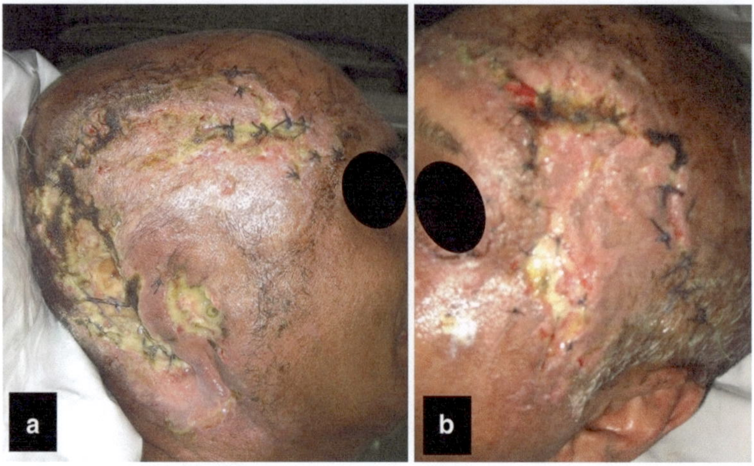

Fig. 10.12 This 33-year-old man had sustained a craniofacial injury following a road-traffic accident. He was initially taken to a local hospital where a primary wound closure was done and was then transferred to our center few days later. Dehiscence and purulent drainage of the cranio-facial wounds were found without evident adjacent cranial bone infection (**a** and **b**) (case number four)

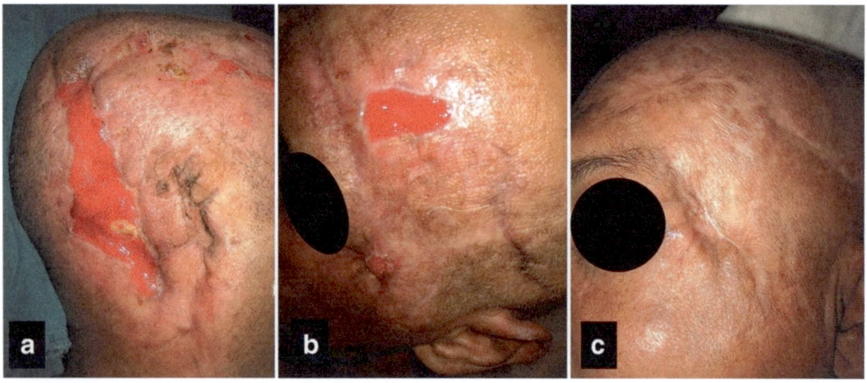

Fig. 10.13 After a soft tissue debridement followed by intravenous antibiotic therapy, this patient was treated with topical application of honey. A semi-permeable dressing containing the honey was applied to keep the honey in contact with the wound bed. The dressing was changed every 2 days and after 3 weeks the wound had a positive granulating surface (**a** and **b**). After the sixth week, the wound had completely healed. On year later, he was admitted for cosmetic surgery (**c**) (case number four)

Complementary Sinogenic Surgery

Frontal sinus may be drained via external and/or endonasal (endoscopic) approach. Limited osteomyelitis due to acute frontal sinusitis has been managed more often with functional endoscopic sinus surgery for drainage of pus [32, 33]. Endoscopic frontal sinusotomy was also performed with wide drainage. Endoscopic intervention has the advantage of the avoidance of facial scars, the preservation of the bony superstructure of the frontal sinus infundibulum and the facilitation of mucociliary clearance [34]. Some patients with limited forms of Pott's puffy tumor were even treated with endoscopic endonasal treatment without supplementary neurosurgical procedure [35, 36]. Recently, Bozdemir et al. reported a successful experience with balloon sinuplasty in three patients with Pott's puffy tumor [37].

More destructive disease processes need an external Lynch Howarth's approach (via the floor of the frontal sinus). In most cases, a conservative bone debridement was done. In cases of involvement of the anterior wall, Riedel's procedure was done by removing the anterior wall of the frontal sinus. Cranialization of the frontal sinus may be necessary during the neurosurgical interventions if inspection of the posterior table reveals bony infection with perforation or necrosis [30, 38]. For some refractory cases, obliteration procedures can be made. In all cases, the pus in the frontal sinus and the subperiosteal abscess was evacuated followed by bone debridement. The diseased sinus mucosa was removed. A draining silastic tube was then placed from the frontal sinus into the nasal cavity [39].

Complementary Otogenic Surgery

Patients with otomastoiditis may need local treatment of the auditory canal including careful cleaning and debridement in addition to topical application of antimicrobial agents. Sequestra and other necrotic tissue should be removed. Initially, treatment may include the application of antimicrobial-impregnated dressings to the canal.

Most destructive lesions may need a post auricular approach under general anesthesia. The skin with the periosteum was elevated over the mastoid and along the external auditory canal. The necrotic cartilage and the osteomyelitic bone segment of the external auditory canal and the mastoid bone were drilled out until healthy bone was present without opening up the whole of the mastoid. A wide meatoplasty can be performed. An antibiotic pack was placed and changed every 2 days until the wound healed [39]. The role of surgery is not very well defined, except for biopsy and local debridement of necrotic tissue and drainage of abscess or formal tympanomastoid procedures such as modified radical or radical mastoidectomy with partial petrous apicectomy and embolectomy for jugular vein thrombosis [40]. Concern exists that surgery may enhance necrotizing otitis externa and skull base osteomyelitis by opening up facial spaces and new soft tissue plane with spreading infection [9].

Post-craniotomy Osteomyelitis

The principles of treatment of post-operative cranial osteomyelitis are grossly the same as those described above; however, certain peculiarities should be considered.

The wound has to be widely opened and specimens are collected for biologic studies (Figs. 10.14, 10.15, 10.16, and 10.17). The bone flap can be removed if needed (Fig. 10.18). An extensive, radical surgical debridement is mandatory: the main goal for managing persistent infective changes in a cranial flap, is the visual removal of all foreign material and all nonviable and grossly infected tissues (Fig. 10.19). The edges of the skull should be rongeured back to healthy bone

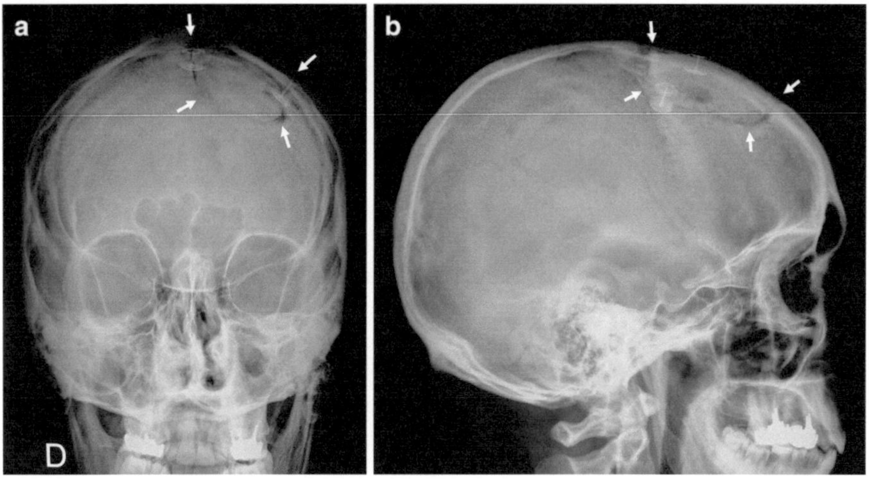

Fig. 10.14 Antero-posterior (**a**) and lateral (**b**) skull radiographies with confirmed post-operative chronic osteomyelitis. This patient was operated on 2 months previously for a malignant glioma with complementary radio and chimiotherapy (case number five)

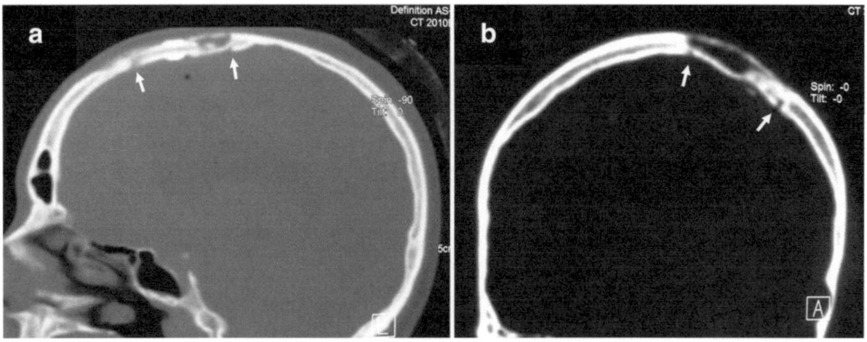

Fig. 10.15 Cranial CT-scan in bone windows: sagittal (**a**) and coronal (**b**) reconstructions demonstrating the chronic bone flap infection (case number five)

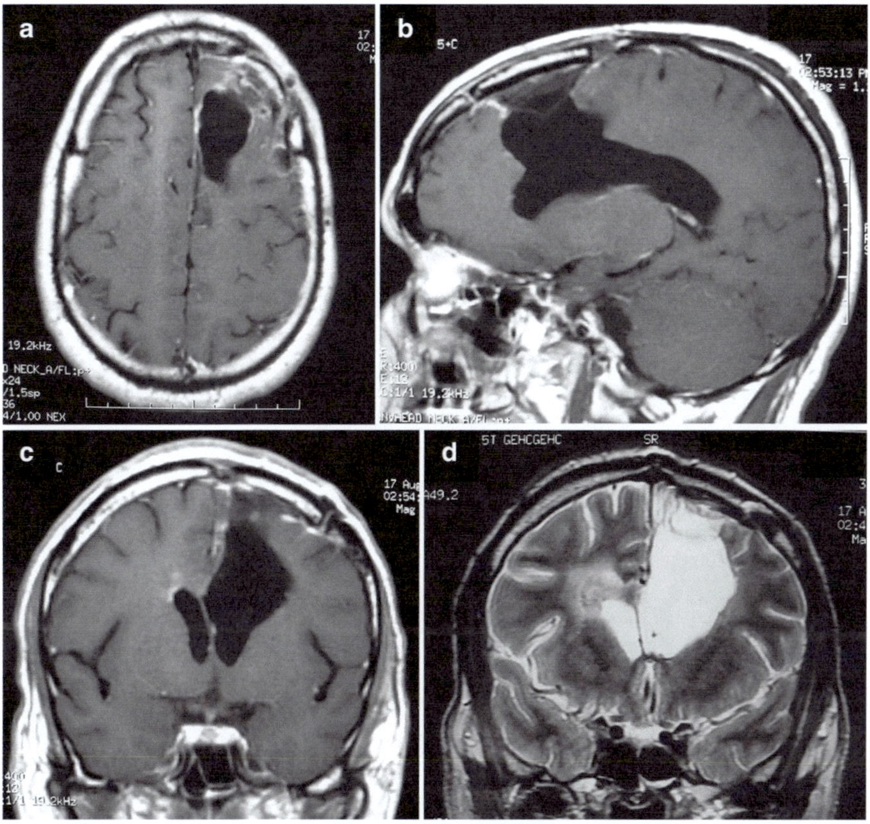

Fig. 10.16 MRI appearance of the chronic bone flap osteomyelitis. Cranial MRI on T1-weighted images after gadolinium injection (axial (**a**), sagittal (**b**), and coronal (**c**) views). Axial T2-weighted image (**d**) (case number five)

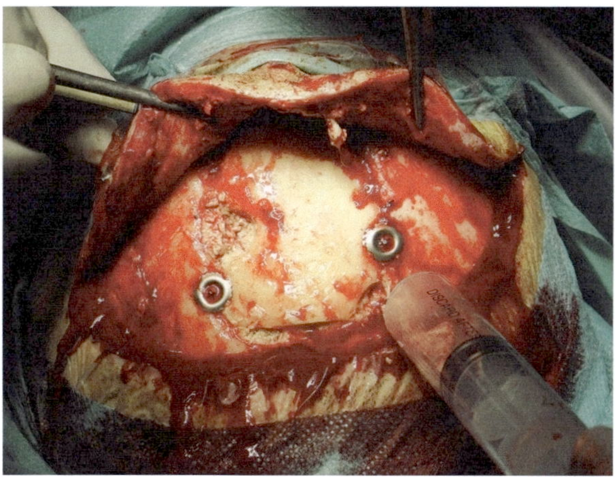

Fig. 10.17 Operative view of the infected bone flap before its removal (case number five)

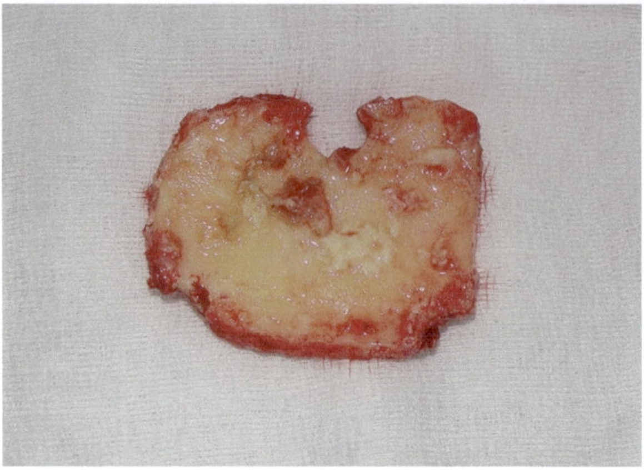

Fig. 10.18 Operative photograph of the cranial bone "moth-eaten" appearance after the bone flap was lifted (case number five)

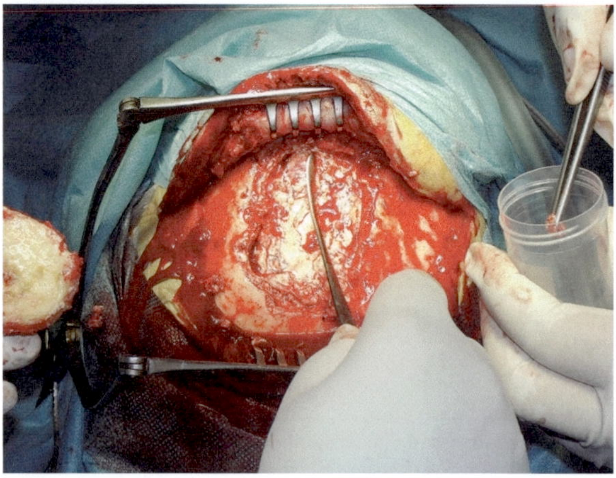

Fig. 10.19 Operative view during surgical debridement of the site infection (case number five)

followed by irrigation with antiseptic solution. It is important to keep in mind that reestablishment of well-perfused tissues enhances antibiotics and anti-microbial defense delivery to potential and actual infected areas. One of our patients developed a mild epidural fronto-epidural empyema 1 month following a pterional approach for intracranial vascular malformation. A 1-week antibiotic therapy was administered without improvement. When re-operated, an undetected infectious granuloma with absorbent cotton fibers (textiloma) was found into the epidural space (Fig. 10.20). Surgeons need to consider seriously the risk of leaving an inert foreign body in the operative field: certainly a factor of subsequent (re)infection [41]. For Boeckx et al., the cause of the continuing infection was owing to the fact that an extensive, radical wound debridement had not been well performed [3]. At the end of the surgical procedure a drain must be placed and the wound closed without additional tension with monofilament nylon or wire. Antibiotic therapy is

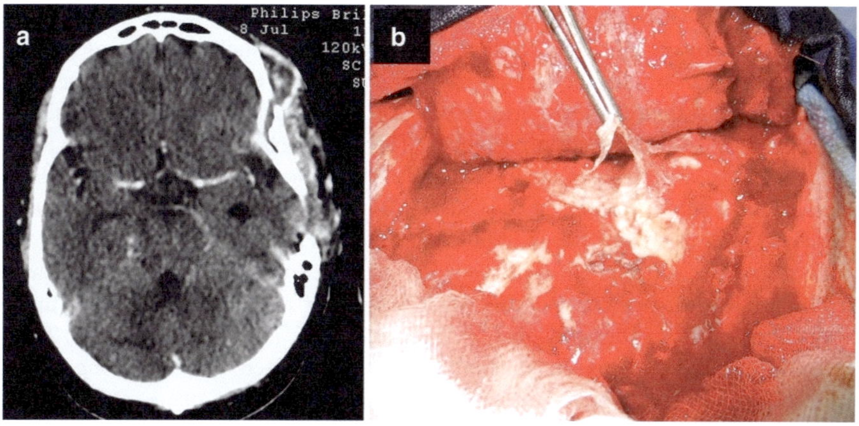

Fig. 10.20 Postoperative cranial CT-scan, axial section after contrast injection revealing left epidural abscess with frontal extracranial collection (**a**). Operative view after bone flap removal (**b**). The infection was likely due to epidural cotton left behind during surgical time

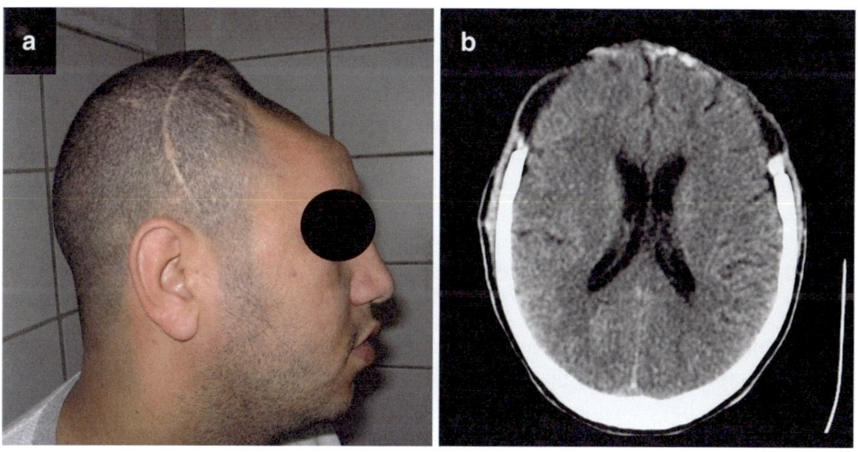

Fig. 10.21 Patient with previous decompressive bifrontal craniectomy. Note the somehow disfiguring deformity (**a**). Axial cranial CT-scan showing the exposed underlying brain (**b**) (case number six)

always considered (see Chap. 11 about antimicrobial and medical therapy) and a delayed cranioplasty can be performed several months later.

When the bone flap is of a significant size, some authors reproach some significant downsides including cosmetic results (disfiguring deformity), increased risk for trauma-related brain injury (unprotected brain), emergence of "*syndrome of the trephined*", and an additional surgery for the delayed cranioplasty [42–45] (Fig. 10.21). Recently, some surgical methods have been suggested to salvage the bone flap in position without requiring a delayed cranioplasty. For Bruce and Bruce, in patients with uncomplicated post-craniotomy infections, simple operative debridement is sufficient and it is not necessary to remove the bone flaps and perform cranioplasties. Even patients with risk factors such as prior surgery or radiotherapy can usually be treated using this strategy. On the contrary, patients who undergo craniofacial surgeries involving the paranasal sinuses are at higher risk and may require bone flap removal. This approach was successful in 11 of 13 patients presented [46]. In more difficult cases, a "*wash-in, wash-out indwelling antibiotic irrigation system*" was used by Auguste and McDermott: this suction/irrigation system contains four drains: one infusion and one suction drain in the epidural space, and one infusion and one suction drain in the subgaleal space. Antibiotic was infused continuously for 5 days along with administration of intravenous antibiotics. The infection resolved in 11 of 12 patients [47]. In 2009, Delgado-López et al. presented another alternative based on "*in situ bone flap sterilization*". The operative technique consisted on three maneuvers: wound debridement, bone flap sterilization (either autoclaved in 130 °C and atmospheric pressure for 20 min or soaked in a sterilizing solution), and insertion of subgaleal/epidural drains for non-continuous antibiotic irrigation (vancomycin 50 mg in 20 cc of saline every 12 h alternating with cefotaxim 100 mg in 20 cc of saline every 12 h). This technique was successful in all five patients managed [42]. With large bone flap infection needing extensive surgical debridement, immediate reconstruction with titanium mesh was also successfully employed by Kshettry et al. in 10 of 12 cases [48]. Although all these procedures may present good option, the number of patients is too small to allow their general approval in the treatment of bone flap infections [43].

Scalp and Cranial Bone Reconstruction

Management of scalp and/or cranial bone defect (either primary or secondary) often requires cooperative neurosurgical and plastic surgical expertise [49]. Reconstructive techniques have a wide range of options from primary closure for small defects to free tissue transfer for defects that are larger and more complex [50].

Scalp Reconstruction

Specific scalp reconstructive options including primary closure, skin grafts, issue expansion, local and regional flaps, and free tissue transfer, exist to provide durable soft tissue coverage, protection of intracranial structures, and control of cerebrospinal leaks [50, 51].

When a scalp defect is only few centimeters in diameter, primary closure is the acceptable form of treatment. Therefore, wide undermining and galeal scoring help in advancement and reduce the tension on the final wound closure. Excessive tension on wound closure should be avoided because the scalp tissue would retract

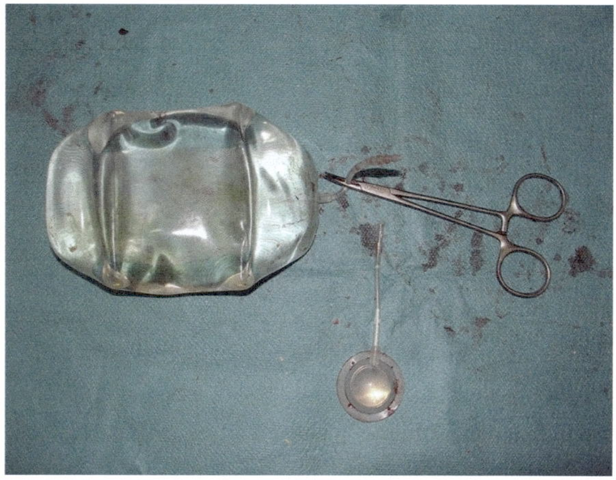

Fig. 10.22 An expandable silicone device (partial inflation of the expander) (case number seven)

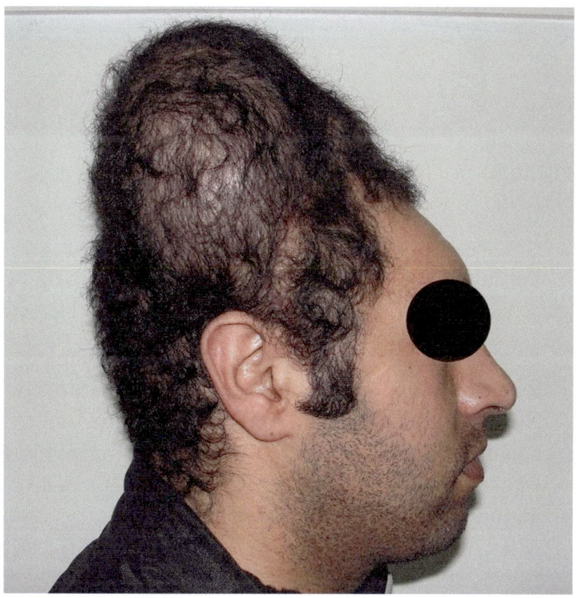

Fig. 10.23 Lateral view of a patient with expander implanted (case number seven)

leaving a scarred contracted soft tissue envelope which can induce an area of denuded cranial bone.

If a scalp defect is too large for primary closure, a primary split-thickness skin graft can be used as long as there is a vascularized bed underneath the scalp affected [52]. Tissue expansion of the surrounding scalp can also be used to permit the surgeon to have a more important quantity of "scalp" for coverage. For this technique, an expandable silicone device (Fig. 10.22) is placed under the adjacent uninjured subgaleal plane and is inflated acutely to help cover smaller defects or chronically (2–3 months) [51] (Figs. 10.23 and 10.24). Defects of 20 × 17 cm or approximately 50 % of the scalp can be reconstructed with expanded scalp tissue [53].

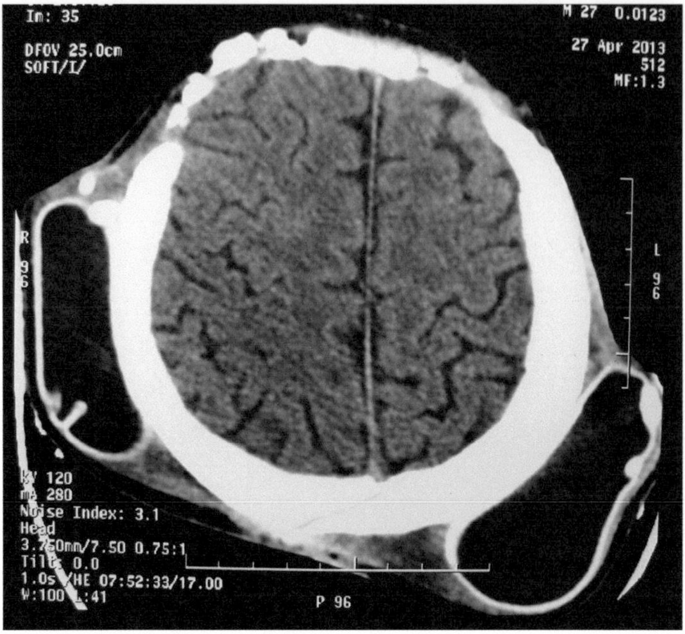

Fig. 10.24 Axial cranial CT-scan showing two expander devices implanted in the subgaleal plane bilaterally (case number seven)

For larger defects of the scalp or when the quality of the scalp is compromised, a great variation of scalp reconstruction methods is used [51, 54, 55]:

- **Local flaps** consist of transposition, advancement, and rotation flaps based on the occipital or superficial temporal artery [56–59].
- **Regional flaps** offer an appropriate alternative to local flaps when there is a hostile wound condition adjacent to the primary scalp defect [60]. The most frequently used regional flaps are the trapezius, latissimus dorsi, pectoralis major, and splenius capitus flaps.
- **Microvascular free tissue transfer** is used for large defect and/or when local tissues are undamaged, or if exposed dura must be covered immediately [49, 61, 62]. An important advantage of free tissue transfer is that it brings well-vascularized soft tissue from a distant site. In addition, free tissue transfer would have provided a more appropriate volume of soft tissue with which to close the potential dead space [63, 64]. Fascio-cutaneous flaps are representing by radial forearm, anterolateral thigh, groing, and scapula. Muscle flaps including latissimus dorsi, serratus anterior, rectus abdominis, or vastus lateralis muscle can be used with or without a skin island [3, 49, 51, 60, 65]. In the setting of infection, the use of muscular free flaps has been classically favored over cutaneous flaps [66, 67]. The omental flap is a good alternative with a rich vascularization, large surface area, and great pliability [3, 51].

Generally, the donor sites are sutured directly or covered with split-thickness skin [55].

Vacuum assisted closure therapy may be useful for the management of difficult cranial wounds. The principles of treatment is exposure of the wound bed to negative pressure, resulting in elimination of edema fluid, enhancement of the blood supply, and stimulation of cellular proliferation of reparative granulation tissue [68]. Many authors reported successful treatment of chronic scalp wounds with exposed dura or cortical brain and chronic infection using vacuum assisted closure therapy. The aims of this procedure are to create a setting for wound closure, secondary healing and skin transplantation [68–71].

Cranial Bone Reconstruction

The main objectives of cranial bone reconstruction (cranioplasty) are to restore the normal barriers protecting the intracranial structures (together with a satisfactory cosmetic result), obtain a permanent or very durable reconstruction using biologically inert materials and to avoid syndrome of the trephined [44, 45].

Many options for cranioplasty are available including alloplastic reconstruction, allergenic or autogenous bone graft. There are various alloplastic cranioplasty materials available that offer protection similar to that of native osseous tissue such as polymethylmethacrylate (Fig. 10.25), hydroxyapatite, polylactic/polyglycolic acid, and polyetheretherketone (PEEK) [72–74]. However, dynamic titanium mesh has the favorable qualities of high tensile strength and biologic inertness. Indeed, multiple studies have demonstrated lower rates of infection with titanium mesh used in cranial surgery [55, 75–77]. More recently, many

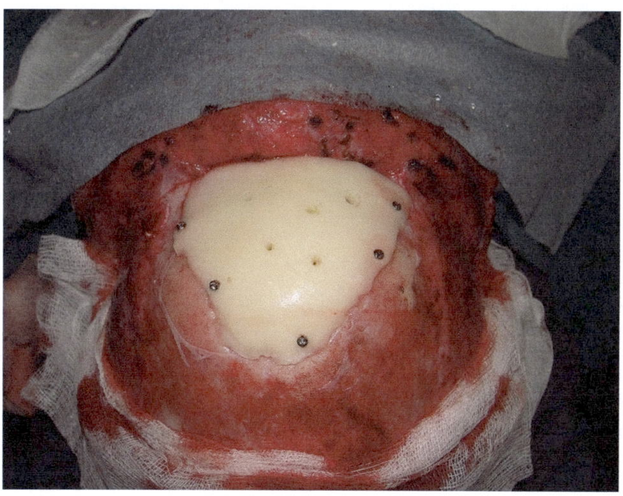

Fig. 10.25 Operative view of a frontal polymethylmethacrylate cranioplasty

techniques have evolved to produce tailored implants preoperatively using CT-scan imaging based data to reduce operative time and avoid risks with heat-curing exposure in the case of polymethylmethacrylate [74, 78–80]. Classic autologous bone can be taken from the adjacent cranial vault, the ribs, or the iliac crest [49, 65, 81, 82]. According to Psillakis et al., the easiest method to obtain a cranial autogenous bone graft is to achieve a full-thickness osteoperiosteal (craniotomy) flap followed by separation of the internal and external surfaces by intradiploic route using a pneumatic saw or a pediatric Gigli saw along the cutting line [83, 84]. For Artico and co-authors, the mechanical, immunologic, and technical-grafting properties of autologous bone, together with its superior esthetic and psychological effects, probably make it the best material for cranioplasty [82]. On the contrary and based on Piitulainen's study of 100 patients who underwent cranioplasty for bone defects [autograft (n = 20), bioactive fiber-reinforced composite (n = 20), hydroxyapatite (n = 31), and other synthetic materials (n = 29)], synthetic materials for cranial bone defect reconstruction exhibit more promising outcomes compared with autograft [81]. In another recent study performing by Wiggins et al., over a 14-year period in which 127 titanium cranioplasties were achieved on 113 patients, 18 infections (16 %) developed (among them three cases after more than 6 years). Infectious complication was significantly more common after titanium cranioplasty for large defects (hemicraniectomy [39 %] and bifrontal craniectomy [28 %]) than after cranioplasty for small defects. In addition, there is a relatively high frequency of reinfection in case of involvement of the frontal sinuses [85]. For Knöringer, the rate of reinfection was 3 % in osteomyelitis of the cranial vault without involvement of the sinuses and 25 % in case of involvement of the frontal sinuses [86]. Vigorous perioperative infection prophylaxis is needed for all procedures of cranioplasty. The long latency period for some chronic cranioplasty infection should be underlined. Some anecdotic cases may be completely asymptomatic. A 52-old-woman had a frontal infected polymethylmethacrylate cranioplasty with surrounding cranial bone infection occurring 25 years (1989–2014) after initial craniotomy for brain tuberculoma (Figs. 10.26, 10.27, 10.28, and 10.29).

Finally, in pediatric population, some patients who had a craniectomy for osteomyelitis did not require a cranioplasty because of a good cosmetic result from new bone formation in situ due to osteogenic potential of dura matter [87].

Timing of Reconstruction

From a practical point of view, acute procedures are limited to soft-tissue reconstruction only, and cranioplasty can be delayed to a second-stage procedure. There is no consensus as to the appropriate time for delayed cranioplasty, and the timing varies from several weeks to as long as a year [88–90]. The traditional

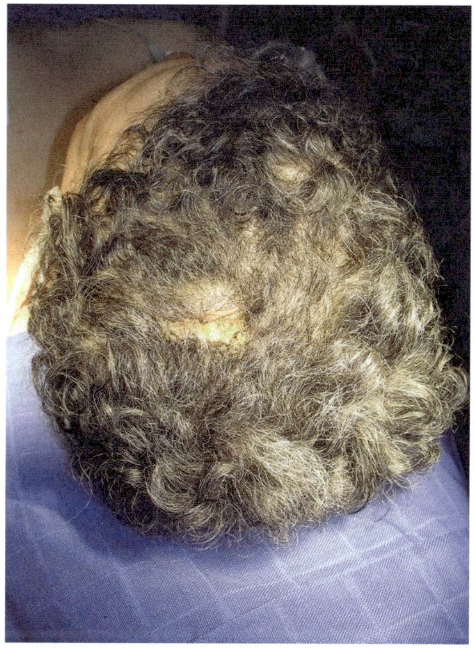

Fig. 10.26 This 47-year-old woman had a polymethylmethacrylate cranioplasty placed 25 years previously after initial craniotomy for brain tuberculoma. The acrylic plate become infected and over time become exposed with surrounding osteomyelitis (case number eight)

neurosurgical dictum stated that "a shorter time from craniectomy to cranioplasty is associated with poor outcome" [91–93]. According to the large series of 1030 cranioplasty procedures reported by Rish et al., cranioplasties taking place 1–6 months after craniectomy had the highest complication rate (7.9 %) and those performed between 12 and 18 months after craniectomy had the lowest complication rate (4.5 %) [90]. The purported advantage of this waiting period includes avoidance of operating on a potentially contaminated wound [90]. However, most authors agree on achievement of antimicrobial therapy and correct healing of the soft tissues without inflammatory symptoms [94]. Based on our experience and that of others, the bone defect is closed following a minimum of 6 months after the healing of the infection. In the opposite, some surgical teams, especially Japanese, use free flaps as composite flaps for simultaneous vascularized bone and soft tissue reconstruction (without any secondary cranioplasty) with excellent results [49, 65, 95, 96]. This method reduces the risk of bone resorption and help in combating possible residual infection. However, the small number of patients limits the strength of any conclusions to be made regarding these data.

Anyway, when scalp and/or bone reconstruction has been performed, a correct *hemostasis* is required and a *drain* must be left in place to avoid epidural hematoma. The presence of large hematoma around the plasty provides a good culture medium for the growth of bacteria and promotes secondary infection.

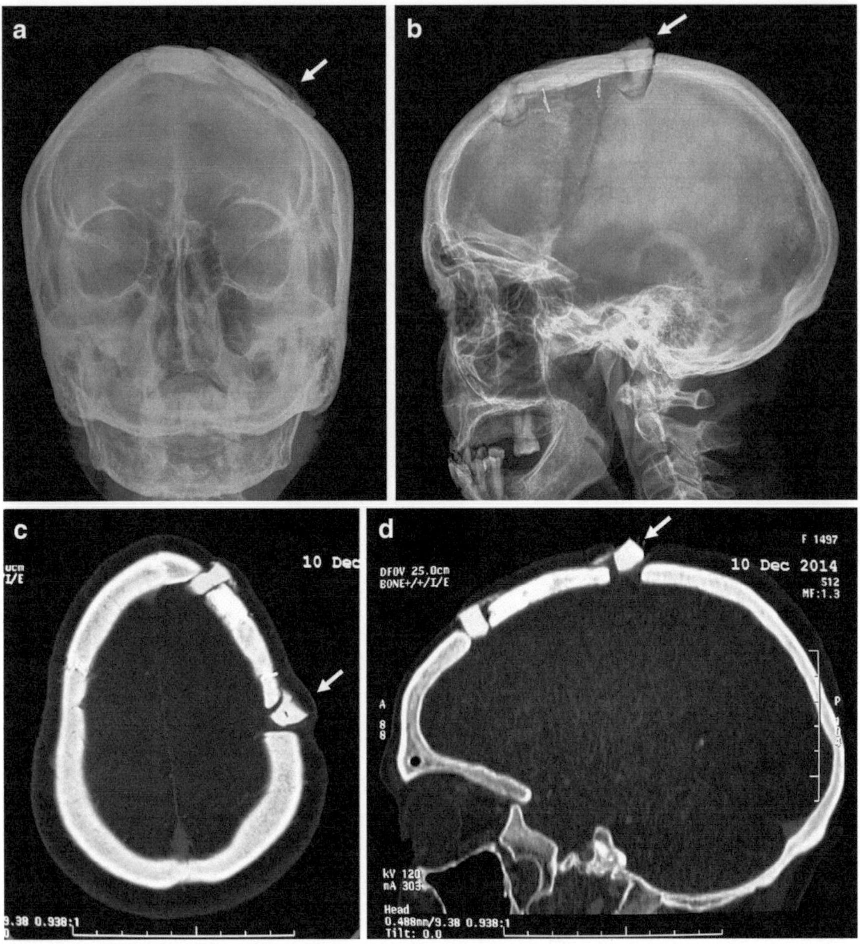

Fig. 10.27 The exposed acrylic plate (cranioplasty). Antero-posterior (**a**) and lateral (**b**) skull radiographies. Cranial CT-scan in bone windows: axial (**c**) and sagittal (**d**) reconstructions (case number eight)

Conservative Versus Surgical Therapy

Surgery in itself is not curative, but it is an important part of treatment in many cases to make conditions that will allow antibiotic drugs to penetrate the infected areas and therefore helping to supply curative therapy. In general, the probability of success is maximized by the removal of as much infectious material as possible. However, it is clear that exact treatment varies according to the cranial bones involved, the severity of the infection and the comorbidities of the patient (Table 10.2).

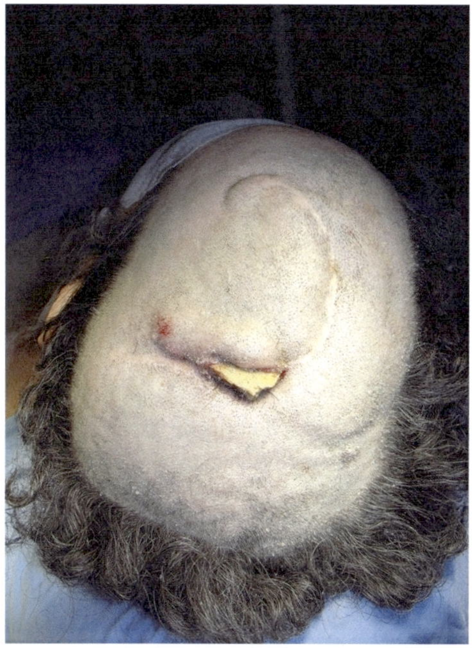

Fig. 10.28 After shaving, we can see the exposed acrylic plate (case number eight)

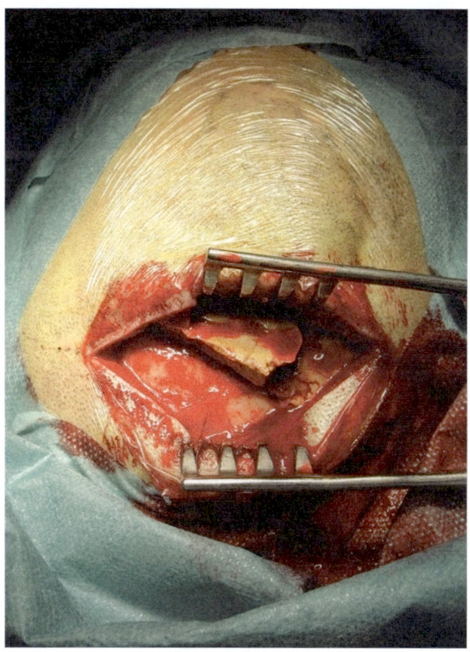

Fig. 10.29 Operative view of the exposed acrylic plate before removal (case number eight)

Table 10.2 Factors that may indicate surgical approach

Factors	Details
Need for diagnosis	Provides tissue for bacteriologic and histopathologic studies
Removal of massive cranial bone erosion	Especially necrotic and non-viable bone
Important intracranial suppurative collections	With brain mass effect or increasing intracranial pressure
Extracranial sinus tracts	Discharging cutaneous or scalp sinuses
Devascularized bone flap	Non-viable bone
Progression or prolonged disease despite adequate antimicrobial therapy	Refractory osteomyelitis
Recurrence of cranial osteomyelitis	

In some cases, cranial osteomyelitis can be managed conservatively without surgical intervention. This choice must be made carefully and with due consideration given to the neuroimaging characteristics of the site of cranial osteomyelitis, its intracranial extension, the neurologic status of the patient and the type of the pathogen suspected. Medical therapy alone can be considered especially for patients with small lesion, very limited disease extension, no intracranial mass effect, no neurologic symptoms or deficits, and an early favorable response to antibiotics. This category of patients must be followed carefully and frequently re-evaluated (clinically, biologically and on neuroimaging basis) and when necessary surgical intervention must be maintained. In addition, conservative management may be suggested in patients with poorly clinical conditions or when comorbidities such as sepsis and coagulopathy require correction before surgery.

In the skull base, surgical therapy is often not recommended because of the high risk of complication [97]. However, surgical procedure can be limited to biopsy, drainage of voluminous abscesses, debridement of soft tissue, and removal of bone sequestrum if possible [98]. For these reasons, some authors advocated that with typical clinical picture and imaging findings jointly with a positive response to ciprofloxacin, the diagnosis of skull base osteomyelitis can be made without the need for biopsies [99]. However, as mentioned by many others, this condition occurs rarely and in varied form clinically and on neuroimaging [98–101]. So, we believe that surgical biopsy (can also be taken endoscopically) is inevitably required to ensure both the absence of malignancy and to help consequent microbiological advice [98, 102]. For a practical point of view, it seems that aggressive surgical debridement is recommended in fungal skull base osteomyelitis but is probably unnecessary in patients with bacterial osteomyelitis of the skull base [103–106].

By contrast, aggressive surgical debridement and resection of devitalized tissue are considered necessary for cure of cranial vault osteomyelitis. In addition, surgical intervention is indicated if the patient did not improve clinically although receiving appropriate intravenous antimicrobial therapy or if an important extracranial or intracranial abscess is formed [107].

Neuroimaging characteristics help greatly on surgical decision by evaluating the consistency of suppurative collections. Commonly, collections that are fluid and thus easily drained tend to be hyperintense on T2-weighted images (WI) and to enhance only peripherally around a central part of hypointensity on T1-WI. More solid organized lesions (granulation tissue) tend to enhance throughout and to appear iso or hypointense on T2-WI. When such lesion is present, small, and the patient is neurologically intact, medical therapy alone may be adequate. If a patient has neuroimaging signs of a fluid collection but lacks any neurologic compromise, the decision is more controversial. Certainly abscesses near the skull base are less surgically strained, whereas those in the cranial vault convexity are more surgically accessible.

As seen above, indications for surgery remain somewhat difficult between acute and chronic forms of cranial osteomyelitis. Routinely, abscess formation from the cranial bone requires drainage and debridement of necrotic material, placement of a drainage catheter, and wound closure. In cases of acute osteomyelitis without suppurative collection or intracranial complications, antibiotherapy alone may be adequate.

When infection persists or progress despite antibiotics or when it recurs, reoperation may be necessary. In this scenario, a search for sequestered and devascularized bone is required, and thus a craniectomy is commonly performed with reconstruction thereafter.

The algorithm for management of patients with associated intracranial suppurative complications has yet to be determined. Literature data continue to support that larger intracranial abscesses (more than 2 cm in diameter) require early neurosurgical drainage when accessible (open surgery or stereotactic approach). Smaller intracranial abscesses (less than 2 cm in diameter) can be treated with initial medical management with intravenous antibiotics and serial radiologic evaluation to assess for improvement or progression of disease [17, 29].

For patients with signs of hydrocephalus or with posterior fossa empyema and/or abscess exerting mass effect on the fourth ventricle (Fig. 10.30), an external

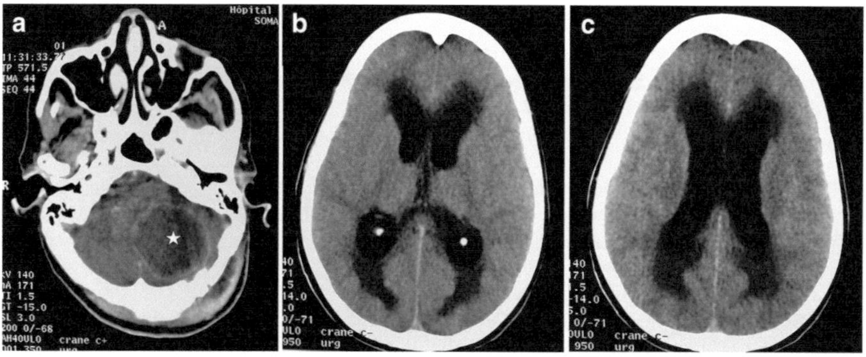

Fig. 10.30 Axial CT-scan with (**a**) and without (**b** and **c**) contrast injection showing an occipital extracranial abscess with adjacent osteomyelitis an left cerebellar abscess (*star*) exerting mass effect on the fourth ventricle. Note the secondary acute hydrocephalus (**b** and **c**)

ventricular drain should be placed to prevent CSF obstruction. The CSF drainage will be either gradually withdrawn over time and removed or replaced by a definitive shunt at a later time. In any case, permanent shunt hardware is not placed until it has been demonstrated that the CSF is sterile on multiple cultures [108].

Finally, HBOT has been described as a valuable adjunct in managing refractory cases of post-surgical cranial osteomyelitis (salvage of skull-bone flaps and acrylic cranioplasties) as well as for invasive malignant external otitis with skull base osteomyelitis (see Chap. 12). Overall, the success rate is between 87.5 and 100 % [109–112]. Moreover, HBOT procedure was particularly useful in patients with impaired immunological defenses.

References

1. Fleming H. Osteomyelitis of the skull. Cal West Med. 1925;23(8):985–8.
2. Phillips K. Osteomyelitis of the skull. J Neurosurg Nurs. 1982;14(5):280–2.
3. Boeckx WD, van der Hulst RR, Nanhekhan LV, De Lorenzi F. The role of free flaps in the treatment of persistent scalp osteomyelitis. Neurosurgery. 2006;59(1 Suppl 1):ONS64–7.
4. Greenberg MS. Osteomyelitis of the skull. In: Greenberg MS, editor. Handbook of neurosurgery. 6th ed. New York: Thieme; 2006.
5. Wilensky AO. Osteomyelitis of the skull. Arch Surg. 1933;27(1):83–158.
6. Johnson AK, Batra PS. Central skull base osteomyelitis: an emerging clinical entity. Laryngoscope. 2014;124(5):1083–7. doi:10.1002/lary.24440.
7. Patmore H, Jebreel A, Uppal S, Raine CH, McWhinney P. Skull base infection presenting with multiple lower cranial nerve palsies. Am J Otolaryngol. 2010;31(5):376–80. doi:10.1016/j.amjoto.2009.04.001.
8. Mani N, Sudhoff H, Rajagopal S, Moffat D, Axon PR. Cranial nerve involvement in malignant external otitis: implications for clinical outcome. Laryngoscope. 2007;117(5):907–10.
9. Amorosa L, Modugno GC, Pirodda A. Malignant external otitis: review and personal experience. Acta Otolaryngol Suppl. 1996;521:3–16.
10. Kraus DH, Rehm SJ, Kinney SE. The evolving treatment of necrotizing external otitis. Laryngoscope. 1988;98(9):934–9.
11. Chandler JR, Grobman L, Quencer R, Serafini A. Osteomyelitis of the base of the skull. Laryngoscope. 1986;96(3):245–51.
12. McCall TD, Fults DW, Schmidt RH. Use of resorbable collagen dural substitutes in the presence of cranial and spinal infections—report of 3 cases. Surg Neurol. 2008;70(1):92–6. doi:10.1016/j.surneu.2007.04.007.
13. Nathoo N, Nadvi SS, van Dellen JR. Cranial extradural empyema in the era of computed tomography: a review of 82 cases. Neurosurgery. 1999;44(4):748–53.
14. Bok AP, Peter JC. Subdural empyema: burr holes or craniotomy? A retrospective computerized tomography-era analysis of treatment in 90 cases. J Neurosurg. 1993;78(4):574–8.
15. Nathoo N, Nadvi SS, Gouws E, van Dellen JR. Craniotomy improves outcomes for cranial subdural empyemas: computed tomography-era experience with 699 patients. Neurosurgery. 2001;49(4):872–7.
16. Tankell A. Subdural empyema, epidural abscess, and suppurative intracranial thrombophlebitis. In: Mandell GL, Bennett JE, Dolin R, editors. Mandell, Douglas, and Bennett's principles and practices of infectious diseases. 6th ed. Philadelphia, PA: Elsevier Churchill Livingstone; 2005.

17. Akhaddar A, Elouennass M, Baallal H, Boucetta M. Focal intracranial infections due to Actinomyces species in immunocompetent patients: diagnostic and therapeutic challenges. World Neurosurg. 2010;74(2–3):346–50. doi:10.1016/j.wneu.2010.05.029.
18. Baer WS. The treatment of chronic osteomyelitis with the maggot (larva of the blow fly). J Bone Joint Surg Am. 1931;13:438–75.
19. McKeever DC. The classic: maggots in treatment of osteomyelitis: a simple inexpensive method. 1933. Clin Orthop Relat Res. 2008;466(6):1329–35. doi:10.1007/s11999-008-0240-5.
20. Galeano M, Ioli V, Colonna M, Risitano G. Maggot therapy for treatment of osteomyelitis and deep wounds: an old remedy for an actual problem. Plast Reconstr Surg. 2001;108 (7):2178–9.
21. Sherman RA, Pechter EA. Maggot therapy: a review of the therapeutic applications of fly larvae in human medicine, especially for treating osteomyelitis. Med Vet Entomol. 1988;2 (3):225–30.
22. Gilead L, Mumcuoglu KY, Ingber A. The use of maggot debridement therapy in the treatment of chronic wounds in hospitalised and ambulatory patients. J Wound Care. 2012;21(2):78. 80, 82–85.
23. French VM, Cooper RA, Molan PC. The antibacterial activity of honey against coagulase-negative staphylococci. J Antimicrob Chemother. 2005;56(1):228–31.
24. Ahmed AK, Hoekstra MJ, Hage JJ, Karim RB. Honey-medicated dressing: transformation of an ancient remedy into modern therapy. Ann Plast Surg. 2003;50(2):143–7.
25. Olusanya AA, Gbolahan OO, Aladelusi TO, Akinmoladun VI, Arotiba JT. Clinical parameters and challenges of managing cervicofacial necrotizing fasciitis in a Sub-Saharan Tertiary Hospital. Niger J Surg. 2015;21(2):134–9. doi:10.4103/1117-6806.162572.
26. Robson V, Dodd S, Thomas S. Standardized antibacterial honey (Medihoney) with standard therapy in wound care: randomized clinical trial. J Adv Nurs. 2009;65(3):565–75. doi:10.1111/j.1365-2648.2008.04923.x.
27. Zeiger B. The use of active Leptospermum honey dressings to re-initiate the wound healing process. Ostomy Wound Manage. 2010;56(1):10.
28. Jull AB, Cullum N, Dumville JC, Westby MJ, Deshpande S, Walker N. Honey as a topical treatment for wounds. Cochrane Database Syst Rev. 2015;3, CD005083. doi:10.1002/14651858.CD005083.pub4.
29. Bondar' VP, Nekhlopochin SN. [Surgical treatment of osteomyelitis of the frontal bone and the walls of the frontal sinus]. Vestn Otorinolaringol 1989;(1):42–5. Russian.
30. van Dijk JM, Wagemakers M, Korsten-Meijer AG, Kees Buiter CT, van der Laan BF, Mooij JJ. Cranialization of the frontal sinus—the final remedy for refractory chronic frontal sinusitis. J Neurosurg. 2012;116(3):531–5. doi:10.3171/2011.11.JNS101849.
31. Lang EE, Curran AJ, Patil N, Walsh RM, Rawluk D, Walsh MA. Intracranial complications of acute frontal sinusitis. Clin Otolaryngol Allied Sci. 2001;26(6):452–7.
32. Germiller JA, Monin DL, Sparano AM, Tom LW. Intracranial complications of sinusitis in children and adolescents and their outcomes. Arch Otolaryngol Head Neck Surg. 2006;132 (9):969–76.
33. DelGaudio JM, Evans SH, Sobol SE, Parikh SL. Intracranial complications of sinusitis: what is the role of endoscopic sinus surgery in the acute setting. Am J Otolaryngol. 2010;31 (1):25–8. doi:10.1016/j.amjoto.2008.09.009.
34. Herrmann BW, Chung JC, Eisenbeis JF, Forsen Jr JW. Intracranial complications of pediatric frontal rhinosinusitis. Am J Rhinol. 2006;20(3):320–4.
35. Jung J, Lee HC, Park IH, Lee HM. Endoscopic endonasal treatment of a Pott's puffy tumor. Clin Exp Otorhinolaryngol. 2012;5(2):112–5. doi:10.3342/ceo.2012.5.2.112.
36. Parida PK, Surianarayanan G, Ganeshan S, Saxena SK. Pott's puffy tumor in pediatric age group: a retrospective study. Int J Pediatr Otorhinolaryngol. 2012;76(9):1274–7. doi:10.1016/j.ijporl.2012.05.018.

37. Bozdemir K, Kutluhan A, Yalçıner G, Cetin H, Bilgen AS, Tarlak B. Treatment of Pott's Puffy tumor with balloon sinuplasty: report of three cases. Kulak Burun Bogaz Ihtis Derg. 2012;22(6):342–7. doi:10.5606/kbbihtisas.2012.065.
38. Lerner DN, Choi SS, Zalzal GH, Johnson DL. Intracranial complications of sinusitis in childhood. Ann Otol Rhinol Laryngol. 1995;104(4 Pt 1):288–93.
39. Prasad KC, Prasad SC, Mouli N, Agarwal S. Osteomyelitis in the head and neck. Acta Otolaryngol. 2007;127(2):194–205.
40. DeCesare GE, Deleyiannis FW-B, Losee JE. Reconstruction of osteomyelitis defects of the craniofacial skeleton. Semin Plast Surg. 2009;23(2):119–31. doi:10.1055/s-0029-1214164.
41. Akhaddar A, Boulahroud O, Naama O, Al-Bouzidi A, Boucetta M. Paraspinal textiloma after posterior lumbar surgery: a wolf in sheep's clothing. World Neurosurg. 2012;77(2):375–80. doi:10.1016/j.wneu.2011.07.017.
42. Delgado-López PD, Martín-Velasco V, Castilla-Díez JM, Galacho-Harriero AM, Rodríguez-Salazar A. Preservation of bone flap after craniotomy infection. Neurocirugia (Astur). 2009;20(2):124–31.
43. Wind JJ, Ohaegbulam C, Iwamoto FM, Black PM, Park JK. Immediate titanium mesh cranioplasty for treatment of postcraniotomy infections. World Neurosurg. 2013;79(1):207. e11–3. doi:10.1016/j.wneu.2011.02.013.
44. Annan M, De Toffol B, Hommet C, Mondon K. Sinking skin flap syndrome (or Syndrome of the trephined): a review. Br J Neurosurg. 2015;29(3):314–8. doi:10.3109/02688697.2015.1012047.
45. Jeyaraj P. Importance of early cranioplasty in reversing the "syndrome of the trephine/motor trephine syndrome/sinking skin flap syndrome". J Maxillofac Oral Surg. 2015;14(3):666–73. doi:10.1007/s12663-014-0673-1.
46. Bruce JN, Bruce SS. Preservation of bone flaps in patients with postcraniotomy infections. J Neurosurg. 2003;98(6):1203–7.
47. Auguste KI, McDermott MW. Salvage of infected craniotomy bone flaps with the wash-in, wash-out indwelling antibiotic irrigation system. Technical note and case series of 12 patients. J Neurosurg. 2006;105(4):640–4.
48. Kshettry VR, Hardy S, Weil RJ, Angelov L, Barnett GH. Immediate titanium cranioplasty after debridement and craniectomy for postcraniotomy surgical site infection. Neurosurgery. 2012;70(1 Suppl Operative):8–14. doi:10.1227/NEU.0b013e31822fef2c. discussion 14–5.
49. Baumeister S, Peek A, Friedman A, Levin LS, Marcus JR. Management of postneurosurgical bone flap loss caused by infection. Plast Reconstr Surg. 2008;122(6):195e–208. doi:10.1097/PRS.0b013e3181858eee.
50. Seitz IA, Adler N, Odessey E, Reid RR, Gottlieb LJ. Latissimus dorsi/rib intercostal perforator myo-osseocutaneous free flap reconstruction in composite defects of the scalp: case series and review of literature. J Reconstr Microsurg. 2009;25(9):559–67. doi:10.1055/s-0029-1236834.
51. Tutela JP, Banta JC, Boyd TG, Kelishadi SS, Chowdhry S, Little JA. Scalp reconstruction: a review of the literature and a unique case of total craniectomy in an adult with osteomyelitis of the skull. Eplasty. 2014;14:e27.
52. Hoffman JF. Management of scalp defects. Otolaryngol Clin North Am. 2001;34(3):571–82.
53. Wieslander JB. Tissue expansion in the head and neck. A 6-year review. Scand J Plast Reconstr Surg Hand Surg. 1991;25(1):47–56.
54. Leedy JE, Janis JE, Rohrich RJ. Reconstruction of acquired scalp defects: an algorithmic approach. Plast Reconstr Surg. 2005;116(4):54e–72.
55. Lu Y, Cen Y, Qing Y, Wang H. [Surgical treatment of chronic osteomyelitis of the skull]. Zhongguo Xiu Fu Chong Jian Wai Ke Za Zhi. 2011;25(5):558–61. Chinese.
56. Beasley NJ, Gilbert RW, Gullane PJ, Brown DH, Irish JC, Neligan PC. Scalp and forehead reconstruction using free revascularized tissue transfer. Arch Facial Plast Surg. 2004;6(1):16–20.

57. Uppal HS, Issa F, Byren I, Johnson D. A case of pancalvarial osteomyelitis: diagnosis and management. J Plast Reconstr Aesthet Surg. 2010;63(2):e159–60. doi:10.1016/j.bjps.2009.05.015.
58. Kim JC, Hadlock T, Varvares MA, Cheney ML. Hair-bearing temporoparietal fascial flap reconstruction of upper lip and scalp defects. Arch Facial Plast Surg. 2001;3(3):170–7.
59. Guerrissi JO. Reconstruction of large defects in the scalp with fasciocutaneous flaps. Scand J Plast Reconstr Surg Hand Surg. 1999;33(2):217–24.
60. Lutz BS. Scalp and forehead reconstruction. Semin Plast Surg. 2010;24(2):171–80. doi:10.1055/s-0030-1255334.
61. Varvares MA, Lin D, Hadlock T, Azzizadeh B, Gliklich R, Rounds M, Rocco J, Deschler DG, Fabian R, Cheney ML. Success of multiple, sequential, free tissue transfers to the head and neck. Laryngoscope. 2005;115(1):101–4.
62. Lin YT, Chen CT, Lai JP. Post-traumatic fronto-ethmoid osteomyelitis treated with free muscle transfer. J Plast Reconstr Aesthet Surg. 2010;63(6):963–9. doi:10.1016/j.bjps.2009.03.017.
63. Newman MI, Hanasono MM, Disa JJ, Cordeiro PG, Mehrara BJ. Scalp reconstruction: a 15-year experience. Ann Plast Surg. 2004;52(5):501–6.
64. Editorial Board of Plastic and Reconstructive Surgery. Management of a complex scalp defect. Plast Reconstr Surg. 2008;122(2):623–5. doi:10.1097/PRS.0b013e31817d7f91.
65. Kurokawa M, Inoue K. One stage reconstruction of the skull defect following chronic osteomyelitis using a serratus anterior muscle rib osteomyocutaneous free flap. Eur J Plast Surg. 1994;17(4):204–7.
66. Chang N, Mathes SJ. Comparison of the effect of bacterial inoculation in musculocutaneous and random-pattern flaps. Plast Reconstr Surg. 1982;70(1):1–10.
67. Fisher J, Wood MB. Experimental comparison of bone revascularization by musculocutaneous and cutaneous flaps. Plast Reconstr Surg. 1987;79(1):81–90.
68. Powers AK, Neal MT, Argenta LC, Wilson JA, DeFranzo AJ, Tatter SB. Vacuum-assisted closure for complex cranial wounds involving the loss of dura mater. J Neurosurg. 2013;118(2):302–8. doi:10.3171/2012.10.JNS112241.
69. Prince N, Blackburn S, Murad G, Mast B, Sapountzis S, Shaw C, Werning J, Singhal D. Vacuum-assisted closure therapy to the brain: a safe method for wound temporization in composite scalp and calvarial defects. Ann Plast Surg. 2015;74 Suppl 4:S218–21. doi:10.1097/SAP.0000000000000374.
70. Ahmed O, Storey CM, Zhang S, Chelly MR, Yeoh MS, Nanda A. Vacuum-assisted closure of necrotic and infected cranial wound with loss of dura mater: a technical note. Surg Neurol Int. 2015;6:11. doi:10.4103/2152-7806.149846.
71. Subotic U, Kluwe W, Oesch V. Community-associated methicillin-resistant Staphylococcus aureus-infected chronic scalp wound with exposed dura in a 10-year-old boy: vacuum-assisted closure is a feasible option: case report. Neurosurgery. 2011;68(5):E1481–3. doi:10.1227/NEU.0b013e318210c7fb.
72. Eppley BL. Biomechanical testing of alloplastic PMMA cranioplasty materials. J Craniofac Surg. 2005;16(1):140–3.
73. Afifi AM, Gordon CR, Pryor LS, Sweeney W, Papay FA, Zins JE. Calcium phosphate cements in skull reconstruction: a meta-analysis. Plast Reconstr Surg. 2010;126(4):1300–9. doi:10.1097/PRS.0b013e3181ead057.
74. Jalbert F, Boetto S, Nadon F, Lauwers F, Schmidt E, Lopez R. One-step primary reconstruction for complex craniofacial resection with PEEK custom-made implants. J Craniomaxillofac Surg. 2014;42(2):141–8. doi:10.1016/j.jcms.2013.04.001.
75. Cabraja M, Klein M, Lehmann TN. Long-term results following titanium cranioplasty of large skull defects. Neurosurg Focus. 2009;26(6):E10. doi:10.3171/2009.3.FOCUS091.
76. Matsuno A, Tanaka H, Iwamuro H, Takanashi S, Miyawaki S, Nakashima M, Nakaguchi H, Nagashima T. Analyses of the factors influencing bone graft infection after delayed cranioplasty. Acta Neurochir (Wien). 2006;148(5):535–40.

77. Joffe J, Harris M, Kahugu F, Nicoll S, Linney A, Richards R. A prospective study of computer-aided design and manufacture of titanium plate for cranioplasty and its clinical outcome. Br J Neurosurg. 1999;13(6):576–80.
78. Lai JB, Sittitavornwong S, Waite PD. Computer-assisted designed and computer-assisted manufactured polyetheretherketone prosthesis for complex fronto-orbito-temporal defect. J Oral Maxillofac Surg. 2011;69(4):1175–80. doi:10.1016/j.joms.2010.05.034.
79. Dean D, Min KJ, Bond A. Computer aided design of large-format prefabricated cranial plates. J Craniofac Surg. 2003;14(6):819–32.
80. Chen ST, Chang CJ, Su WC, Chang LW, Chu IH, Lin MS. 3-D titanium mesh reconstruction of defective skull after frontal craniectomy in traumatic brain injury. Injury. 2015;46(1):80–5. doi:10.1016/j.injury.2014.09.019.
81. Piitulainen JM, Kauko T, Aitasalo KM, Vuorinen V, Vallittu PK, Posti JP. Outcomes of cranioplasty with synthetic materials and autologous bone grafts. World Neurosurg. 2015;83 (5):708–14. doi:10.1016/j.wneu.2015.01.014.
82. Artico M, Ferrante L, Pastore FS, Ramundo EO, Cantarelli D, Scopelliti D, Iannetti G. Bone autografting of the calvaria and craniofacial skeleton: historical background, surgical results in a series of 15 patients, and review of the literature. Surg Neurol. 2003;60(1):71–9.
83. Psillakis JM, Nocchi VL, Zanini SA. Repair of large defect of frontal bone with free graft of outer table of parietal bones. Plast Reconstr Surg. 1979;64(6):827–30.
84. Psillakis JM, Grotting JC, Casanova R, Cavalcante D, Vasconez LO. Vascularized outer-table calvarial bone flaps. Plast Reconstr Surg. 1986;78(3):309–17.
85. Wiggins A, Austerberry R, Morrison D, Ho KM, Honeybul S. Cranioplasty with custom-made titanium plates—14 years experience. Neurosurgery. 2013;72(2):248–56. doi:10.1227/NEU.0b013e31827b98f3.
86. Knöringer P. [Treatment of bone infection in the area of the skull]. Unfallchirurgie. 1986;12 (2):81–92. German.
87. Gupta S, Vachhrajani S, Kulkarni AV, Taylor MD, Dirks P, Drake JM, Rutka JT. Neurosurgical management of extraaxial central nervous system infections in children. J Neurosurg Pediatr. 2011;7(5):441–51. doi:10.3171/2011.2.PEDS09500.
88. Josan VA, Sgouros S, Walsh AR, Dover MS, Nishikawa H, Hockley AD. Cranioplasty in children. Childs Nerv Syst. 2005;21(3):200–4.
89. Lee C, Antonyshyn OM, Forrest CR. Cranioplasty: indications, technique, and early results of autogenous split skull cranial vault reconstruction. J Craniomaxillofac Surg. 1995;23 (3):133–42.
90. Rish BL, Dillon JD, Meirowsky AM, Caveness WF, Mohr JP, Kistler JP, Weiss GH. Cranioplasty: a review of 1030 cases of penetrating head injury. Neurosurgery. 1979;4 (5):381–5.
91. Shaffrey ME, Persing JA, Shaffrey CI, Delashaw JB, Jane JA. Craniofacial reconstruction. In: Apuzzo MLJ, editor. Brain surgery: complication and avoidance management. New York: Churchill Livingstone; 1993.
92. Prolo DJ. Cranial defects and cranioplasty. In: Wilkins RH, Rengachary SS, editors. Neurosurgery. 2nd ed. New York: McGraw-Hill; 1996.
93. Foster RD, Antonyshyn OM, Lee C, Holland M, Fazl M. Cranioplasty: indications, techniques, and results. In: Schmideck HH, editor. Schmidek and sweet operative neurosurgical techniques. Philadelphia: WB Saunders; 2000.
94. Kshettry VR, Angelov L. Technical note regarding immediate titanium mesh cranioplasty for postcraniotomy infections. World Neurosurg. 2014;81(3–4):e16. doi:10.1016/j.wneu.2013.08.057.
95. Hirase Y, Kojima T, Kinoshita Y, Bang HH, Sakaguchi T, Kijima M. Composite reconstruction for chest wall and scalp using multiple ribs-latissimus dorsi osteomyocutaneous flaps as pedicled and free flaps. Plast Reconstr Surg. 1991;87(3):555–61.
96. Ueda K, Harashina T, Inoue T, Tanaka I, Harada T. Microsurgical scalp and skull reconstruction using a serratus anterior myo-osseous flap. Ann Plast Surg. 1993;31(1):10–4.

97. Lee SJ, Weon YC, Cha HJ, Kim SY, Seo KW, Jegal Y, Ahn JJ, Ra SW. A case of atypical skull base osteomyelitis with septic pulmonary embolism. J Korean Med Sci. 2011;26 (7):962–5. doi:10.3346/jkms.2011.26.7.962.
98. Clark MP, Pretorius PM, Byren I, Milford CA. Central or atypical skull base osteomyelitis: diagnosis and treatment. Skull Base. 2009;19(4):247–54. doi:10.1055/s-0028-1115325.
99. Cavel O, Fliss DM, Segev Y, Zik D, Khafif A, Landsberg R. The role of the otorhinolaryngologist in the management of central skull base osteomyelitis. Am J Rhinol. 2007;21 (3):281–5.
100. Cunningham M, Yu VL, Turner J, Curtin H. Necrotizing otitis externa due to Aspergillus in an immunocompetent patient. Arch Otolaryngol Head Neck Surg. 1988;114(5):554–6.
101. Ridder GJ, Breunig C, Kaminsky J, Pfeiffer J. Central skull base osteomyelitis: new insights and implications for diagnosis and treatment. Eur Arch Otorhinolaryngol. 2015;272 (5):1269–76. doi:10.1007/s00405-014-3390-y.
102. Cunningham C. Transanal endoscopic microsurgery. Recent Results Cancer Res. 2014;203:31–8. doi:10.1007/978-3-319-08060-4_4.
103. Stodulski D, Kowalska B, Stankiewicz C. Otogenic skull base osteomyelitis caused by invasive fungal infection. Case report and literature review. Eur Arch Otorhinolaryngol. 2006;263(12):1070–6.
104. Blyth CC, Gomes L, Sorrell TC, da Cruz M, Sud A, Chen SC. Skull-base osteomyelitis: fungal vs. bacterial infection. Clin Microbiol Infect. 2011;17(2):306–11. doi:10.1111/j.1469-0691.2010.03231.x.
105. Laccourreye L, Halimi P, Bonfils P, Laccourreye O. Atypical pseudotumoral osteomyelitis of the skull base. Otolaryngol Head Neck Surg. 2007;137(3):524–5.
106. Ducic Y. Management of osteomyelitis of the anterior skull base and craniovertebral junction. Otolaryngol Head Neck Surg. 2003;128(1):39–42.
107. Adcock PM, Marshall GS. Osteomyelitis of the axial skeleton and the flat and small bones. Semin Pediatr Infect Dis. 1997;8:234–41.
108. Akhaddar A. Infective complications. In: Di Rocco C, Turgut M, Jallo G, Martinez-Lage DJF, editors. Complications of CSF shunting in hydrocephalus. Switzerland: Springer International; 2015.
109. Larsson A, Engström M, Uusijärvi J, Kihlström L, Lind F, Mathiesen T. Hyperbaric oxygen treatment of postoperative neurosurgical infections. Neurosurgery. 2002;50(2):287–95.
110. Martel J, Duclos JY, Darrouzet V, Guyot M, Bébéar JP. [Malignant or necrotizing otitis externa: experience in 22 cases]. Ann Otolaryngol Chir Cervicofac. 2000;117(5):291. French.
111. Narozny W, Kuczkowski J, Mikaszewski B. Infectious skull base osteomyelitis—still a life-threatening disease. Otol Neurotol. 2006;27(7):1047–8.
112. Davis JC, Gates GA, Lerner C, Davis MG, Mader JT, Dinesman A. Adjuvant hyperbaric oxygen in malignant external otitis. Arch Otolaryngol Head Neck Surg. 1992;118(1):89–93.

Chapter 11
Antimicrobial and Medical Therapy

Contents

Abbreviations

CSF Cerebrospinal fluid
MRSA Methicillin-resistant *Staphylococcus aureus*
VRSA Vancomycin-resistant *Staphylococcus aureus*

Medical therapy, especially antimicrobial therapy, is generally concomitant to surgical procedure. Antimicrobial agents require in particular a good penetration into the cranial bone, the meninges and the brain parenchyma. Antimicrobial treatment can be further divided into empirical and targeted treatment. As in other sites of the body, the duration of treatment of cranial osteomyelitis is not standardized. It mainly depends on the duration and extent of the infection, the rapidity of the clinical and laboratory response to treatment, and the quality of the initial surgical debridement. However, it is important to know that insufficient treatment duration leads to recurrence and increase the spread of antibiotic-resistant pathogens.

Additionally, various concomitant therapies may be added depending on potential comorbidities, the location of the cranial suppuration, and severity of the disease. It is important for the treating physician to consider host compromise

A. Akhaddar, *Cranial Osteomyelitis*, DOI 10.1007/978-3-319-30268-3_11

and treat any compromising condition, when feasible, concomitantly with the infection.

Anyway, consultation with microbiologists, infectious disease specialists and pharmacologists is advised to help guide antibiotic selection and duration for patients with cranial osteomyelitis.

Choice of Antimicrobial Agents

The high success rates of antimicrobial therapy in most infectious diseases have not yet been achieved in bone infections due to the physiological and anatomical characteristics of osseous tissue in general and cranial bones in particular. A comprehensive discussion of antibiotics is well beyond the scope of this chapter; however, several principles should be kept in mind when prescribing antibiotics for cranial osteomyelitis.

Osteomyelitis habitually requires prolonged antibiotic therapy, with a course lasting a matter of weeks or months. Peripherally inserted or tunneled central venous catheter may be very useful, avoiding excessive repeated insertions of peripheral intravenous. However, central venous catheter can be associated with catheter-related complications such as catheter malfunction, thrombosis and catheter associated bloodstream infections [1–3].

Unfortunately, there is no consensus about the best antibiotic regimen for skull osteomyelitis. Empiric antimicrobial therapy should include broad-spectrum drugs with activity against aerobic and anaerobic cocci and bacilli and infectious pathogens most frequently isolated. These drugs should achieve both therapeutic concentrations in the involved tissues (soft tissue, bone and central nervous system) and have low local rates of microbial resistance. The age of the patient, underlying medical conditions, associated source of infection, and extension of the disease should also be taken into consideration (Table 11.1). The appropriate antibiotics chosen should be started as soon as an adequate specimen is obtained for culture (empirical treatment). The antibiotic regimen is then adapted to the specific pathogen once antibiotic susceptibilities are established (targeted treatment) [4, 5]. Unnecessary antibiotics must be discontinued to prevent the emergence of resistant strains. In cases with negative cultures or if no specimen can be sampled, continuation of empirical broad-spectrum antimicrobials against the most probable microorganisms is recommended.

In general, the standard empiric antibiotic regimen includes vancomycin, metronidazole and a third generation cephalosporin. An antistaphylococcal activity should always be considered. As mentioned previously, *Staphylococcus aureus* remains the most important pathogen isolated in skull bone osteomyelitis. *S. aureus* is susceptible to amoxicillin/clavulanic acid or flucloxacillin (if - penicillin-allergic, consider clindamycin). The rise of resistance in the prevalence of methicillin-resistant *Staphylococcus aureus* (MRSA) is well documented [6–8]. Vancomycin was developed with the intention that it would be highly

Table 11.1 Suggested empiric antibiotics against the most frequent bacteria involved in osteomyelitic cranial bones

Origin	Suggested antibiotic therapy
Paranasal sinuses	Vancomycin[a] + metronidazole + third or fourth generation cephalosporin
Otogenic	Vancomycin[a] + metronidazole + third generation cephalosporin
Surgical site infection	Vancomycin[a] + third generation cephalosporin
Head trauma	Oxacillin + metronidazole + third generation cephalosporin
Hematogenous	Vancomycin[a] + metronidazole + cefotaxime

[a]If methicillin-resistant *Staphylococcus aureus* (MRSA) or vancomycin-resistant *Staphylococcus aureus* (VRSA) consider Linezolid

resistant to the developement of bacterial resistance. However, some strains of *Staphylococcus aureus* vancomycin-resistant (VRSA) were isolated. The new antibiotic named linezolid is in the first line in the treatment of infections resistant to vancomycin [9, 10]. Disadvantages of linezolid are its high cost and some serious side effects including reversible bone marrow suppression, optic neuropathy and nonreversible peripheral neuropathy [11]. The increasing development of antibiotic resistance will probably make conservative treatment even less successful than it is now.

When intracranial infection is suspected, the third generation of cephalosporin (such as cefotaxime or ceftriaxone) is a good choice [12–14]. Antibiotics that penetrate the cerebro-spinal fluid (CSF) and achieve therapeutic concentrations within the subdural structures include chloramphenicol, metronidazole, penicillin, methicillin, nafcillin, vancomycin, trimethoprim-sulfamethoxazole and some of the third generation cephalosporins [15]. Anyway, treatment should be optimized according to the results of the susceptibility testing of the microorganism isolated.

Intravenous antimicrobial treatment is continued until the acute sepsis syndrome is controlled; after which, continued recovery should be assessed on oral antibiotics on an outpatient basis. The oral antibiotic should have the same spectrum of coverage as the parenteral drug.

Metronidazole is used to cover anaerobic bacteria. However, high dose metronidazole may cause peripheral (irreversible) neuropathies [16]. In case of fungal infection, antifungal drug such as amphotericin B, voriconazole or posaconazole is required. Antifungal agent toxicity should be taken in consideration, especially the side effects of amphotericin B (in particular nephrotoxicity and morbidity of prolonged venous access) [17]. Voriconazole and posaconazole have fewer side effects with acceptable bioavailability [18, 19]. Anti-tuberculous chemotherapy comprised four drugs (isoniazid, rifampicin, pyrazinamide and streptomycin or ethambutol) [20]. For skull syphilis, penicillin is the antibiotic of choice but doxycycline will be an alternative in case of penicillin allergy [21]. Antihelminthic drugs (such as albendazole or mebendazole) are effective against hydatid cyst [22]. More specific information about antimicrobial therapies for specific organisms is given in Chap. 14.

Classically, ciprofloxacin is the most important antibiotic treatment for otogenic skull base osteomyelitis [23, 24], although some studies advised increasing acquisition of resistances [25–29]. According to Patmore et al., double antibiotic coverage is required to provide adequate antipseudomonal activity: ciprofloxacin with carbapenems seems to be a good synergistic association [30]. Given the possibility of MRSA, empiric therapy with vancomycin must also be considered [31]. For refractory skull base osteomyelitis, Yamazaki and colleagues suggested that intraarterial antibiotherapy raised the antibiotic concentration in infectious tissue. They conducted successfully intraarterial antibiotic infusion in the external carotid artery of two subjects with intractable malignant otitis externa deteriorating after long-term intravenous antibiotic administration with surgical debridement [32].

Sometimes, there were serious cases of drug-related toxicity necessitating the withdrawal/change-over of the drug.

Duration of Antimicrobial Therapy

The length of antibiotic treatment is important because the early cessation of treatment will often lead to the recurrence of infection, aid transition from acute to chronic forms of osteomyelitis and may expose the patient to the risk of antibiotic resistance [33].

The duration of antibiotherapy has not been standardized and the literature does not provide a clear recommendation of the duration. According to some authors, the length of antibiotic treatment should be individualized on the basis of severity illness, location of infection and clinical response. So, antibiotic regimens may vary among centers but at least 2 weeks of high-dose intravenous therapy followed by 6–12 weeks of supplemental oral therapy is commonly used [4]. The change to oral antibiotics is generally made when fever, pain and signs of local inflammation have resolved and laboratory values are normalizing. Treatment for acute infection is usually for 4–6 weeks and chronic infection for at least 12 weeks [34, 35].

Habitually, patients with less significant degrees of bone infection and who are immunocompetent can clear with 6–8 weeks of antibiotic therapy. When significant cranial osteomyelitis is present with or without intracranial extension or when patient is immunocompromised, 8 weeks of antibiotherapy or longer is the recommended duration. Patients with concomitant brain suppurations or skull base osteomyelitis might need longer courses. For osteomyelitis of the skull base, duration of antimicrobial therapy vary among authors between 6 and 20 weeks. This relative long duration was justified to provide a good antipseudomonal activity in diabetic patients [24, 26, 30, 36, 37]. Indeed, this population of patients may require longer duration therapy because vasculopathy compromises antibiotic drugs passage and absorption.

In common practice, the duration of antibiotherapy was rarely influenced by the nature of the pathogen with a few exceptions, that is, those proven to require long-lasting antimicrobial treatment for eradication such as mycobacteria, actinomycosis, fungi and some parasitosis [20, 38–40] (see Chap. 14).

Monitoring Response to Treatment

Patients should be monitored closely for evidence of therapy success. The effectiveness of such therapy is gauged by reductions in pain and fever, resolution of signs of local inflammation, and normalization of laboratory values. However, as seen in Chap. 7, biologic parameters are not entirely reliable as markers for infection, and some patients show continued elevations in spite of clinical improvement (elevation of the CRP level can persist for up to 4 weeks). In such cases, it is reasonable to extend the length of antibiotic treatment. When the infection does not respond sufficiently (suggestive of treatment failure), the management should be asked and adjustments must be made, including repeated cultures to ensure correct antimicrobial therapy, more extensive surgical debridement and possibly adjuvant hyperbaric oxygen therapy.

Repeated computed tomography-scan (CT-scan) or magnetic resonance imaging (MRI) is a poor predictor of outcome after treatment has started and may become visible worse than pre-treatment imaging. However, MRI may be indicated if the neurologic symptoms deteriorate to rule out new or worsening intracranial lesions. In skull base, resolution of infection is better documented by nuclear medicine studies especially with gallium nucleotic scan [23]. For many authors [41, 42], follow-up assessment with imaging is best performed with In-111 white blood cell and Tc-99m MDP bone imaging since this imaging technique reverts to normal sooner than CT-scan, MRI and Gallium-67 imaging [42, 43].

The optimal use of antibiotics is important in managing patients and in preventing development and spread of antibiotic-resistant strains. Despite the availability of several classes of antimicrobial agents with various mechanisms of action, resistance will regularly develop due to wide antibiotic use and can extend rapidly within the hospital environment. Microbial resistance must be suspected in patients with deteriorating clinical features (increasing headache, fever, new focal neurologic deficit or cranial nerve palsies) or rising levels of inflammatory markers. If the treatment fails, then repeated culturing are indicated and should include a search for less common causative agents, such as fungal and mycobacteria [44–46] (for more information please refer to Chap. 14). For this reason, patients are followed with biologic and neuroimaging surveillance every 4–8 weeks until the lesions have resolved completely. Out-patient follow-up should be for a minimum of 1 year. Predisposing factors that are modifiable should be addressed on a long-term basis. Moreover, regular laboratory testing is usually indicated to monitor for antimicrobial toxicity.

Supportive Therapy

Besides surgical procedures, antimicrobial drugs and hyperbaric oxygen therapy, many other adjunctive therapies may be necessary. These concomitant therapies vary with location and severity of the disease.

Initial Resuscitation and Severe Infection Issues

Acute management of sepsis and septic shock may be necessary for some patients with serious condition [47–50]. Supportive treatment includes intubation and mechanical ventilation when needed and the correction of any electrolyte disturbances when present. Early and aggressive fluid resuscitation is sometimes recommended to optimize care as well as proper nutrition [51]. When an infectious source is identified, it should be treated aggressively. Other medical therapies vary with location and severity of infections, and include hyperosmotic compounds, and cerebrospinal fluid diversion with monitoring of intracranial pressure [52].

Anticonvulsants

Valproate, carbamazepine and phenytoin are the most frequently used drugs. Anticonvulsants may be used in the early stages of treatment of cranial osteomyelitis with intracranial extension (particularly with lesions close to the brain cortical surface) to prevent seizures, although strong evidence for their benefit is lacking and there is no consensus on the duration of treatment. Treatment is mandatory if seizures occur. Anticonvulsant drugs can be stopped if patients remain seizure free for more than 1 year and the electroencephalography findings do not show any evidence of seizure disorder.

Corticosteroids

Corticosteroids may be helpful (especially dexamethasone at doses ranging from 6 to 16 mg/day or even higher doses), but they should be initiated after appropriate antibiotics. They can be initiated in patients with significant surrounding intracerebral swelling secondary to the vasogenic edema causing increased intracranial pressure. On CT-scan, grey-white matter differentiation is maintained and the edema involves mainly white matter, extending in finger-like fashion. On MRI, edema will appear hyperintense on T2 weighted images and fluid attenuation inversion recovery (FLAIR) signals which do not show restricted diffusion.

A rapid response is usually obtained and most patients improve their condition in a matter of hours or a few days. However, symptom relapses may occur at the time of corticosteroid interruption so gradual tapering of these drugs should be considered. Corticosteroids benefits are offset somewhat by the fact that steroids decrease antibiotic penetration into the suppurative sites and may slow encapsulation of the abscess site. Corticosteroids have also immune-suppressive effects.

Anticoagulation

Anticoagulation with heparin is beneficial in septic sinus thrombosis (superior sagittal sinus, cavernous sinus or transverse sinus), particularly if used early, and should be strongly considered [47]. Risk of intracerebral bleeding is small and it is not an absolute contraindication to heparin therapy [53, 54]. Thrombolysis has been suggested in septic intracranial thrombosis, however its efficacy has not been adequately evaluated [54]. Most reviews agree that vigorous heparin therapy followed by warfarin is the treatment of choice [50, 55–57]; however, there is no consensus about the initial type of heparin to use: unfractionated heparin or low molecular weight heparin. Generally, Warfarin treatment was continued with a target International Normalized Ratio (INR) being between 2 and 3, without hemorrhagic complications, over 1 year [26].

There is not sufficient information on the use of anticoagulation or antiaggregants for the thromboembolic events due to carotid artery infection. In one patient, cavernous sinus and right carotid artery involvement caused middle cerebral artery (MCA) infarct, resulting in left hemiparesis, aphasia, homonym hemianopsia, and the treatment used antibiotherapy and aspirin. Hemiparesis and homonym hemianopsia improved but the aphasia remained [58]. Another patient with skull base osteomyelitis causing right internal carotid artery (ICA) bifurcation complete occlusion and right MCA infarct, resulting in left hemiparesis, right XIth to XIIth nerve paralyses and right Horner syndrome, was treated only with antibiotherapy [59]. One more patient with meningitis underwent cerebral angiography after the development of IIIrd to VIth cranial nerve paralyses. Severe narrowing was observed in the bilateral ICA cavernous segment along with mural thrombus, which suggested cavernous sinus thrombosis. Antibiotherapy and 4 months of warfarin treatment was given. The sixth month follow-up angiography showed that the left ICA narrowness has improved but the right side remained unchanged [60].

Analgesics and Antipyretics

They may be used as symptomatic treatment. Headache should be appropriately assessed to rule out intracranial hypertension. If no signs of intracranial hypertension exist, common analgesics should be used to obtain appropriate pain control.

However, anti-inflammatory non-steroidal (AINS) drugs should be avoided, because they can reduce symptoms and delay diagnosis.

Comorbidities

It is important for the treating physician to consider host compromise and treat any medical comorbidities (such as diabetes, immunocompromised status, and poor nutrition), when feasible, concomitantly with the infection. Consultation with the appropriate medical specialist will be helpful in resolving many of these underlying medical problems.

Functional Rehabilitation

Recovery from neurologic and cranial nerves dysfunction is variable. A complementary aiding therapy such as functional neurology, speech-language and orthoptic therapy may be requested in the aftercare of the patient.

References

1. Benak MA, Kent 3rd RB. Simultaneous placement of long-term central venous catheters and surgical debridement for treatment of osteomyelitis. Am Surg. 2001;67(8):790–2.
2. Schmid MW. Risks and complications of peripherally and centrally inserted intravenous catheters. Crit Care Nurs Clin North Am. 2000;12(2):165–74.
3. Ruebner R, Keren R, Coffin S, Chu J, Horn D, Zaoutis TE. Complications of central venous catheters used for the treatment of acute hematogenous osteomyelitis. Pediatrics. 2006;117 (4):1210–5.
4. Akova M, Akalı̇n HE, Korten V, Ozgen T, Erbengi A. Treatment of intracranial abscesses: experience with sulbactam/ampicillin. J Chemother. 1993;5(3):181–5.
5. Savitz MH, Dickinson T. Drug therapy for intracranial suppuration. Am Fam Physician. 1988;37(2):341–4.
6. Tomovic S, Friedel ME, Liu JK, Eloy JA. Community-acquired methicillin-resistant Staphylococcus aureus skull base osteomyelitis with occipital condylar cerebrospinal fluid leak in an immunocompetent patient. Laryngoscope. 2012;122(5):977–81. doi:10.1002/lary.23253.
7. Menif K, Bouziri A, Borgi A, Khaldi A, Ben Hassine L, Ben JN. Community acquired methicillin-resistant Staphylococcus aureus preseptal cellulitis complicated by zygomatic osteomylitis, cavernous sinus thrombosis and meningitis in a healthy child. Fetal Pediatr Pathol. 2011;30(4):252–6. doi:10.3109/15513815.2011.555810.
8. Laurens MB, Becker RM, Johnson JK, Wolf JS, Kotloff KL. MRSA with progression from otitis media and sphenoid sinusitis to clival osteomyelitis, pachymeningitis and abducens nerve palsy in an immunocompetent 10-year-old patient. Int J Pediatr Otorhinolaryngol. 2008;72(7):945–51. doi:10.1016/j.ijporl.2008.02.025.

9. Nam JR, Kim MS, Lee CH, Whang DH. Linezolid treatment for osteomyelitis due to Staphylococcus epidermidis with reduced vancomycin susceptibility. J Korean Neurosurg Soc. 2008;43(6):307–10. doi:10.3340/jkns.2008.43.6.307.
10. Rayner CR, Baddour LM, Birmingham MC, Norden C, Meagher AK, Schentag JJ. Linezolid in the treatment of osteomyelitis: results of compassionate use experience. Infection. 2004;32 (1):8–14.
11. Garazzino S, Tovo PA. Clinical experience with linezolid in infants and children. J Antimicrob Chemother. 2011;66 Suppl 4:iv23–41. doi:10.1093/jac/dkr074.
12. Osborn MK, Steinberg JP. Subdural empyema and other suppurative complications of paranasal sinusitis. Lancet Infect Dis. 2007;7(1):62–7.
13. Hall WA, Truwit CL. The surgical management of infections involving the cerebrum. Neurosurgery. 2008;62 Suppl 2:519–30. doi:10.1227/01.neu.0000316255.36726.5b.
14. Heth JA. Neurosurgical aspects of central nervous system infections. Neuroimaging Clin N Am. 2012;22(4):791–9. doi:10.1016/j.nic.2012.05.005.
15. Tunkel AR. Brain abscess. In: Mandell GL, Bennett JE, Dolin R, editors. Principles and practice of infectious diseases. 6th ed. New York: Churchill Livingstone; 2005.
16. Uçkay I, Jugun K, Gamulin A, Wagener J, Hoffmeyer P, Lew D. Chronic osteomyelitis. Curr Infect Dis Rep. 2012;14(5):566–75. doi:10.1007/s11908-012-0286-0.
17. Parize P, Chandesris MO, Lanternier F, Poirée S, Viard JP, Bienvenu B, Mimoun M, Méchai F, Mamzer MF, Herman P, Bougnoux ME, Lecuit M, Lortholary O. Antifungal therapy of Aspergillus invasive otitis externa: efficacy of voriconazole and review. Antimicrob Agents Chemother. 2009;53(3):1048–53. doi:10.1128/AAC.01220-08.
18. Lass-Flörl C. Triazole antifungal agents in invasive fungal infections: a comparative review. Drugs. 2011;71(18):2405–19. doi:10.2165/11596540-000000000-00000.
19. Lodge BA, Ashley ED, Steele MP, Perfect JR. Aspergillus fumigatus empyema, arthritis, and calcaneal osteomyelitis in a lung transplant patient successfully treated with posaconazole. J Clin Microbiol. 2004;42:1376–8.
20. Ramdurg SR, Gupta DK, Suri A, Sharma BS, Mahapatra AK. Calvarial tuberculosis: uncommon manifestation of common disease—a series of 21 cases. Br J Neurosurg. 2010;24 (5):572–7. doi:10.3109/02688697.2010.495166.
21. Elopre L, Morell V, Bosshardt C, Geisler WM. A case of syphilitic osteitis in a patient with HIV infection. Int J STD AIDS. 2014;25(10):765–7. doi:10.1177/0956462414522031.
22. Eckert J, Deplazes P. Biological, epidemiological, and clinical aspects of echinococcosis, a zoonosis of increasing concern. Clin Microbiol Rev. 2004;17(1):107–35.
23. Spielmann PM, Yu R, Neeff M. Skull base osteomyelitis: current microbiology and management. J Laryngol Otol. 2013;127 Suppl 1:S8–12. doi:10.1017/S0022215112002356.
24. Cavel O, Fliss DM, Segev Y, Zik D, Khafif A, Landsberg R. The role of the otorhinolaryngologist in the management of central skull base osteomyelitis. Am J Rhinol. 2007;21 (3):281–5.
25. Mani N, Sudhoff H, Rajagopal S, Moffat D, Axon PR. Cranial nerve involvement in malignant external otitis: implications for clinical outcome. Laryngoscope. 2007;117(5):907–10.
26. Lee SJ, Weon YC, Cha HJ, Kim SY, Seo KW, Jegal Y, Ahn JJ, Ra SW. A case of atypical skull base osteomyelitis with septic pulmonary embolism. J Korean Med Sci. 2011;26(7):962–5. doi:10.3346/jkms.2011.26.7.962.
27. Djalilian HR, Shamloo B, Thakkar KH, Najme-Rahim M. Treatment of culture-negative skull base osteomyelitis. Otol Neurotol. 2006;27(2):250–5.
28. Bernstein JM, Holland NJ, Porter GC, Maw AR. Resistance of pseudomonas to ciprofloxacin: implications for the treatment of malignant otitis externa. J Laryngol Otol. 2007;121 (2):118–23.
29. Le Clerc N, Verillaud B, Duet M, Guichard JP, Herman P, Kania R. Skull base osteomyelitis: incidence of resistance, morbidity, and treatment strategy. Laryngoscope. 2014;124 (9):2013–6. doi:10.1002/lary.24726.

30. Patmore H, Jebreel A, Uppal S, Raine CH, McWhinney P. Skull base infection presenting with multiple lower cranial nerve palsies. Am J Otolaryngol. 2010;31(5):376–80. doi:10.1016/j.amjoto.2009.04.001.
31. Johnson AK, Batra PS. Central skull base osteomyelitis: an emerging clinical entity. Laryngoscope. 2014;124(5):1083–7. doi:10.1002/lary.24440.
32. Yamazaki H, Kikuchi M, Shinohara S, Naito Y, Fujiwara K, Kanazawa Y, Tona R. Intra-arterial administration of antibiotics for refractory skull base osteomyelitis. Auris Nasus Larynx. 2014;41(4):380–3. doi:10.1016/j.anl.2013.12.003.
33. Moser R, Schweintzger G, Uggowitzer M, Urban C, Stammberger H, Eder H, Kerbl R. Recurrent Pott's puffy tumor—atypical presentation of a rare disorder. Wien Klin Wochenschr. 2009;121(21–22):719–22. doi:10.1007/s00508-009-1268-6.
34. Lew DP, Waldvogel FA. Osteomyelitis. N Engl J Med. 1997;336(14):999–1007.
35. Lew DP, Waldvogel FA. Osteomyelitis. Lancet. 2004;364(9431):369–79.
36. Ng J, Connolly DJ, Rittey CD, Mordekar SR. Skull base osteomyelitis leading to lateral medullary syndrome in a child. Eur J Paediatr Neurol. 2007;11(2):111–4.
37. Lee S, Hooper R, Fuller A, Turlakow A, Cousins V, Nouraei R. Otogenic cranial base osteomyelitis: a proposed prognosis-based system for disease classification. Otol Neurotol. 2008;29(5):666–72. doi:10.1097/MAO.0b013e318179972f.
38. Dawar P, Satyarthee GD, Sharma BS. Total resolution of large scalp swelling due to calvarial tuberculosis with medical management only: case report and review of the literature. Turk Neurosurg. 2015;25(2):313–6. doi:10.5137/1019-5149.JTN.7937-13.1.
39. Akhaddar A, Elouennass M, Baallal H, Boucetta M. Focal intracranial infections due to Actinomyces species in immunocompetent patients: diagnostic and therapeutic challenges. World Neurosurg. 2010;74(2–3):346–50. doi:10.1016/j.wneu.2010.05.029.
40. Walsh TJ, Anaissie EJ, Denning DW, Herbrecht R, Kontoyiannis DP, Marr KA, Morrison VA, Segal BH, Steinbach WJ, Stevens DA, van Burik JA, Wingard JR, Patterson TF, Infectious Diseases Society of America. Treatment of aspergillosis: clinical practice guidelines of the Infectious Diseases Society of America. Clin Infect Dis. 2008;46(3):327–60. doi:10.1086/525258.
41. Seabold JE, Simonson TM, Weber PC, Thompson BH, Harris KG, Rezai K, Madsen MT, Hoffman HT. Cranial osteomyelitis: diagnosis and follow-up with In-111 white blood cell and Tc-99m methylene diphosphonate bone SPECT, CT, and MR imaging. Radiology. 1995;196(3):779–88.
42. Epstein JS, Ganz WI, Lizak M, Grobman L, Goodwin WJ, Dewanjee MK. Indium 111-labeled leukocyte scintigraphy in evaluating head and neck infections. Ann Otol Rhinol Laryngol. 1992;101(12):961–8.
43. Parker KM, Nicholson JK, Cezayirli RC, Biggs PJ. Aspergillosis of the sphenoid sinus: presentation as a pituitary mass and postoperative gallium-67 imaging. Surg Neurol. 1996;45(4):354–8.
44. Yocum J, Seligson D. Blastomycosis of the knee and skull after arthroscopy. Am J Sports Med. 1991;19(6):670–2.
45. Wilkinson EP, Robinson RA, Trask DK. Skull base thrombotic mycosis. Ear Nose Throat J. 2007;86(3):137.
46. Mukherjee KK, Kaushik R, Nada R, Khosla VK, Khandelwal N, Kak VK. Calvarial tuberculosis. Surg Neurol. 2002;57(3):195–202.
47. Peer Mohamed B, Carr L. Neurological complications in two children with Lemierre syndrome. Dev Med Child Neurol. 2010;52(8):779–81. doi:10.1111/j.1469-8749.2010.03718.x.
48. Kao CH, Wang SJ. Spread of infectious complications of odontogenic abscess detected by technetium-99m-HMPAO-labeled WBC scan of occult sepsis in the intensive care unit. J Nucl Med. 1992;33(2):254–5.
49. Nakwan N, Nakwan N, Wannaro J, Dissaneevate P, Kritsaneepaiboon S, Chokephaibulkit K. Septicemia, meningitis, and skull osteomyelitis complicating infected cephalhematoma

caused by ESBL-producing Escherichia coli. Southeast Asian J Trop Med Public Health. 2011;42(1):148–51.

50. He J, Lam JC, Adlan T. Clival osteomyelitis and hypoglossal nerve palsy-rare complications of Lemierre's syndrome. BMJ Case Rep. 2015;2015:pii: bcr2015209777. doi:10.1136/bcr-2015-209777.
51. Dellinger RP, Levy MM, Rhodes A, Annane D, Gerlach H, Opal SM, Sevransky JE, Sprung CL, Douglas IS, Jaeschke R, Osborn TM, Nunnally ME, Townsend SR, Reinhart K, Kleinpell RM, Angus DC, Deutschman CS, Machado FR, Rubenfeld GD, Webb SA, Beale RJ, Vincent JL, Moreno R, Surviving Sepsis Campaign Guidelines Committee including the Pediatric Subgroup. Surviving sepsis campaign: international guidelines for management of severe sepsis and septic shock: 2012. Crit Care Med. 2013;41(2):580–637. doi:10.1097/CCM.0b013e31827e83af.
52. Pradilla G, Ardila GP, Hsu W, Rigamonti D. Epidural abscesses of the CNS. Lancet Neurol. 2009;8(3):292–300. doi:10.1016/S1474-4422(09)70044-4.
53. Bhatia K, Jones NS. Septic cavernous sinus thrombosis secondary to sinusitis: are anticoagulants indicated? A review of the literature. J Laryngol Otol. 2002;116(9):667–76.
54. Bousser MG. Cerebral venous thrombosis: nothing, heparin, or local thrombolysis? Stroke. 1999;30(3):481–3.
55. Stam J. Thrombosis of the cerebral veins and sinuses. N Engl J Med. 2005;352(17):1791–8.
56. Masuhr F, Mehraein S, Einhaupl K. Cerebral venous and sinus thrombosis. J Neurol. 2004;251 (1):11–23.
57. Crawford SC, Digre KB, Palmer CA, Bell DA, Osborn AG. Thrombosis of the deepvenous drainage of the brain in adults. Analysis of seven cases with review of the literature. Arch Neurol. 1995;52(11):1101–8.
58. Bentham JR, Pollard AJ, Milford CA, Anslow P, Pike MG. Cerebral infarct and meningitis secondary to Lemierre's syndrome. Pediatr Neurol. 2004;30(4):281–3.
59. Huang KL, Lu CS. Skull base osteomyelitis presenting as Villaret's syndrome. Acta Neurol Taiwan. 2006;15(4):255–8.
60. Jones TH, Bergvall V, Bradshaw JP. Carotid-artery stenoses and thrombosis secondary to cavernous sinus thromboses in fusobacterium-necrophorum meningitis. Postgrad Med J. 1990;66(779):747–50.

Chapter 12
Adjuvant Hyperbaric Oxygen Therapy

Contents

Abbreviations

HBOT Hyperbaric oxygen therapy

Definition and Principles of Hyperbaric Oxygen

Hyperbaric oxygen is defined in the European Code of Good Practice (http://www.oxynet.org/) as oxygen at high pressure (a level higher than atmospheric pressure). Air contains nearly 21 % oxygen, and more than 78 % nitrogen. In hyperbaric oxygen therapy (HBOT), the oxygen percentage breathed by the patient is nearly or actually 100 %, almost five times more than in air. The pressure of the oxygen breathed by the patient in hyperbaric oxygen is usually more than 1.5 times (and can be as much as three times) greater than atmospheric pressure. So, HBOT can deliver to the patient nearly 15 times as much oxygen as there is in air at normal pressure.

The extra oxygen is breathed in through the lungs, and dissolved in the blood plasma: it is then delivered to any part of the body with a good blood supply. The effects of this extra oxygen are different in several parts of the body: in some medical conditions it can save life, and in others it can promote healing and tissue repair. A hyperbaric chamber is needed for this reason (Fig. 12.1). It is defined as a pressure vessel able of accepting one (monoplace) or more persons (multiplace) with the purpose of providing medical treatment (Fig. 12.2). Like any other

A. Akhaddar, *Cranial Osteomyelitis*, DOI 10.1007/978-3-319-30268-3_12

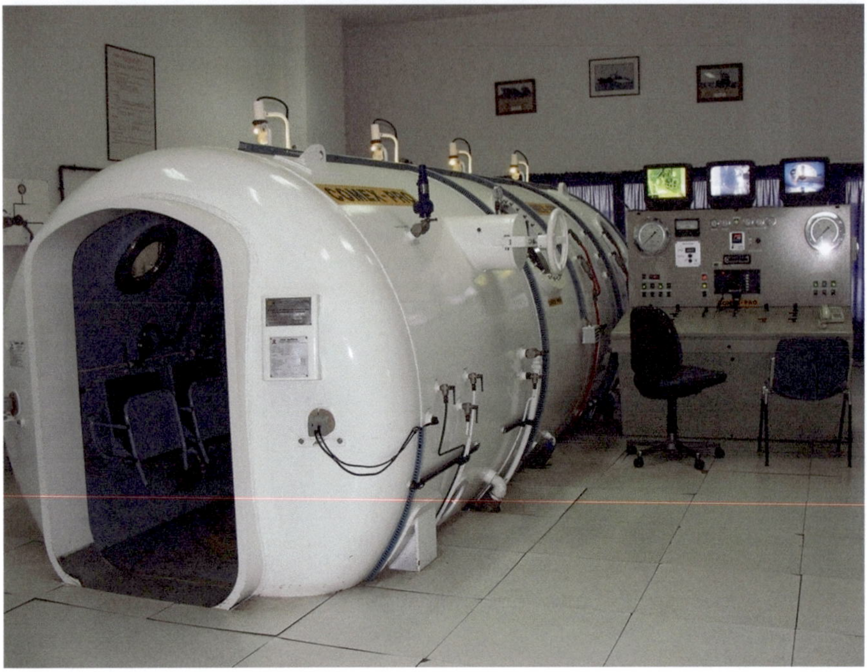

Fig. 12.1 Multiplace hyperbaric oxygen chamber (multiple occupancy). It is a large vessel made of steel and looks like a submarine. The chamber is pressurized with air and the patients breathe 100 % oxygen through clear hoods (Courtesy of Najib El Omari MD, Department of Hyperbaric Medicine, Mohammed V Military Teaching Hospital, Rabat, Morocco)

medicine or drug, hyperbaric oxygen can lead to unwanted effects [1]. However, HBOT is not always readily available in many developing countries.

Therapeutic Uses of Hyperbaric Oxygen

Hyperbaric oxygen therapy is used as primary and/or adjunctive therapy in the treatment of various clinical conditions complicated by local hypoxia. In a number of medical emergencies situations, where the patient might also need intensive care, HBOT is used such as in air or gas embolism, decompression illness, carbon monoxide poisoning, clostridial myonecrosis (gas gangrene), some other aggressive infections (Fournier's gangrene and necrotizing fasciitis), crush injury, burns, sudden deafness, severe hemorrhagic anemia and near-hanging. There are also a number of other situations where HBOT is used and where courses of treatment tend to be longer than for emergency referrals like ischemic skin flaps and grafts, refractory osteomyelitis, radiation bone and soft tissue damage, and problem wounds healing [2, 3].

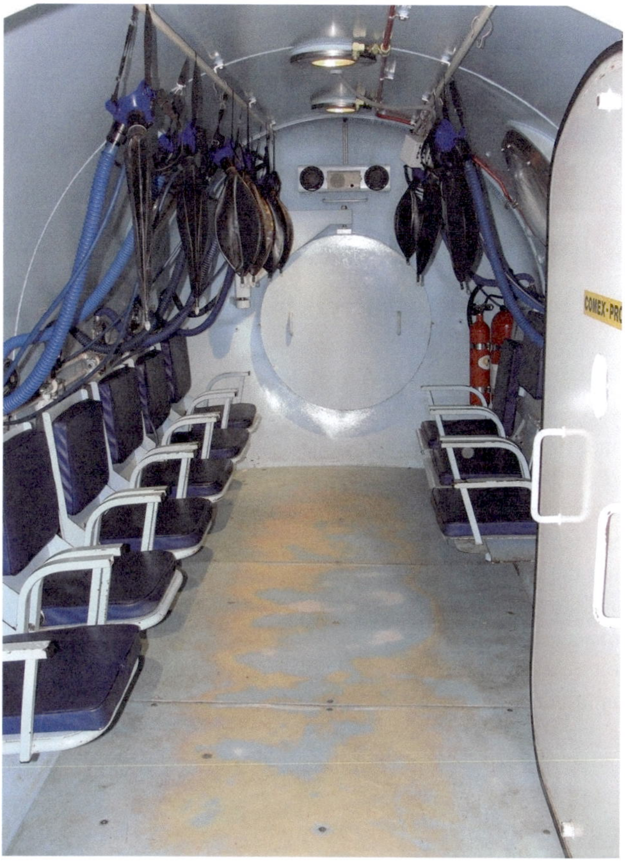

Fig. 12.2 Inside view of the multiplace hyperbaric oxygen chamber. Patients can be seated or situated in a lying position on stretchers if needed (Courtesy of N. El Omari MD, Department of Hyperbaric Medicine, Mohammed V Military Teaching Hospital, Rabat, Morocco)

Oxygen Tolerance in Bacteria

Before addressing the topic of infection, it is important to know that bacteria can be divided into five major groups depending on their susceptibility to oxygen [4]:

- **Strictly aerobic bacteria**. These bacteria absolutely need oxygen to develop (Like *Neisseira spp.* and *Pseudomonas spp.*).
- **Microaerophils**. These bacteria need oxygen, but develop best in concentrations of oxygen lower than in air (Like *Helicobacter spp.* and *Campylobacter spp.*).
- **Aero-anaerobes** or **facultative anaerobes**. These bacteria can develop with or without oxygen (Like *Staphylococcus spp.* or *Enterobacteriaceae spp.*).

- **Aerotolerant anaerobes**. These bacteria can grow with oxygen but develop better without oxygen (Like *Streptococcus spp.* and *Enterococcus spp.*).
- **Strictly anaerobes**. These bacteria can only develop without oxygen (Like *Bacteroides spp.*, *Clostridium spp.*, or *Peptostreptococcus spp.*).

However, the toxic effects of molecular oxygen vary from some bacteria to others even within the same group.

Biochemical and Cellular Effects in Infected Tissues

In the field of infectious disease, hyperbaric oxygen provides normal or above-normal pressures of oxygen in hypoxic infected tissues [5]. Therefore it has a direct action on anaerobic bacteria, an indirect action of cellular defense mechanisms of the body and finally a synergistic effect on antibiotic activity [4, 6–8]. Hyperbaric oxygen was also shown to be effective in the treatment of mucormycosis as it decreases the local acidosis which promotes fungal growth [9].

Concerning the wound healing processes, hyperbaric oxygenation can stimulate fibroblast proliferation and differentiation, increase collagen formation and enhance neovascularization as well as stimulation of microbial killing by leukocytes. Hypoxic wounds also benefit from increased oxygen supply through improved maintenance of energy metabolism and reduction of edema [10].

HBOT has been also established as a useful adjunct to antibiotics and surgery for the treatment of infected wound complications after surgery in the irradiated head and neck [11].

Hyperbaric Oxygenation Therapy in Osteomyelitis

In 1965, Slack et al. were the first to report the efficacy of HBOT in chronic osteomyelitis of humans [12]. Since then, many authors described the HBOT as an adjuvant therapy for refractory osteomyelitis. Beside the previously mentioned effects of HBOT in general, this adjunctive treatment modality is useful in osteomyelitis in promoting osteoblast and osteoclast activities. It is well known that the resorption of necrotic bone by osteoclast is oxygen-dependent [13].

Overall and on the base of experimental studies, the following conclusions were selected [14, 15]:

- Osteomyelitic bone and the surrounding area have a decreased blood flow and are hypoxic.
- Hypoxia reduces host defense mechanisms by impairing the oxygen-dependent killing of bacteria by polymorphonuclear leukocytes.
- Hypoxia diminishes fibroblast proliferation and collagen production, the basis of bone repair.

- Decreased oxygen tension in osteomyelitic bone and surrounding tissue can be elevated to normal or above normal by HBOT.
- HBOT has a synergistic effect with certain antibiotics and antifungal agents.
- Experimental treatment of osteomyelitis caused by *Staphylococcus aureus* was equally effective when using HBOT as when giving antibiotics.

In most clinical studies which used surgical and hyperbaric oxygen therapies of chronic refractory osteomyelitis, success rates range from 64 to 86 % [16–22]. Aitasalo and coauthors demonstrated sustained resolution of chronic osteomyelitis of the mandible and maxilla in 79 % of 33 patients [23]. According to Handschell et al. who made a review of 27 patients with secondary chronic osteomyelitis of the jaw that had been treated with HBOT, adjuvant HBOT therapy was successful in the treatment of patients with chronic osteomyelitis which could avoid ablative surgery in some instances [24].

HBOT is world-wide recommended as adjuvant therapy in cases of persistent osteomyelitis when previous appropriate antimicrobial therapy for 6 weeks, together with at least one surgical therapy, has failed. Treatment protocols should use treatment pressure of 200–250 kPa with treatment time varying from 90 to 120 min depending on the clinical situation. Utilization review is recommended after 40 hyperbaric treatments [14]. However, the surgery (like the removal of infected implants and dead bone) cannot be avoided just because HBOT is being used. The timing of surgery and the use of the right antibiotics should be planned at the same time as the HBOT.

Hyperbaric Oxygenation Therapy in Cranial Osteomyelitis

Hyperbaric oxygen therapy has been reported to be a valuable adjunct in the treatment of refractory cranial osteomyelitis [15]. To our knowledge, the first clinical report on patients with cranial osteomyelitis described success in one case with malignant external otitis and mastoid involvement. He was treated with a combination of appropriate antibiotics and HBOT (20 sessions) without needing surgical debridement [25]. Since this first publication in 1982, less than 80 cases were reported in English literature, generally with skull base invasion. An overview of the papers on HBOT in cranial osteomyelitis is given in Table 12.1 [25–39]. There is effectively sparse neurosurgical literature on this subject and few publications explain clearly their inclusion criteria and therapeutic protocol.

One of the best clinical studies so far comes from Larsson et al. [32]. In a retrospective study of postoperative neurosurgical infections they report a series of patients previously failing to resolve skull osteomyelitis with antibiotic therapy. Prior to start of HBOT, none of these patients had undergone attempts at surgical debridement. Overall, cranial infection resolved in 30 of 31 patients (96.7 %). Interestingly, only one of four bone flaps (25 %) and three of six acrylic flaps (50 %) were removed. The authors found HBOT efficient to salvage skull-bone

Table 12.1 Summary of reported publications in English literature relevant to hyperbaric oxygen therapy and skull bone osteomyelitis

Authors	Year	Country	No. of cases	Location	Microorganism	Treatment	No. of HBOT sessions	Evolution
Mader[a] [25]	1982	USA	1	Skull base MOE	*Pseudomonas aeruginosa*	Antibiotic	20	Resolved
Shupak [26]	1989	Israel	2	Skull base MOE	*Pseudomonas aeruginosa*	Antibiotic Debridement	27 and 29	All resolved
Schweitzer [27]	1990	USA	1	Temporal	*Staphylococcus spp.*	Antibiotic	n/a	Resolved
Davis [28]	1992	USA	14	Skull base MOE	*Pseudomonas aeruginosa*	Antibiotic Debridement or mastoidectomy	30	All resolved 100 %
Seabold [29]	1995	USA	1	Mastoid and Petrous	*Pseudomonas aeruginosa* *Pseudomonas pickettii*	Antibiotic	n/a	Resolved
Kountakis [30]	1997	USA	1	Skull base	*Aspergillus flavus*	Antifungal Mastoidectomy	n/a	Resolved
Genden [31]	1998	USA	1	Skull base	*Escherichia coli*	Antibiotic Mastoidectomy	n/a	Resolved
Larsson [32]	2002	Sweden	31	Bone flap	Mainly *S. epidermidis* (10 cases) *and S. aureus* (8 cases)	Antibiotic with/without bone flap removed	Mostly 40	30 of 31 resolved (96.7 %)
Singh [33]	2005	Sultanate of Oman	2	Skull base	n/a	Antibiotic	34	Case 1: resolved Case 2: died
Stodulski [34]	2006	Poland	1	Otogenic Skull base	*Aspergillus flavus*	Antifungal	16	Died

Prasad [35]	2007	India	1	Skull base	n/a	Debridement	n/a	Resolved
Vasoo [36]	2008	Singapore	1	Skull base	*Scedosporium apiospermum*	Antibiotic	30	Failure Diagnostic error
Blyth [37]	2010	Australia	2	Skull base	Fungi	Antifungal Surgery	n/a	n/a
Leahy [38]	2011	Australia	1	Skull base MOE	*Pseudomonas aeruginosa*	Antimicrobial	2 × 54	Resolved
Personal case	2012	Morocco	1	Frontal (bone flap with extradural empyema	*Staphylococcus aureus*	Antibiotic Bone flap removed	10	Resolved
Johnson [39]	2013	USA	1	Skull base	*n/a*	Antimicrobial Surgical debridement	n/a	n/a

[a]This case was reported again by Davis
Nb number, *n/a* no data available, *MOE* Malignant Otitis Externa

flaps and acrylic cranioplasties, mostly without removal of fixation systems. This effect was particularly useful in patients with impaired immunological defenses. For Larsson, cost of HBOT averaged 7,100 $US per patient, this relatively high cost must be taken into consideration against the risks and costs related with repeat craniotomy [32].

In our own experience, one of our patients with frontal bone flap osteomyelitis and extradural empyema was successfully treated with antibiotics, surgical debridement (bone flap removed) and ten sessions of HBOT. In the setting of antibiotic refractory skull osteomyelitis and prior to sustaining major cranial debridement, a trial of HBOT should be considered [40].

Skull base osteomyelitis is represented essentially by the invasive form of malignant external otitis. This otitis-associated skull base infection was rarely encountered in neurosurgical practices, mainly seen in otorhinolaryngology. However, as seen previously, the terminology describing osteomyelitis in the temporal bone, bony extension versus soft tissue involvement and the number of cases requiring surgical debridement was confusing [39, 41]. In addition, no clear evidence exists to demonstrate the efficacy of hyperbaric oxygen therapy when compared to treatment with antibiotics and/or surgery. Until now, no data were found to compare rates of complication between the different treatment modalities in malignant external otitis [42]. However, HBOT has been described as a valuable adjunct in managing refractory cases of invasive malignant external otitis. Narozny et al. demonstrated sustained resolution in seven of eight patients (87.5 %) [43]. Only one patient required simultaneous surgical debridement and this single treatment failure was associated with *Aspergillus spp.* agent. In a large series of 14 cases with skull base involvement, a success rate of 100 % with adjuvant HBOT of previously refractory osteomyelitis was reported by Davis and colleagues [28]. All patients were diabetics and culture yielded *Pseudomonas aeruginosa.* This curative success persisted without recurrence throughout more than 1 year follow-up period. Martel et al. report a success rate of 95 % in 22 retrospectively examined cases without the need for surgery by combining HBOT with antibiotics [44]. However, these cases were not reported as being previously refractory to antibiotics. There are quite a number of interesting reports in the German literature on HBOT of skull base osteomyelitis with malignant external otitis; unfortunately, they are not easily accessible [45–48].

Based on the results of these previously publications, treatment of cranial osteomyelitis with the combination of antimicrobial drugs, surgical debridement and HBOT appears to maximize the potential for infection clearance. HBOT cannot be recommended as a solitary treatment modality in the management of skull bone infection. However, HBOT should be considered as adjuvant therapy for the treatment of refractory osteomyelitis of the skull combined with antimicrobial therapy prior to sustaining major cranial debridement. No specific recommendations can be prescribed for the total number of HBOT sessions. This duration must be judged depending on the clinical outcome of each patient (usually between 20 and 40 sessions, five to seven times per week).

References

1. Doherty MJ, Hampson NB. Partial seizure provoked by hyperbaric oxygen therapy: possible mechanisms and implications. Epilepsia. 2005;46(6):974–6.
2. Wattel F, Mathieu D. Methodology for assessing hyperbaric oxygen therapy in clinical practice. In: Mathieu D, editor. Handbook on hyperbaric medicine. Netherlands: Springer; 2006.
3. Tibbles PM, Edelsberg JS. Hyperbaric-oxygen therapy. N Engl J Med. 1996;334(25):1642–8.
4. Mathieu D, Wattel F. Physiologic effects of hyperbaric oxygen on microorganisms and host defenses against infection. In: Mathieu D, editor. Handbook on hyperbaric medicine. Netherlands: Springer; 2006.
5. Mader JT, Brown GL, Guckian JC, Wells CH, Reinarz JA. A mechanism for the amelioration by hyperbaric oxygen of experimental staphylococcal osteomyelitis in rabbits. J Infect Dis. 1980;142(6):915–22.
6. Park MK, Myers RAM, Marzella L. Oxygen tensions and infections : modulation of microbial growth, activity of antimicrobial agents, and immunologic responses. Clin Infect Dis. 1992;14 (3):720–40.
7. Park MK, Muhvich KH, Myers RA, Marzella L. Hyperoxia prolongs the aminoglycoside-induced postantibiotic effect in *Pseudomonas aeruginosa*. Antimicrob Agents Chemother. 1991;35(4):691–5.
8. Mendel V, Simanowski HJ, Scholz HC. Synergy of HBO2 and a local antibiotic carrier for experimental osteomyelitis due to *Staphylococcus aureus* in rats. Undersea Hyperb Med. 2004;31(4):407–16.
9. Segal E, Menhusen MJ, Shawn S. Hyperbaric oxygen in the treatment of invasive fungal infections: a single center experience. Isr Med Assoc J. 2007;9(5):355–7.
10. Niinikoski J. Physiologic effects of hyprbaric oxygen on wound healing processes. In: Mathieu D, editor. Handbook on hyperbaric medicine. Netherlands: Springer; 2006.
11. Neovius EB, Lind MG, Lind FG. Hyperbaric oxygen therapy for wound complications after surgery in the irradiated head and neck: a review of the literature and a report of 15 consecutive patients. Head Neck. 1997;19(4):315–22.
12. Slack WK, Thomas DA, Perrins D. Hyperbaric oxygenation chronic osteomyelitis. Lancet. 1965;1(7395):1093–4.
13. Barth E, Sullivan T, Berg E. Animal model for evaluating bone repair with and without adjunctive hyperbaric oxygen therapy (HBO): comparing dose schedules. J Invest Surg. 1990;3(4):387–92.
14. Kemmer A, Stein T, Hierholzer C. Persistent osteomyelitis. In: Mathieu D, editor. Handbook on hyperbaric medicine. Netherlands: Springer; 2006.
15. Steinhart H, Schulz S, Mutters R. Evaluation of ozonated oxygen in an experimental animal model of osteomyelitis as a further treatment option for skull base osteomyelitis. Eur Arch Otorhinolaryngol. 1999;256:153–7.
16. Davis JC. Refractory osteomyelitis of the extremities and axial skeleton. In: Davis JC, Hunt TK, editors. Hyperbaric oxygen therapy. Bethesda, MD: Undersea Medical Society; 1977.
17. Davis JC, Heckman JD, DeLee JC, Buckwold FJ. Chronic non-hematogenous osteomyelitis treated with adjuvant hyperbaric oxygen. J Bone Joint Surg Am. 1986;68(8):1210–7.
18. Chen CY, Lee SS, Chan YS, Yen CY, Chao EK, Ueng SW. Chronic refractory tibia osteomyelitis treated with adjuvent hyperbaric oxygen: a preliminary report. Changgeng Yi Xue Za Zhi. 1998;21(2):165–71.
19. Chen CE, Shih ST, Fu TH, Wang JW, Wang CJ. Hyperbaric oxygen therapy in the treatment of chronic refractory osteomyelitis: a preliminary report. Chang Gung Med J. 2003;26 (2):114–21.
20. Skeik N, Porten BR, Isaacson E, Seong J, Klosterman DL, Garberich RF, Alexander JQ, Rizvi A, Manunga Jr JM, Cragg A, Graber J, Alden P, Sullivan T. Hyperbaric oxygen

treatment outcome for different indications from a single center. Ann Vasc Surg. 2015;29 (2):206–14. doi:10.1016/j.avsg.2014.07.034.
21. Ahmed R, Severson MA, Traynelis VC. Role of hyperbaric oxygen therapy in the treatment of bacterial spinal osteomyelitis. J Neurosurg Spine. 2009;10(1):16–20. doi:10.3171/2008.10. SPI08606.
22. Kawashima M, Tamura H, Nagayoshi I, Takao K, Yoshida K, Yamaguchi T. Hyperbaric oxygen therapy in orthopedic conditions. Undersea Hyperb Med. 2004;31(1):155–62.
23. Aitasalo K, Niinikoski J, Grénman R, Virolainen E. A modified protocol for early treatment of osteomyelitis and osteoradionecrosis of the mandible. Head Neck. 1998;20(5):411–7.
24. Handschel J, Brüssermann S, Depprich R, Ommerborn M, Naujoks C, Kübler NR, Meyer U. Evaluation of hyperbaric oxygen therapy in treatment of patients with osteomyelitis of the mandible. Mund Kiefer Gesichtschir. 2007;11(5):285–90. German.
25. Mader JT, Love JT. Malignant external otitis. Cure with adjunctive hyperbaric oxygen therapy. Arch Otolaryngol. 1982;108(1):38–40.
26. Shupak A, Greenberg E, Hardoff R, Gordon C, Melamed Y, Meyer WS. Hyperbaric oxygen for necrotizing (malignant) otitis externa. Arch Otolaryngol Head Neck Surg. 1989;115 (12):1470–5.
27. Schweitzer VG. Hyperbaric oxygen management of chronic staphylococcal osteomyelitis of the temporal bone. Am J Otol. 1990;11(5):347–53.
28. Davis JC, Gates GA, Lerner C, Davis MG, Mader JT, Dinesman A. Adjuvant hyperbaric oxygen in malignant external otitis. Arch Otolaryngol Head Neck Surg. 1992;118(1):89–93.
29. Seabold JE, Simonson TM, Weber PC, Thompson BH, Harris KG, Rezai K, Madsen MT, Hoffman HT. Cranial osteomyelitis: diagnosis and follow-up with In-111 white blood cell and Tc-99 m methylene diphosphonate bone SPECT, CT, and MR imaging. Radiology. 1995;196 (3):779–88.
30. Kountakis SE, Kemper Jr JV, Chang CY, DiMaio DJ, Stiernberg CM. Osteomyelitis of the base of the skull secondary to Aspergillus. Am J Otolaryngol. 1997;18(1):19–22.
31. Genden EM, Goebel JA. Escherichia coli osteomyelitis of the skull base. Otolaryngol Head Neck Surg. 1998;118(6):853–5.
32. Larsson A, Engström M, Uusijärvi J, Kihlström L, Lind F, Mathiesen T. Hyperbaric oxygen treatment of postoperative neurosurgical infections. Neurosurgery. 2002;50(2):287–95.
33. Singh A, Al Khabori M, Hyder MJ. Skull base osteomyelitis: diagnostic and therapeutic challenges in atypical presentation. Otolaryngol Head Neck Surg. 2005;133(1):121–5.
34. Stodulski D, Kowalska B, Stankiewicz C. Otogenic skull base osteomyelitis caused by invasive fungal infection. Case report and literature review. Eur Arch Otorhinolaryngol. 2006;263(12):1070–6.
35. Prasad KC, Prasad SC, Mouli N, Agarwal S. Osteomyelitis in the head and neck. Acta Otolaryngol. 2007;127(2):194–205.
36. Vasoo S, Yeo SB, Lim PL, Ang BS, Lye DC. Efficacy of voriconazole for Scedosporium apiospermum skull base osteomyelitis: case report and literature review. Int J Antimicrob Agents. 2008;31(2):184–5.
37. Blyth CC, Gomes L, Sorrell TC, da Cruz M, Sud A, Chen SC. Skull-base osteomyelitis: fungal vs. bacterial infection. Clin Microbiol Infect. 2011;17(2):306–11. doi:10.1111/j.1469-0691. 2010.03231.x.
38. Leahy TW, Sader C. A rare case of bilateral malignant otitis externa and osteomyelitis with lower cranial nerve sequelae. BMJ Case Rep. 2011;2011:pii: bcr0320113957. doi:10.1136/bcr. 03.2011.3957.
39. Johnson AK, Batra PS. Central skull base osteomyelitis: an emerging clinical entity. Laryngoscope. 2014;124(5):1083–7. doi:10.1002/lary.24440.
40. Hart B. Refractory osteomyelitis. Hyperbaric oxygen therapy indications. 12th ed. Durham, NC: Undersea and Hyperbaric Medical Society; 2008.

41. Rothholtz VS, Lee AD, Shamloo B, Bazargan M, Pan D, Djalilian HR. Skull base osteomyelitis: the effect of comorbid disease on hospitalization. Laryngoscope. 2008;118 (11):1917–24. doi:10.1097/MLG.0b013e31817fae0d.
42. Phillips JS, Jones SE. Hyperbaric oxygen as an adjuvant treatment for malignant otitis externa. Cochrane Database Syst Rev. 2013;5:CD004617. doi:10.1002/14651858.CD004617.pub3.
43. Narozny W, Kuczkowski J, Mikaszewski B. Infectious skull base osteomyelitis—still a life-threatening disease. Otol Neurotol. 2006;27(7):1047–8.
44. Martel J, Duclos JY, Darrouzet V, Guyot M, Bébéar JP. Malignant or necrotizing otitis externa: experience in 22 cases. Ann Otolaryngol Chir Cervicofac. 2000;117(5):291. French.
45. Sandner A, Henze D, Neumann K, Kösling S. Value of hyperbaric oxygen in the treatment of advanced skull base osteomyelitis. Laryngorhinootologie. 2009;88(10):641–6. German.
46. Tisch M, Maier H. Malignant external otitis. Laryngorhinootologie. 2006;85(10):763–9, 770–3. German.
47. Hehl K, Tisch M, Lampl L, Draf W, Stussak G, Frey G. Bilateral Gradenigo syndrome—on the value of an integrated therapy concept including hyperbaric oxygenation and chronic destructive inflammation of the skull base. HNO. 1992;40(8):318–21. German.
48. Pilgramm M, Frey G, Schumann K. Hyperbaric oxygenation—a sensible adjunctive therapy in malignant external otitis. Laryngol Rhinol Otol (Stuttg). 1986;65(1):26–8. German.

Chapter 13
Outcomes and Prognoses

Contents

Abbreviations

CSBO Central skull base osteomyelitis
SBO Skull base osteomyelitis

General Concerns

The prognosis of cranial osteomyelitis has improved with the advancement of imaging and biologic tools, the development of more potent antimicrobial agents and a refinement of surgical techniques. Misdiagnosis and lack of antibiotics were the main reason for a high mortality rate in the past [1, 2]. Nowadays, as seen in our experience and others, excellent prognosis in otherwise uncomplicated cases is possible with the appropriate treatment. However, the outcome of cases of acute and chronic cranial osteomyelitis is only documented scarcely in the literature. Overall, it is clear that the severity of infection, the anatomic site of the disease, the coexistence of intracranial extension, the underlying medical condition, and the delay in diagnosis play an important role in the outcomes of cranial bone infections. Factors associated with excellent and poor prognosis in cranial osteomyelitis are given in Table 13.1.

Delay in medical treatment with or without surgical intervention has been associated with prolonged hospitalization. Ridder et al. found a significant longer postoperative and post-inpatient medicamentous treatment in patients with fungal

A. Akhaddar, *Cranial Osteomyelitis*, DOI 10.1007/978-3-319-30268-3_13

Table 13.1 Factors associated with good/excellent and poor prognosis in cranial osteomyelitis

Factors associated with a good/excellent prognosis	Poorer prognosis is often associated with the following factors
– Young age of patient – Timely diagnosis – No altered mental status – Absence of severe neurologic deficit on initial presentation – Absence of neurologic deterioration during initial management – No comorbid factors – Good general condition – Cranial vault osteomyelitis – Sinogenic focus – Localized infection – Quick response to appropriate treatment – No resistant bacteria	– Advanced age of patient – Delay in diagnosis – Poor neurologic status on initial presentation – Co-existence of serious intracranial complications – Deterioration during initial management with altered mental status, signs of intracranial hypertension, or new neurologic deficit – Immunocompromised hosts or severe underlying disease – Poor general condition – Skull base osteomyelitis – Hematogenous spread/sepsis – Fungal pathogens – Extensive infection – Microorganisms resistance – Refractory osteomyelitis

skull base osteomyelitis (SBO) compared with bacterial infection. They also saw by trend a higher improvement rate of cranial nerve palsies in patients with sinugenic SBO than otogenic ones. Additionally, length of inpatient treatment and number of hospital stays are more important in patients with pseudomonas than no-pseudomonas SBO infection [3]. According to a systematic study performed by Johnson et al., diabetes did not statistically impact the number of courses of therapy, length of therapy, or morbidity/mortality, indicating that central skull base osteomyelitis (CSBO) may be less influenced by concurrent diabetes than isolated malignant otitis externa [4]. In the opposite, cranial vault has a favorable prognosis if diagnosed promptly and treated appropriately. For example, complete clinical recovery is predictable in most patients with Pott's puffy tumor [5–7]. However, we should always take into account that coexistent intracranial complications (brain abscess, meningitis, parameningeal suppuration and sinus venous thrombosis) still represent a non-negligible problem, both in terms of morbidity and mortality.

Despite the fact that the follow-up period in the vast majority of cases did not exceed 1 year, long term control may be required for some cases. Unlike biologic inflammatory markers, both computed tomography-scan (CT-scan) and magnetic resonance imaging (MRI) may take months to years to return to normal following the resolution of osteomyelitis. Healing of osteomyelitis on CT-scan is based on remineralization of bone following the complete recovery of infection. So, a large time interval must pass before this can occur (see Chaps. 8 and 10). Interestingly, Indium-labeled white blood cell-scan has been found to be more sensitive and specific returning to normal within a month following successful treatment [8, 9]. Healed osteomyelitis often leaves a region of increased sclerosis behind. This can be observed in radiographs and is referred to as bone scar. In bone scans these "scars" tend to show a physiological to slightly increased activity. We think that persisting of some areas of osteolysis in the absence of clinical symptoms must not be interpreted as active regions which require therapeutic (surgical) intervention. We recommend to carefully follow-up this group of patients.

It is interesting to note that patients who underwent a bone flap cranioplasty should be informed of the possibility of surgical site infection [10]. About 10 % of patients may present with deep infections, particularly autogenous cranioplasty infection (about 23 % of all cases with deep infections) that necessitated flap removal and antimicrobial treatment [10]. A high index of suspicion is necessary because late presentations are possible [11]. As seen previously, one of our patients presented with a parietal cranial osteomyelitis 11 years following a craniotomy for an acute subdural hematoma. Another patient, a 52-year-old woman, presented with infected frontal cranioplasty (methylmethacrylate) with contiguous cranial osteomyelitis revealing by purulent drainage from scalp sinus tract (see Figs. 10.26–10.29). These complications have occurred 25 years after cranioplasty following a brain tuberculoma resection.

In our own patient data, 72 % (21 cases) of the treated patients with cranial osteomyelitis was free of symptoms at the end of the follow-up period. In 17 % (5 cases) of the treated patients residual symptoms such as mild headache, reduced visual acuity, local discomfort and/or hypoesthesia were noted. Closer inspection of this patient group, however, revealed that these symptoms were often related to postsurgical effects rather than the infection itself. Three patients died (10 %): the first case is about a 61-year old diabetic man who had a frontal osteomyelitis with multiple brain abscesses related to a recurrent otitis media. The second patient is a 34-year-old immuno-competent woman who developed a bone flap osteomyelitis with epidural abscess 2 months following surgical removal of a cranial meningioma. The last patient, a 44-year-old man, survived to his bone flap infection but he died about 6 months later of recurrent malignant brain tumor.

Recurrence

Cranial bone infection may rarely recur in a delayed fashion after apparently successful treatment [12–15]. However, the recurrence rate of skull base osteomyelitis is reported as 15–20 % [14, 16]. On the opposite, only very rare cases of recurrence were reported in the cranial vault [12]. For these reasons, patients are followed with surveillance clinic, biologic and neuroimaging every 4–8 weeks until the lesions have resolved completely. Out-patient follow-up should be for a minimum of 1 year. Predisposing factors that are modifiable should be addressed on a long-term basis. In addition, insufficient treatment duration leads also to recurrence.

Many specific and non-specific pathogens had a potential for recurrence, however hydatidosis is the most important among them. This parasitic infection should be considered as a "locally aggressive tumor", the treatment of which ideally should be radical excision of all affected osseous tissues with a margin of healthy tissue [17, 18]. Technically, this is very improbable to be achieved because of the absence of distinct anatomic planes, containment within small spaces having bony limitations, and the existence of neural structures in close area particularly in the skull base [19]. Therefore, the management of echinococcal cysts usually involves a combination of surgical resection and antihelminthic therapy to avoid recurrence [17–19]. Therefore, a long follow-up period is required.

Malignancy as Late Complication

Malignancy occurring at the site of previous chronic osteomyelitis elsewhere in the body has been frequently documented in the orthopedic literature [20–22]. There was generally a long history of intermittent drainage from a sinus tract with multiples surgical interventions prior to the onset of the malignant tumor. A causal relationship between chronic inflammation and later development of malignancy was highly supported [21]. Only two previous cases were reported in the skull [23, 24]. Sercarz et al. reported a 34-year-old man who required multiple operations for fronto-ethmoid sinusitis and mucocele. He developed, few months soon after, an extensive osteomyelitis of the frontal ethmoid and sphenoid bones. A poorly differentiated squamous cell carcinoma of the adjacent skull base was diagnosed 12 years after the onset of osteomyelitis. The patient was treated with radiotherapy to the nasopharynx, skull base, and neck. There was minimal response and he died 5 years later with persistent local and regional tumoral disease [24]. Interestingly, one other patient was cited among 24 patients treated surgically by Lu and colleagues for chronic osteomyelitis of the skull [23]. This patient with chronic osteomyelitis of the skull had a concomitant localized squamous carcinoma diagnosed only on histopathological examination. No more details could be found about this case [23].

Sequelae

Recovery from neurologic and cranial nerves dysfunction is variable. A complementary aiding therapy such as functional neurology, speech-language and orthoptic therapy may be requested in the aftercare of the patient. Unfortunately, permanent nervous system damage can occur.

Some patients who healed from cranial vault osteomyelitis, may have long-term sequels including hemiparesis, chronic seizure disorder, decreased cognitive function (e.g. aphasia), and rarely residual cranial nerve deficiencies. Chronic osteomyelitis and facial/esthetic scar might also occur [5, 25–30]. Neurologic sequelae are more frequent and serious in patients following skull base osteomyelitis. For example, cranial nerve abnormalities persisted in all 18 patients with skull base osteomyelitis reported by Blyth et al. [31]. Others described ocular nerves paresis (diplopia) and lower cranial nerves palsy manifesting as definitive dysphagia and dysphonia [14, 32, 33]. Even more importantly, patients with CSBO will have permanent hemiparesis, monoparesis, tetraparesis, visual impairment, behavioural problems, learning difficulties (especially in child), and seizure [34].

Mortality

Overall mortality rate associated with cranial osteomyelitis has fallen from 52 to 100 % in the preantibiotic era [1, 2] to virtually 0 % [3, 11, 29, 35]. Misdiagnosis was the main reason for this high mortality rate in the past. However, it is obvious that the case-fatality rates differ greatly based on the cause of the infection, its location, the extension of the disease and the underlying medical condition of the host.

Cranial bone infections arising from adjacent paranasal sinusitis or previous craniotomy appear to carry lower mortality rates than those caused by metastatic hematogenous spread or those localizing in the skull base. To the best of our knowledge, only two patients died secondary to a Pott's puffy tumor and both patients had serious intracranial complications [36, 37]. Hematogenous cranial osteomyelitis tends to occur more often in patients with serious systemic disease [38–41]. Furthermore, the diagnosis may be delayed when the cause of infection is distant from the skull. Post-surgical cranial osteomyelitis is a real nightmare for the neurosurgeon. Fortunately, most cases improve without sequelae [42–49]. Despite its nosocomial aspect, this favorable outcome of post-surgical osteomyelitis is probably due to the close follow-up of the recently operated patients.

Skull base osteomyelitis is a well-known life-threatening condition [50–53]. In 1972 Chandler et al. reported a mortality rate of 50 % [54]. Since that time the mortality rate has dropped, but many authors still report mortality rates as high as 15 % [4, 31, 55, 56]. For Blyth and coauthors, risk factors for death include fungal pathogens and immunosuppression [31]. Some studies, especially those that include patients with malignant external otitis only, indicate lower mortality rates, as for example Rothholz et al. in 2008 with 1.1 % [57]. In contrast, no patient died (among 20 patients) in Ridder's study exclusively focused on CSBO. The higher danger of skull base osteomyelitis probably results from its special location (deeper, adjacent to temporal lobe and posterior fossa) and otogenic abscess flora that was more often resistant to antibiotics, necessitating more frequent antibiotics changes [58]. On the other hand, it is clear that mortality is lower in patients with isolated cranial osteomyelitis than when an intracranial complication occurs [2, 59].

Although most authors observe no important influence of bacteriology, an increased mortality rate has been occasionally reported with fungal and *pseudomonas spp.* [53, 54, 60–64]. While knowing that fungal cranial osteomyelitis is predominantly seen in the immunocompromised state and have a different prognosis than the typical cases of cranial osteomyelitis [61]. A number of pathogens of cranial osteomyelitis has been associated with very low mortality rates such as tuberculosis and syphilis [35, 65, 66].

References

1. Wilensky AO. Osteomyelitis of the skull. Arch Surg. 1933;27(1):83–158.
2. Eisenstein VW, Friedman ED, Davison C. Brain abscess of uncommon origin-relation to osteomyelitis of the skull: a clinicopathologic study. Ann Surg. 1942;115(3):336–55.
3. Ridder GJ, Breunig C, Kaminsky J, Pfeiffer J. Central skull base osteomyelitis: new insights and implications for diagnosis and treatment. Eur Arch Otorhinolaryngol. 2015;272 (5):1269–76. doi:10.1007/s00405-014-3390-y.
4. Johnson AK, Batra PS. Central skull base osteomyelitis: an emerging clinical entity. Laryngoscope. 2014;124(5):1083–7. doi:10.1002/lary.24440.
5. Parida PK, Surianarayanan G, Ganeshan S, Saxena SK. Pott's puffy tumor in pediatric age group: a retrospective study. Int J Pediatr Otorhinolaryngol. 2012;76(9):1274–7. doi:10.1016/j.ijporl.2012.05.018.
6. Salomão JF, Cervante TP, Bellas AR, Boechat MC, Pone SM, Pone MV, de A Pereira B. Neurosurgical implications of Pott's puffy tumor in children and adolescents. Childs Nerv Syst. 2014;30(9):1527–34. doi:10.1007/s00381-014-2480-x.
7. Akiyama K, Karaki M, Mori N. Evaluation of adult Pott's puffy tumor: our five cases and 27 literature cases. Laryngoscope. 2012;122(11):2382–8. doi:10.1002/lary.23490.
8. Epstein JS, Ganz WI, Lizak M, Grobman L, Goodwin WJ, Dewanjee MK. Indium 111-labeled leukocyte scintigraphy in evaluating head and neck infections. Ann Otol Rhinol Laryngol. 1992;101(12):961–8.
9. Seabold JE, Simonson TM, Weber PC, Thompson BH, Harris KG, Rezai K, Madsen MT, Hoffman HT. Cranial osteomyelitis: diagnosis and follow-up with In-111 white blood cell and Tc-99m methylene diphosphonate bone SPECT, CT, and MR imaging. Radiology. 1995;196 (3):779–88.
10. Bhaskar IP, Inglis TJ, Lee GY. Clinical, radiological, and microbiological profile of patients with autogenous cranioplasty infections. World Neurosurg. 2014;82(3–4):e531–4. doi:10.1016/j.wneu.2013.01.013.
11. Blumenkopf B, Hartshorne MF, Bauman JM, Cawthon MA, Patton JA, Friedman AH. Craniotomy flap osteomyelitis: a diagnostic approach. J Neurosurg. 1987;66(1):96–101.
12. Moser R, Schweintzger G, Uggowitzer M, Urban C, Stammberger H, Eder H, Kerbl R. Recurrent Pott's puffy tumor—atypical presentation of a rare disorder. Wien Klin Wochenschr. 2009;121(21–22):719–22. doi:10.1007/s00508-009-1268-6.
13. Radosavljević R, Zivković V, Mojsilović Z. [Chronic recurrent Hematogenous osteomyelitis of the skull bones and other sites]. Med Pregl. 1984;37(1–2):47–9. Croatian.
14. Leahy TW, Sader C. A rare case of bilateral malignant otitis externa and osteomyelitis with lower cranial nerve sequelae. BMJ Case Rep. 2011. pii: bcr0320113957. doi: 10.1136/bcr.03.2011.3957.
15. Lin YT, Chen CT, Lai JP. Post-traumatic fronto-ethmoid osteomyelitis treated with free muscle transfer. J Plast Reconstr Aesthet Surg. 2010;63(6):963–9. doi:10.1016/j.bjps.2009.03.017.
16. Singh A, Al Khabori M, Hyder MJ. Skull base osteomyelitis: diagnostic and therapeutic challenges in atypical presentation. Otolaryngol Head Neck Surg. 2005;133:121–5.
17. Limaiem F, Bellil S, Bellil K, Chelly I, Mekni A, Kallel J, Haouet S, Zitouna M, Kchir N. Hydatid cyst of the cranial vault. J Infect Dev Ctries. 2009;3(10):807–10.
18. Kanaka TS, Balasubramaniam V, Meenakshisundaram E, Varadarajan M. Hydatid of the skull. Indian J Surg. 1970;32:200–3.
19. Yazdani N, Basam A, Heidarali M, Kashani SS, Hasibi M, Mokhtari Z. Infratemporal hydatid cyst: a case presenting with blindness. J Laryngol Otol. 2010;124(4):456–9. doi:10.1017/S0022215109991927.
20. McGrory JE, Pritchard DJ, Unni KK, Ilstrup D, Rowland CM. Malignant lesions arising in chronic osteomyelitis. Clin Orthop Relat Res. 1999;362:181–9.

21. Sankaran-Kutty M, Corea JR, Ali MS, Kutty MK. Squamous cell carcinoma in chronic osteomyelitis. Report of a case and review of the literature. Clin Orthop. 1985;198:264–7.
22. Panteli M, Puttaswamaiah R, Lowenberg DW, Giannoudis PV. Malignant transformation in chronic osteomyelitis: recognition and principles of management. J Am Acad Orthop Surg. 2014;22(9):586–94.
23. Lu Y, Cen Y, Qing Y, Wang H. [Surgical treatment of chronic osteomyelitis of the skull]. Zhongguo Xiu Fu Chong Jian Wai Ke Za Zhi. 2011;25(5):558–61. Chinese.
24. Sercarz JA, Wang MB, Calcaterra TC. Skull base malignancy following long-term sinus mucocele and osteomyelitis. Ann Otol Rhinol Laryngol. 1991;100(2):137–41.
25. Uren RF, Howman-Giles R. Pott's puffy tumor. Scintigraphic findings. Clin Nucl Med. 1992;17(9):724–7.
26. Feder Jr HM, Cates KL, Cementina AM. Pott puffy tumor: a serious occult infection. Pediatrics. 1987;79(4):625–9.
27. Bannon PD, McCormack RF. Pott's puffy tumor and epidural abscess arising from pansinusitis. J Emerg Med. 2011;41(6):616–22. doi:10.1016/j.jemermed.2008.04.050.
28. Kaabia N, Abdelkafi M, Bellara I, Khalifa M, Bahri F, Letaief A. Pott's puffy tumor. A case report. Med Mal Infect. 2007;37(6):350–3.
29. Nisa L, Landis BN, Giger R. Orbital involvement in Pott's puffy tumor: a systematic review of published cases. Am J Rhinol Allergy. 2012;26(2):e63–70. doi:10.2500/ajra.2012.26.3746.
30. Pandey AS, Surana A. Tuberculous osteomyelitis of the bone flap following craniotomy. Indian J Tuberc. 2011;58(3):129–31.
31. Blyth CC, Gomes L, Sorrell TC, da Cruz M, Sud A, Chen SC. Skull-base osteomyelitis: fungal vs. bacterial infection. Clin Microbiol Infect. 2011;17(2):306–11. doi:10.1111/j.1469-0691.2010.03231.x.
32. Patel B, Souqiyyeh A, Ali A. A case of transient, isolated cranial nerve VI palsy due to skull base osteomyelitis. Case Rep Infect Dis. 2014;2014:369867. doi:10.1155/2014/369867.
33. Kim CW, Lee JJ, Kim HS, Won JY. Skull base osteomyelitis following a mastoidectomy. Auris Nasus Larynx. 2013;40(6):584–6. doi:10.1016/j.anl.2012.12.002.
34. Chang PC, Fischbein NJ, Holliday RA. Central skull base osteomyelitis in patients without otitis externa: imaging findings. AJNR Am J Neuroradiol. 2003;24(7):1310–6.
35. Ramdurg SR, Gupta DK, Suri A, Sharma BS, Mahapatra AK. Calvarial tuberculosis: uncommon manifestation of common disease—a series of 21 cases. Br J Neurosurg. 2010;24(5):572–7. doi:10.3109/02688697.2010.495166.
36. Ketenci I, Unlü Y, Tucer B, Vural A. The Pott's puffy tumor: a dangerous sign for intracranial complications. Eur Arch Otorhinolaryngol. 2011;268(12):1755–63. doi:10.1007/s00405-011-1660-5.
37. Tsai BY, Lin KL, Lin TY, Chiu CH, Lee WJ, Hsia SH, Wu CT, Wang HS. Pott's puffy tumor in children. Childs Nerv Syst. 2010;26(1):53–60. doi:10.1007/s00381-009-0954-z.
38. Panos GZ, Karydis I, Velakoulis SE, Falagas ME. Multi-skeletal Pneumocystis jiroveci (carinii) in an HIV-seropositive patient. Int J STD AIDS. 2007;18(2):134–7.
39. Mazor Y, Sprecher H, Braun E. Mycobacteria kansassi disseminated disease. Isr Med Assoc J. 2010;12(2):121–2.
40. Capdevila O, Zurita A, Domingo E, Corbella X, Alcaide F, Monfort JL, Fernández-Viladrich P. Multiple cranial osteolytic lesions due to Mycobacterium kansasii in a patient with AIDS. Scand J Infect Dis. 1998;30(3):305–6.
41. Blom NA, Vreede WB. Infected cephalhematomas associated with osteomyelitis, sepsis and meningitis. Pediatr Infect Dis J. 1993;12(12):1015–7.
42. Abu Hamdeh S, Lytsy B, Ronne-Engström E. Surgical site infections in standard neurosurgery procedures—a study of incidence, impact and potential risk factors. Br J Neurosurg. 2014;28(2):270–5. doi:10.3109/02688697.2013.835376.
43. Nisbet M, Briggs S, Ellis-Pegler R, Thomas M, Holland D. Propionibacterium acnes: an under-appreciated cause of post-neurosurgical infection. J Antimicrob Chemother. 2007;60(5):1097–103.
44. Larsson A, Engström M, Uusijärvi J, Kihlström L, Lind F, Mathiesen T. Hyperbaric oxygen treatment of postoperative neurosurgical infections. Neurosurgery. 2002;50(2):287–95.

45. Olsen JJ, Bingaman KD. Cranial bone flap infections and osteomyelitis of the skull. In: Osenbach RK, Zeidman SM, editors. Infections in neurological surgery diagnosis and management. Philadelphia, PA: Lippincott-Ravan; 1999.
46. Bruce JN, Bruce SS. Preservation of bone flaps in patients with postcraniotomy infections. J Neurosurg. 2003;98(6):1203–7.
47. Auguste KI, McDermott MW. Salvage of infected craniotomy bone flaps with the wash-in, wash-out indwelling antibiotic irrigation system. Technical note and case series of 12 patients. J Neurosurg. 2006;105(4):640–4.
48. Delgado-López PD, Martín-Velasco V, Castilla-Díez JM, Galacho-Harriero AM, Rodríguez-Salazar A. Preservation of bone flap after craniotomy infection. Neurocirugia (Astur). 2009;20 (2):124–31.
49. McClelland III S, Hall WA. Postoperative central nervous system infection: incidence and associated factors in 2111 neurosurgical procedures. Clin Infect Dis. 2007;45(1):55–9.
50. Asimakopoulos P, Supriya M, Kealey S, Vernham GA. A case-based discussion on a patient with non-otogenic fungal skull base osteomyelitis: pitfalls in diagnosis. J Laryngol Otol. 2013;127(8):817–21. doi:10.1017/S002221511300145X.
51. Unnikrishnan R, Faizal BP, Pillai MGK, Paul G. Villaret's syndrome—a rare presentation of skull base osteomyelitis. Amrita J Med. 2013;9(2):32–4.
52. Senegor M, Lewis HP. Salmonella osteomyelitis of the skull base. Surg Neurol. 1991;36 (1):37–9.
53. Ong A, Blyth CC, Bency R, Vicaretti M, Harun A, Meyer W, Shingde M, Gilroy N, Chapman J, Chen SC. Fatal mycotic aneurysms due to Scedosporium and Pseudallescheria infection. J Clin Microbiol. 2011;49(5):2067–71. doi:10.1128/JCM.02615-10.
54. Chandler JR, Grobman L, Quencer R, Serafini A. Osteomyelitis of the base of the skull. Laryngoscope. 1986;96(3):245–51.
55. Ducic Y. Skull base osteomyelitis. South Med J. 2006;99(10):1051.
56. Spielmann PM, Yu R, Neeff M. Skull base osteomyelitis: current microbiology and management. J Laryngol Otol. 2013;127 Suppl 1:S8–12. doi:10.1017/S0022215112002356.
57. Rothholtz VS, Lee AD, Shamloo B, Bazargan M, Pan D, Djalilian HR. Skull base osteomyelitis: the effect of comorbid disease on hospitalization. Laryngoscope. 2008;118 (11):1917–24. doi:10.1097/MLG.0b013e31817fae0d.
58. Soga Y, Oka K, Sato M, Kabata T, Kawasaki T, Kawano H, Hayano M. Cavernous sinus thrombophlebitis caused by sphenoid sinusitis—report of autopsy case. Clin Neuropathol. 2001;20(3):101–5.
59. Cohen I. Osteomyelitis of the Skull. Ann Surg. 1933;97(5):733–48.
60. Reinig JW, Hungerford GD, Mohrmann ME, Vera CL. Case report 268. Diagnosis: cryptococcal osteomyelitis of the calvaria. Skeletal Radiol. 1984;11(3):221–3.
61. Abril V, Ortega E, Segarra P, Pedro F, Sabater V, Herrera A. Rhinocerebral mucormycosis in a patient with AIDS: a complication of diabetic ketoacidosis following pentamidine therapy. Clin Infect Dis. 1996;23(4):845–6.
62. Carr MM, Cusimano MD, Muller PJ, Bilbao J. Aspergillosis of the cranial base. Skull Base Surg. 1994;4(3):159–63.
63. Menachof MR, Jackler RK. Otogenic skull base osteomyelitis caused by invasive fungal infection. Otolaryngol Head Neck Surg. 1990;102(3):285–9.
64. Stodulski D, Kowalska B, Stankiewicz C. Otogenic skull base osteomyelitis caused by invasive fungal infection. Case report and literature review. Eur Arch Otorhinolaryngol. 2006;263(12):1070–6.
65. Dawar P, Satyarthee GD, Sharma BS. Total resolution of large scalp swelling due to calvarial tuberculosis with medical management only: case report and review of the literature. Turk Neurosurg. 2015;25(2):313–6. doi:10.5137/1019-5149.JTN.7937-13.1.
66. Park KH, Lee MS, Hong IK, Sung JY, Choi SH, Park SO, Shin MJ, Chung HW, Lee SH. Bone involvement in secondary syphilis: a case report and systematic review of the literature. Sex Transm Dis. 2014;41(9):532–7. doi:10.1097/OLQ.0000000000000164.

Part V
Special Conditions in Cranial Osteomyelitis

Chapter 14
Unusual Pathogens

Contents

Abbreviations

FNAC Fine needle aspiration cytology
HIV Human immunodeficiency virus
PCR Polymerase chain reaction

Changes in our societies and advances in medicine are liable for an increasing number of infections secondary to tuberculosis, fungi and parasites. Although still uncommon in daily practice, it is important to be attentive of these diseases and to consider them in the differential diagnosis of appropriate cases because early diagnosis and treatment have a significant impact on improved outcome.

Tuberculosis

Tuberculosis is one of the few infectious diseases that have resisted eradication even with the development of effective chemotherapeutic drugs. Though the incidence has considerably declined in the developed countries in the early twentieth century, it continues to be a significant health problem in many developing

A. Akhaddar, *Cranial Osteomyelitis*, DOI 10.1007/978-3-319-30268-3_14

countries. However, the profile of tuberculosis has changed again in recent years in view of a gradual re-emergence of this infection as a public health problem in Europe and North America. This is mainly due to the increase in travel and migration, poorer socio-economic status and living conditions experienced by certain population groups and emergence of immunodeficiency syndromes, in particular *human immunodeficiency virus* (HIV) infection [1–4].

The causative organism of tuberculosis is *Mycobacterium tuberculosis* which is rarely seen in organs other than the lungs. Skeletal lesions occur in approximately 1 % of all cases of tuberculosis [5]. Bone is infected through hematogenous or lymphatic dissemination of bacilli from an active focus, commonly in the lungs. Infection can smolder for months/years before clinical signs are apparent. The most usually involved bones are the vertebrae (spondylitis) and the long bones. Cranial tuberculosis is rare, occurring in only 0.2–1.3 % of all types of skeletal tuberculosis [6] and approximately 1/10,000 cases of tuberculosis [7] with the cranial vault being more commonly involved than the skull base. The relative paucity of lymphatic systems in the skull has been considered to explain the rare tuberculosis infections of the skull bones. The first one who describe cranial bone localization as a consequence of tuberculosis was Reid in 1842 [8]. There were other limited presentations in the literature of tuberculosis of the skull bone (in 1933 by Strauss, in 1942 by Meng and Wu, in 1981 by Mohanty et al., in 1999 by Jadhav and Palande and in 2010 by Ramdurg et al.) [5, 6, 9, 10]. Mukherjee et al. reviewed 365 reported cases of skull tuberculosis between 1842 and 2000. Overall, 91 cases of calvarial tuberculosis were reported between 1954 and 2000 [11].

Young males are most commonly affected, 50 % of patients under the age of 10 years and 70–90 % under the age of 20 years [5, 9, 10]. Many authors have stressed the importance of trauma as a predisposing factor in the formation of bony lesions (increasing vascularity, decreased resistance and unmasking of a latent infection secondary to injury). For others, the role of trauma is probably coincidental rather than causal [10, 12]. *Mycobacterium tuberculosis* appears to fit into the diploë, then the infection causes capillary obliteration and replacement of osseous trabeculae by granulation tissue. When the process is not contained, further extension can occur through the inner and/or outer table of the cranium. Outer table is associated with formation of subgaleal swelling and/or discharging sinus [10]. Whereas, formation of underlying epidural granulation lesions are seen when the inner table is involved. However, it is not uncommon that both tables are affected. Skull sutures do not prevent the spread of granulation tissue and widespread destruction can occur before a sinus or swelling manifests [13]. With extensive intracranial lesions, neurologic deficits and seizure may appear. As seen in Chap. 5, the common sites of involvement are frontal and parietal bones and clinical manifestations are non specific, mainly as a progressive cranial mass lesion without or with mild local cardinal signs of inflammation [14]. Some patients may present with a classic Pott's puffy tumor [15, 16].

Systemic manifestations are uncommon, but inflammatory biomarkers are raised and the tuberculin tests are found positive [10, 11]. False negativity should be read with prudence due to the immunocompromised status in some patients. Imaging

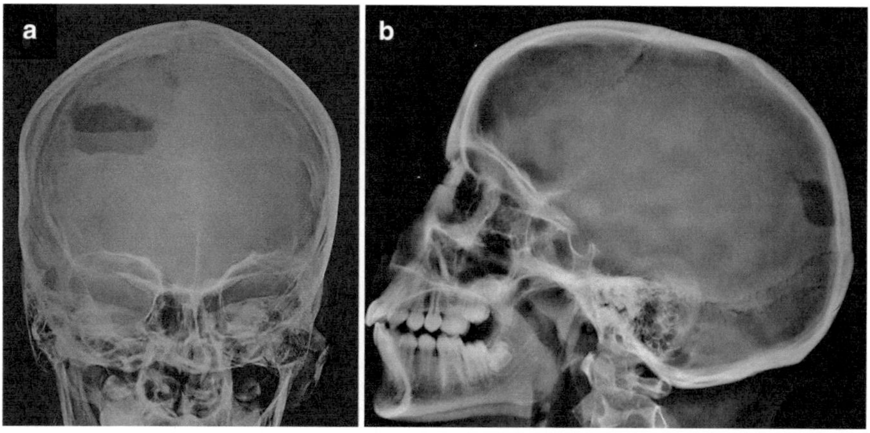

Fig. 14.1 Plain radiographs of the skull in antero-posterior (**a**) and lateral view (**b**). Calvarial tuberculosis. There is a solitary calvarial defect (osteolytic lesion) on the right posterior parietal region

features may be variable and lack of specificity. The commonest lesion is a solitary calvarial defect surrounded by area of increased density (Fig. 14.1). An osseous sequestrum or "bone sand" may be seen within the lesion [17]. LeRoux and Mukherjee emphazise the bony defect aspect on computed tomography-scan (CT-scan): wider at the inner table and forming a "cone" appearance [11, 13]. The lesion is often diffuse and hypodense with enhancing margins and central hypodensity [18] (Figs. 14.2 and 14.3). Magnetic resonance imaging (MRI) characteristics can lead to a conclusive diagnosis. T2-weighted images show a high signal intensity soft tissue mass within the bone defect. This may project into the subgaleal and/or epidural spaces with peripheral capsular enhancement after gadolinium injection [19]. MRI is also very useful in demonstrating intracranial associated lesions such as brain tuberculoma and dural sinus thrombosis [2, 19, 20]. Differential diagnosis includes other infectious osteomyelitis, metastases, vascular and cystic tumors, eosinophilic granuloma and histiocytosis [1, 21].

Skull base tuberculosis disease is extremely rare and may be spread to the ethmoid, orbit, sellar regions as well as posterior fossa and upper cervical spine [12, 22–29].

The definitive diagnosis remains on demonstration of acid-fast bacilli in the lesion/culture or histologic confirmation by the presence of epithelioid-giant cell granulomas with caseating necrosis. Recently, more sensitive special techniques have been developed such as polymerase chain reaction (PCR) and QuantiFERON-TB Gold [30, 31]. For some authors, fine needle aspiration cytology (FNAC) is a logical investigation in lesions with intact overlying scalp and may obviate the need for surgery [32]. However, FNAC should be interpreted with caution when co-infection occurs [11, 19]. The following pathogens are previously isolated with cranial tuberculosis: *Proteus vulgaris*, *Serratia liquefaciens*,

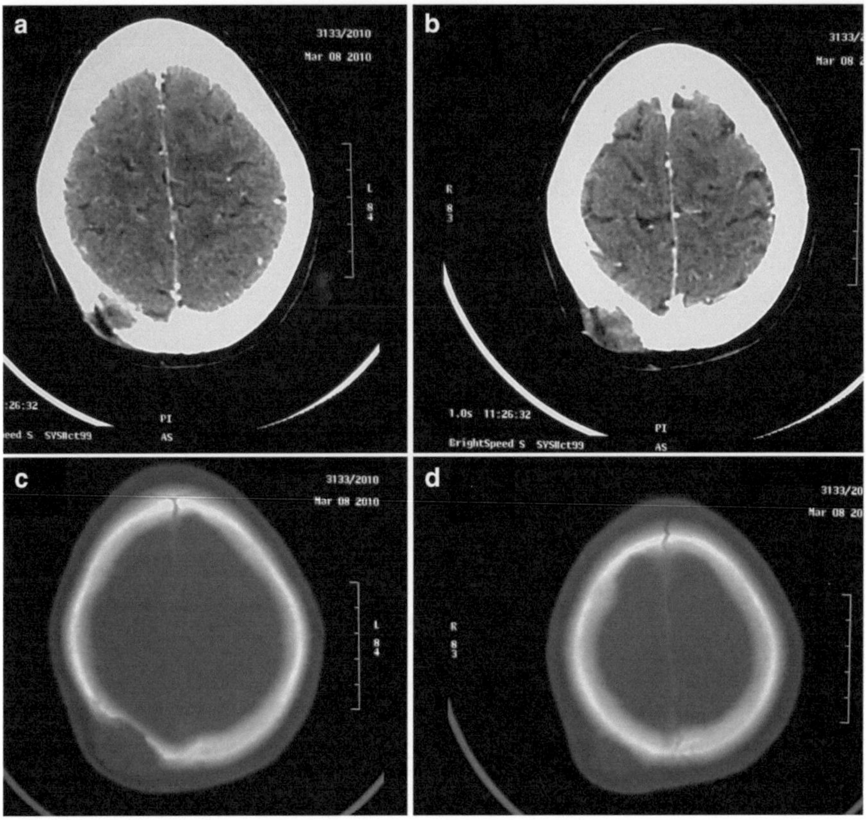

Fig. 14.2 Axial CT-scan of the skull in parenchymatous (**a** and **b**) and bone windows (**c** and **d**) showing hypodense parietal bone lesion with extracranial extension

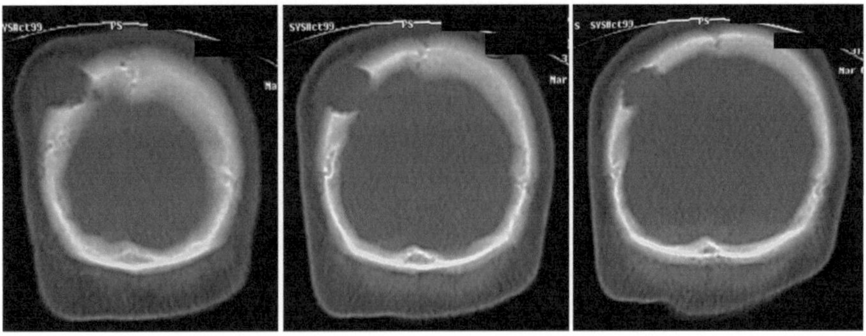

Fig. 14.3 Coronal CT-scan of the skull in bone windows. Parietal global bone defect: the lesion eroded both the inner and outer tables

Acinetobacter species, *Aspergillus flavus* and *Fonsecaea pedrosoi* [11, 19, 22, 33, 34].

As the presentation of cranial bone tuberculosis can be very variable, it is important to maintain a high index of suspicion especially in front of any skull osteolytic lesion that fails to respond to classic antibiotic therapy [9, 11]. Although unusual, it is also important to consider tuberculosis as a cause of post-traumatic [35, 36] or postoperative with bone flap osteomyelitis [37, 38]. Cranial bone tuberculosis may be primary or secondary. Secondary forms are commonly associated with tuberculous infection elsewhere in the body [29, 39–44]. Additionally, some cases of cranial osteomyelitis were complication of otorhinologic tuberculosis [44, 45].

The management of cranial bone tuberculosis includes surgery and anti-tuberculous therapy. However, the role of surgery has declined manifestly with the advent of effective anti-tuberculous drugs. For many authors, surgery is indicated only for diagnosis purposes, for removal of epidural collections and/or large sequestra, and for patients with discharging sinuses, intracranial extensions, or large collections of caseating material causing mass effect or an increase in intracranial pressure [1, 12, 13]. For others, debridement of osteolytic lesion not only provides tissue for biopsy but also helps in accelerated healing [9, 10]. Epidural granulation tissue and involved bone should be removed till normal bone is encountered but dura matter must be left intact.

Tuberculous osteomyelitis is an insidious process requiring long-term therapy. Anti-tuberculous chemotherapy comprised four drugs (isoniazid, rifampicin, pyrazinamide and streptomycin or ethambutol) for 2 months followed by two drugs (isoniazid and rifampicin) for 10 months. In India, patients receive up to 2 years of antibacillar drug therapy [10]. Sometimes, there were serious cases of drug-related toxicity necessitating the withdrawal/change-over of the drug. Additionally, the emergence of new strain of drug resistance should be taken into consideration and managed with second line of therapy. Regular follow-up is necessary for a complete cure.

Prognosis of tuberculous cranial osteomyelitis depends on the state of general health, the extent of local lesion, the early establishment of diagnosis and the response to therapy. Overall, this prognosis is usually favorable and mortality due to cranial bone tuberculosis is very rare.

Some sites of extrapulmonary tuberculosis and focal complications of brucellosis are very difficult to differentiate clinically, radiologically, and even histopathologically [46]. In differential diagnosis of skull osteomyelitis, consumption of unpasteurized cheese, dealing with husbandry, sweating, arthralgia, hepatomegaly and elevated alanine transaminase, may be predictors of brucellosis. Two cases of cranial vault *Brucella species* were previously reported. A 14-year-old boy with an erythematous, non-tender mass over the left mid-forehead area had Brucella osteomyelitis of the left frontal bone with an epidural abscess [47]. Sohn et al. reported a 47-year-old man, who was a stockbreeder, complained of myalgia with fever and chills for 2 weeks. Alanine aminotransferase (50 IU/L) was elevated. The serology titers and blood cultures for brucellosis were positive. Bone scintigraphy demonstrated a focally increased uptake in the left supraorbital area. Plain radiographs and MRI showed a frontal osteolytic lesion suggestive of a bone abscess. The patient underwent a craniotomy. The biopsy confirmed a chronic granulomatous infection caused by *Brucella species*. He received antibiotic therapy [48]. Brucellosis should be remembered in the differential diagnosis of tuberculous osteomyelitis.

Syphilis

Syphilis is a chronic systemic infectious disease caused by the spirochete *Treponema pallidum*. It is a contagious venereal disease which leads to many structural and cutaneous lesions [49]. Acquired syphilis is transmitted by direct contact whereas congenital syphilis is transmitted in utero [50]. Acquired syphilitic infection, if not treated, has three distinct clinical stages after an initial incubation period lasting about 2–3 weeks. The primary stage consists of a nonpainful skin lesion (chancre) of the mouth or genital area that is usually associated with regional lymphadenopathy and initial bacteremia. The secondary stage begins 5–10 weeks after the occurrence of chancres and consists of diffuse eruptions on skin and mucous membrane. This rash may be accompanied by swollen lymph nodes throughout the body, a sore throat, weight loss, malaise, headache and loss of hair. The secondary stage can also damage the eyes, liver, kidneys and other organs. Latent syphilis, having no clinical manifestations, is detected only by reactive serologic tests. The tertiary-stage lesions may not appear for several years to decades after the onset of the disease. In this stage of syphilis, ascending aorta, central nervous system, skin, liver and skeletal systems show gummatous destruction which is a soft, gummy tumor that resembles granulation tissue [49]. Although such syphilitic lesions have not been described for decades, there has recently been an increase in the number of osteitis cases reported, especially in patients with HIV infection [51–60].

Bone involvement is rare, identified in less than 0.2 % of patients diagnosed as having early (primary and secondary) syphilis [50, 61]. Thompson and Preston performed skull radiographs on 80 patients with secondary syphilis and found 7 cases with cranial osteolytic lesions, only 4 of whom had symptomatic headache [62]. In a recent systematic review performed by Park et al. from 1964 to 2013, 21 cases (57 %) of skull localization were found among 37 patients of secondary syphilis with bone involvement [63]. Clinical manifestations vary greatly and are non specific since this disease has long been labeled as "The great medical imitator". Bony lesions may appear as early as 1 month after the primary chancre [64]. In the skull, chronic headache is routinely found particularly in the frontotemporal area, more rarely skull vault swelling [55, 58].

Cranial vault bones seem the only ones affected. Radiography, CT-scan and MRI are not specific and often show osteolytic lesion. The outer table worm-eaten appearance on plain radiography is suggestive [51]. MRI findings demonstrate a focal enhancing cranial vault lesion and contiguous soft tissue abnormality in the scalp [53]. As mentioned in Chap. 9, the differential diagnosis for osteolytic lesion is very extensive, then serologic tests as venereal disease research laboratory (VDRL) test, rapid plasma reagin (RPR) or *Treponema pallidum* hemagglutination assay (TPHA) should be enough to eliminate syphilis. Intracranial extensions are unusual [53, 63]. Curiously, a patient developed progressive intracranial hypertension with papilloedema secondary to thrombosis of the superior sagittal sinus by extension of a calvarial syphilitic lesion [65]. Recently, Son et al. reported a patient whose initial presentation of neurosyphilis was painful calvarial lesions [59]. Bone involvement is usually multifocal, which is evident in bone scintigraphy [52, 54, 60, 66, 67].

Histopathologic study often revealed a plasma cell and lymphocytic perivascular infiltration in the bone and surrounding tissue. Vasculitis with a predominance of mononuclear and plasma cells surrounding the involved vessels is also typical of syphilitic involvement [57, 68]. Identification of *Treponema pallidum* in the osseous lesion with dark-field microscope, silver stain, immunoperoxidase stain, or PCR was exceptionally reported in the skull bone [66, 69].

Skull syphilis is a treatable medical entity. Penicillin is the antibiotic of choice but doxycycline will be an alternative in case of penicillin allergy [57]. In general practice, intramuscular benzathine penicillin 2.4 million Units weekly for 2–4 weeks may be a useful therapeutic option for syphilitic bone lesions [63]. Surgical debridement is not mandatory. One patient underwent excision of frontal bone due to uncertain diagnosis [53]. Although symptomatic relief after therapy is typically rapid, the osseous lesions in early-phase syphilis resolve more slowly and can persist for up to 7–11 months [53, 63, 66, 68]. The coexistence of HIV infection must be taken into consideration because about one third of patients with skull syphilis combine HIV infection [63, 70].

Salmonellosis

Salmonella species is a rod-shaped bacterium of the Enterobacteriaceae family. Salmonella infection most commonly causes gastroenteritis and enteric fever due to ingestion of contaminated food. They can be divided into two groups: typhoidal and nontyphoidal Salmonella [71]. Extra-intestinal manifestations are unusual especially osseous infection which constitutes 0.8 % of all salmonella infections and 0.45 % of all types of osteomyelitis [72]. The skull is rarely infected by *Salmonella species*. In 1996, Kamarulzamane et al. described two patients with salmonella osteomyelitis and reviewed ten cases previously described in the literature [73]. Since then, we found seven more cases including one of our patients [74–79]. It is more often seen in adults than in children, and males and females are equally affected.

Generally, the clinical presentation of cranial osteomyelitis caused by *Salmonella species* does not differ from that caused by other pathogens. The most common presenting complaint was headache, fluctuant mass, seizure and focal neurological deficits. Approximately half of these patients had underlying intracranial abscesses. Fever was not a common symptom, despite the presence of an underlying suppurative collection.

Neuroimaging study (CT-scan and MRI) are useful in diagnosing osteomyelitis of the skull and in detecting underlying intracranial complications such as epidural abscess, subdural empyema and brain abscess [73, 74, 78, 79]. Skull base localization was found in only one case [80]. Pathogens include *S. typhimurium*, *S. typhi*, *S. paratyphi A*, *S. paratyphi B and S. enteritidis*. Data of histopathologic study are no specific however Salmonella infection may produce tuberculoid granules with variable central necrosis [81].

Six of the 17 well-documented patients are not found to have any associated illness. Two patients are receiving immunosuppressive therapy and another two patients are diabetics. Non-typhoidal salmonella infections are recognized with increasing frequency in HIV-infected individuals [82, 83] but Involvement of cranial bones in this group of patients who are most susceptible to salmonella osteomyelitis was described in only two cases [78, 84]. Concerning late reactivation of previous infection, Meyer et al. presented a case of skull osteomyelitis due to *Salmonella typhi* 40 years after gastrointestinal primary infection [75]. One newborn had a cephalhematoma due to *Salmonella typhimurium* [76]. Curiously, four patients have a post-surgical site infection following craniotomy [74, 85, 86]. One of our patients, a 36-year-old man without specific medical history, presented with a left parietal brain glioma which was treated with extensive surgical resection. At 4-week follow-up, he reported an inflammatory swelling above the scalp closure, but denied any neurological symptoms. This surgical site infection was radiologically and bacteriologically diagnosed to be a subgaleal abscess with bone flap osteomyelitis due to *Salmonella enteritidis*. The patient treated successfully with antibiotherapy alone. Treatment was started with ciprofloxacin, gentamicin and metronidazole and patient was discharged to home 1 month later for 4-week course of ciprofloxacin with a good outcome.

A combination of surgery and prolonged antibiotic therapy are used for 12 of the 17 well-documented cases. Eleven of the 12 patients recovered and one diabetic patient with skull base infection died [80]. Four patients received antibiotherapy alone and one patient was treated with surgery alone in the preantibiotic area. Third-generation cephalosporins and quinolones are currently the drugs of choice in the treatment of systemic salmonella disease. A good outcome can be expected with the combination of surgery and prolonged antibiotic therapy.

Actinomycosis

Actinomycosis is a rare chronic granulomatous disease caused by *Actinomyces species*. This anaerobic filamentous Gram-positive bacteria-like fungus generally colonizes the human mouth and gastrointestinal/urogenital tracts. Infection can occur anywhere in the body, but two-thirds of all cases occur in the cervicofacial region [87–90]. In the skeleton, the mandible is the most affected bone [88], whereas involvement of the cranial bones is quite rare, with no more than 20 cases reported in the English-language literature until now [90–102]. *Actinomyces israelii* is the most prevalent species isolated in human infections, rarely *A. odontolicus, A. bovis, A. naeslundi or A. viscosus* [94, 103]. In the skull, the portal of entry is generally the oral cavity or the paranasal sinuses [92, 94]. However, infection may spread by the hematogenous route from a distant primary site. If the lesion progresses slowly, little suppuration takes place. Then, it frequently mimics malignancy, tuberculosis, or nocardiosis, as it spreads continuously and progressively, and often forms a cold abscess. However, in more acute forms, abscesses are formed and discharge pus containing yellow granules (or sulfur granules) through multiple skin sinuses [100]. Actinomyces organisms are often underestimated as causes of infectious diseases because they are not looked for routinely and are difficult to detect. Both cranial vault and skull base are interested, as well as pediatric and adult populations. Some favorable factors must be taken in consideration such as head trauma, previous surgery, other otorhinolaryngeal infections, cardiac malformations, and diseases of the immune system [96]. In contrast to most fungi, cranial osteomyelitis due to actinomycosis are unusual in immunocompromised hosts. As other systemic localization, the definitive diagnosis of actinomycosis was made after the disease was rather advanced [97, 101]. Traditionally, osteomyelitis attributable to *Actinomyces species* often results in recurrent disease and inconsistent responses to antimicrobial agents [103]. In the skull, actinomycosis is frequently associated with intracranial lesions such as epidural abscess, subdural empyema and brain abscess [89, 96, 98–100, 102, 104]. Two cases are previously reported with craniocervical dissemination [92, 101].

Swelling over the head, headache and focal neurologic signs are the most common findings, however high fever is usually absent [93]. The mean duration of symptoms prior to diagnosis was more than 3 months, longer than with most causes of bacterial osteomyelitis. Neuroimaging explorations do not provide a specific diagnosis, but they allow an accurate definition of the dimensions and extension of the infection especially intracranial involvement [98]. To detect these unusual bacteria, several specimens should be obtained and then expeditiously transported to the laboratory in media supportive of anaerobic growth. Differentiation from nocardiosis, tuberculosis and malignant neoplasms is crucial to the selection of appropriate antimicrobial therapy [105].

Adequate surgical debridement would appear to be the cornerstone of therapy because increased oxygen tension in infected tissue has a direct bactericidal effect on *Actinomyces* organisms [94, 103]. The traditional antibiotic treatment is high-dose penicillin for a prolonged period (6 months to 1 year or longer) [89, 92, 106]. However, there is no evidence that prolonged courses of antibiotic therapy increase the chance of cure or that intravenously administered antibiotics offer any advantage over orally administered antibiotics. In 2010, we reported five immunocompetent patients with focal intracranial infections due to *Actinomyces species*. Interestingly, four of our patients were treated with intravenous ciprofloxacin (at least 4 weeks) with an excellent outcome and all our patients were discharged with a 2-month regimen of oral antibiotic (ciprofloxacin or erythromycin) and were cured with full recovery [104]. Finally, Nomura et al. emphasize the role of the serum level CRP and Fluorodeoxyglucose positron emission tomography (FDG-PET) in the follow-up of the efficacy of antibiotic therapy [92].

Aspergillosis

Despite advancements in surgical techniques and the accessibility of more effective antifungal therapeutic antimicrobial agents, craniocerebral invasive fungus remains an increasingly more common and challenging clinical entity [107]. Diagnosis is frequently delayed and often considered only following failure of antibacterial therapy. Blyth et al. noted that 55 % of patients with fungal skull base osteomyelitis were treated with antibacterial drugs for a median of 5 weeks prior to diagnosis [108], knowing that a delay in antifungal therapy results in increased mortality [109–111].

Most cases of fungal infection result from *Aspergillus species* which are ubiquitous in the environment and mostly noninvasive. Several species have been described as pathogens, *A. fumigatus* is the usual cause of clinical aspergillosis, followed by *A. flavus* and *A. niger*, rarely *A. terreus*. Invasive aspergillosis can occur in most organs, with the lung being the main target of this opportunistic infection [112]. Among the extrapulmonary locations, bone is rarely involved but Aspergillus osteomyelitis is a debilitating and severe form of invasive aspergillosis. The most common sites are spine, ribs and cranium.

Overall, cranial osteomyelitis due to aspergillosis is rare [113]. In a recent literature review performed by Gamaletsou et al., there were 180 cases of Aspergillus osteomyelitis in the English-language literature between 1947 and 2013. Among the 41 cases of cranial localisation, 28 (68 %) had direct invasion from contiguous infection, including 15 patients with Aspergillus malignant externa otitis, middle ear infection, and mastoiditis. Eight other patients had prior surgery or previous trauma, which served as the focus of infection, while the remaining patients had systemic immunological impairments, including diabetes mellitus, neutropenia, corticosteroids, HIV infection, primary immunodeficiency, transplantation, solid tumors and hematologic malignancy [114]. Skull bone aspergillosis occurs predominantly in males (71 %). Pediatric patients constitute 20 % of the population. Thirty-one patients (76 %) have prior broad spectrum antibiotics. The majority of patients (68 %) were managed with both surgery and prolonged antifungal agents. Surgical intervention consists of debridement in 29 patients (71 %) and drainage in 6 cases (15 %). Ten (29 %) patients received antifungal therapy alone and two patients were treated with surgery alone probably in the preantibiotic area. Median duration of therapy was 90 days. The therapeutic effect of antifungal therapy with or without surgery was as fellow: complete response (58 %), partial response (32 %), relapse (12 %) and 13 patients (32 %) died [114].

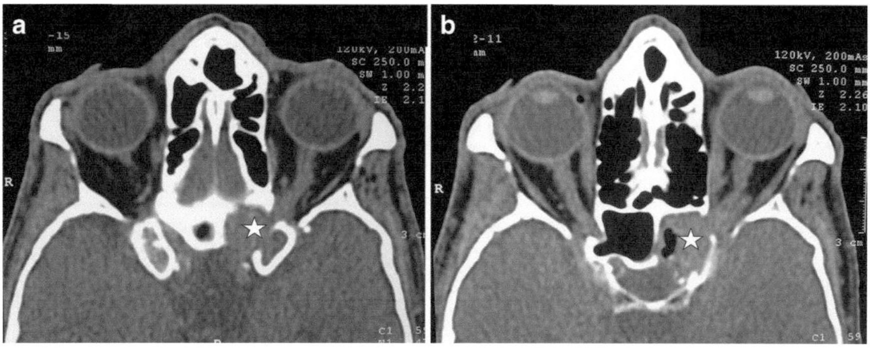

Fig. 14.4 Axial CT-scan of the skull base (bone windows) (**a** and **b**) demonstrating bony destruction of the sphenoid walls and left clinoid (*star*)

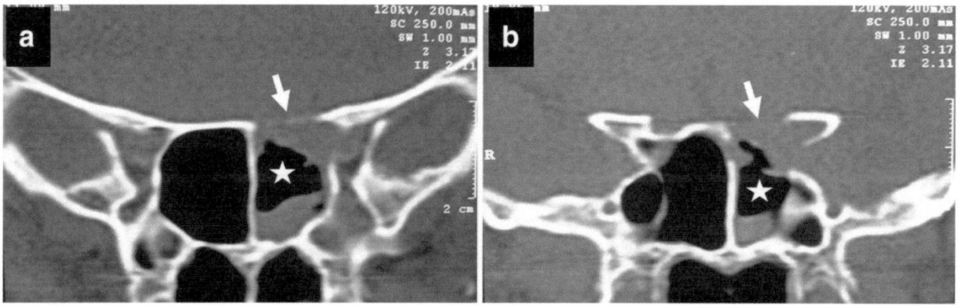

Fig. 14.5 Coronal CT-scan reconstructions (bone windows) (**a** and **b**) showing left sphenoiditis (*star*) with erosion of the left optic canal and superior wall of the sphenoid sinus (*arrow*)

Skull base is more often affected than the cranial vault [113, 115, 116]. Some bacteria may be mixed with *Aspergillus* species such as *Staphylococcus aureus* and *Serratia marcescens* and this co-infection has significant therapeutic implications and treatment failure [117, 118]. Association with other fungal agent has also been reported [111].

Clinical presentation and physical findings are not too different from those with bacterial cranial osteomyelitis. A recent single institution review highlights the difficulty in differentiating bacterial from fungal skull base osteomyelitis on clinical or radiological grounds [108]. Overall, bacterial skull base osteomyelitis was more likely than fungal infection to have arisen from an otogenic focus of infection, whereas fungal skull base osteomyelitis was more likely to have originated from the sinuses [108]. The diagnostic imaging features of osteolysis (Figs. 14.4 and 14.5), bone destruction, and increased MRI T2-weighted signal intensity are compatible with an infectious bony process but not for aspergillosis. Besides CT-scan and MRI (Fig. 14.6), nuclear medicine techniques are very sensitive for skull base infection and are an excellent positive indicator although they may remain "hot" for months following resolution of infection [119]. Recent biopsy and culture of lesions are required for definitive diagnosis and pathogen-directed therapy. Histopathologic

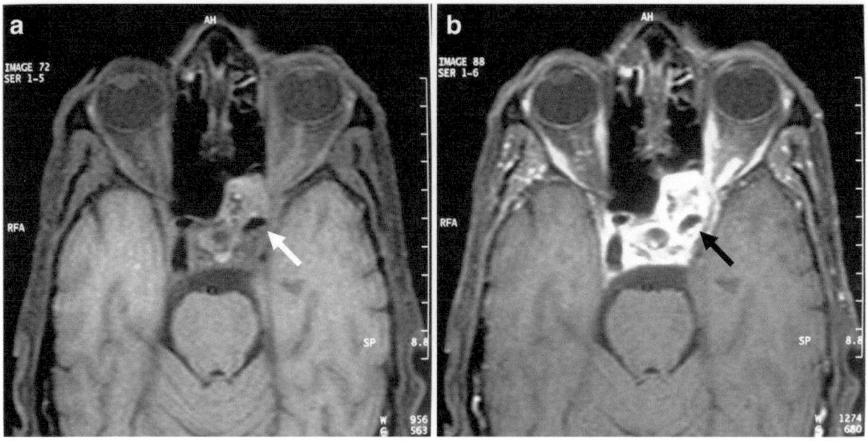

Fig. 14.6 Axial T1-weighted MRI before (**a**) and after (**b**) gadolinium enhancement showing granulomatous invasive fungal ethmoido-sphenoidal sinusitis with intracranial extension on the left side. The left internal carotid is seen within the inflammatory process (*arrow*)

examination shows vascular thrombosis that is surrounded by extensive coagulative necrosis and hemorrhage. Granulomatous inflammation with septate hyphae with acute-angle, dichotomous branching at regular intervals indicates aspergillus infection [107, 113].

Cavernous sinus aspergillosis should be considered in patient with skull base infection, presenting with cranial nerve palsies [113, 120]. In 2008, we described the first recorded patient with sino-orbitocranial infection with cavernous sinus invasion due to *Aspergillus terreus*, a relatively drug-resistant and uncommon *Aspergillus species*. We emphasized the recent increasing frequency of infection by *A. terreus* and the need for accurate speciation to initiate appropriate antifungal therapy [107]. Skull base osteomyelitis may also be associated with findings such as cerebral abscess, meningoencephalitis and infarcts [115, 121].

Cranial bone Aspergillosis secondary to direct inoculation from a scalp wound infection is a very rare condition, reported only twice in the literature. Yuen et al. described a case of scalp necrotizing fasciitis combined with osteomyelitis of the calvarium involving Aspergillus infection [122]. Curiously, another case was reported in which an adult immunocompetent patient presented with *Aspergillus fumigatus* cranial infection secondary to accidental cranial injury. The patient had a dirty wound in the right parietal area with an underlying cranial fracture [123].

Previous studies have stressed the importance of radical surgery in combination with an anti-fungal agent in treating Aspergillus skull base osteomyelitis and neuroaspergillosis [124, 125]. The anti-fungal agent of choice has changed over the past decade, with randomised studies demonstrating the greater efficacy of voriconazole over amphotericin B in such cases [126]. Voriconazole now represents the recommended first-line treatment for invasive aspergillosis [127–129]. Additionally, antifungal agent toxicity should be taken in consideration, especially the side effects of amphotericin B (in particular nephrotoxicity and morbidity of prolonged venous access) which may require interruption of antifungal drugs or a decrease in dosage [129]. Voriconazole and posaconazole have fewer side effects with acceptable bioavailability [130, 131]. Voriconazole also has been used as salvage therapy for refractory Aspergillus osteomyelitis [132–134]. For many authors, hyperbaric oxygen therapy should be considered post-operatively against this life threatening fungal infection with significant high mortality [108, 113, 125, 135, 136].

Cryptococosis

Cryptococcosis is a systemic mycosis caused by the encapsulated yeasts *Cryptococcus neoformans* or *Cryptococcus gattii*, organisms found in soil and often associated with pigeon droppings or eucalyptus trees. The portal of entry of Cryptococcus is the lung from where it disseminates systemically most commonly to the central nervous system [137]. It rarely causes skeletal infection in humans, but when it does, it tends to affect immunocompromised hosts with obvious disease processes [138]. Involvement of bone has been reported in 5–10 % of cases as part of a systemic infection and usually presents with osteolytic lesions. In 2010, a review of the English-language literature indicates that less than 80 cases of cryptococcal infections with bone involvement have been reported [139]. The spine, pelvis, ribs, tibia and femur are most commonly affected.

To date, skull involvement has been reported in less than 20 cases [139–155]. Mechanisms involving cryptococcal infections of the skull include disseminated infections, skull trauma, and embolic phenomena [146]. Skull osteomyelitis due to cryptococcosis rarely occurs in immunocompetent individuals without underlying disease; only four cases were previously described [140, 144, 146, 151]. Conversely, none of the patients were HIV-positive and only one patient had concomitant pulmonary cryptococcal pneumonia [147]. The significant morbidity of reported cases includes corticoid therapy, organ transplantation, leukemia, T-cell deficiency and diabetes mellitus.

The most commonly described clinical presentation was soft tissue swelling and pain developing as an insidious infection. Fever was not a common feature. However, about half of patients presented skin tenderness. The cranial vault is most often affected. Interestingly, temporal bone involvement with cryptococcal disease is documented in five cases, among them four cases were associated with cryptococcal meningitis with VIIth and VIIIth cranial nerves neuropathy [145].

Multifocal skeletal lesions were seen in two patients: skull/patella in one and frontal/mandible in the other [152, 153]. A combination of skull and lung infection was also reported by Luhr and Svane [147].

Neuroimaging data are not specific for cryptococcosis, and radiological findings are similar to those of tuberculosis. The osteolytic cranial lesion is irregular and half of them showed dura matter involvement after contrast enhancement. The diagnosis of skeletal cryptococcosis is mainly made by the identification of *Cryptococcus neoformans* organisms from pathologic sections and culture of specimens obtained through surgical biopsy. Some authors advanced that Mucicarmine stains can help distinguish *Cryptococcus species* from other fungal infections [146].

Most of the cases, being reported, were treated successfully with medical treatment alone (including intravenous amphotericin B or fluconazole, followed by oral fluconazole or 5-flucytosine) or the combination of medical treatment and surgical debridement. To our knowledge, 2 of the 20 patients with skull osteomyelitis died during hospitalization [148, 154]. It seems that Cryptococcal osteomyelitis of the skull has a worse outcome compared to other skeletal localizations [155].

This fungal infection should be considered in an insidious growing soft mass or scalp abscess of undetermined origin as well as any osteolytic lesion with granulomatous reaction.

Mucormycosis

Mucormycosis or zygomycosis is an opportunistic fulminant fungal infection, which mainly infects immunocompromised patients. This deadly affection is increasingly emerging, considered the third most common opportunistic fungal infection in immunocompromised and diabetic patients [156–158]. *Rhizopus species* are the most common causative organisms, followed by Mucor and Absidia from the order of Mucorales. The pathognomonic feature is the presence of invasive aseptate mycelia that are larger than other filamentous fungi with the hyphae exhibiting right angle and haphazard branching [159, 160]. The infection usually involves the lungs, gastrointestinal tract, skin, or less commonly other organ systems but may involve any area [161, 162]. Of all the types of mucormycosis, rhino-facial-cranial area is among the rarest and also the most lethal opportunistic infection [163]. The infection begins in the nose and paranasal sinuses due to inhalation of fungal spores. Then, the infection can spread to orbital and intracranial structures either by direct invasion or through the blood vessels. The fungus invades the arteries leading to thrombosis that subsequently causes soft tissues and bony necrosis [164].

Cranial bone involvement is rare, mainly seen in the skull base [159, 165–167]. As other forms of fungal skull osteomyelitis, mucormycosis is often considered only following failure of antibacterial therapy [168]. The significant morbidity of skull mucormycosis is consisted with previous localization of this opportunistic fungus including diabetes mellitus, chronic leukemia, chronic renal failure, viral hepatitis, severe malnutrition or any other state of immune suppression [158, 159, 163, 168, 169]. Importantly, however, skull osteomyelitis due to mucormycosis may also occur in immunocompetent individuals [170, 171]. Fortun et al. described an unusual case of chronic frontal osteomyelitis after bilateral rhino-orbital mucormycosis of posttraumatic origin in a previously healthy man [170]. Additionally, a temporo-maxillary mycormycosis was reported in a 7-month pregnant woman without evidence of any underlying immune deficiency except that which may be attributed to pregnancy [171].

The initial symptoms are consistent with those of chronic sinusitis, periorbital cellulitis and symptoms attributable to invasive paranasal sinusitis (especially sphenoidal) but with a relative paucity of features attributable to ear infection [159, 169, 171]. Signs and symptoms that suggest intracranial invasion (rhinocerebral mycomycosis) include headache, multiple cranial nerve palsies, orbital apex syndrome, meningitism and focal neurological deficits [157, 167].

CT-scan and MRI shows hyperdense material in the paranasal sinus affected with nodular mucosal thickenings. Proptosis of the orbit is due to enhancement of the soft tissue into the orbital apex. MRI especially the non-enhanced T1 weighted sequence is quite sensitive to minor pathologic abnormalities in skull base. The characteristic finding is high signal intensivity of the skull base marrow fat on T1-weighted images [169]. MR angiography may be used for diagnosing cerebrovascular complications. Intracranial findings include infarcts related to vascular thrombosis, mycotic emboli, and frontal lobe abscesses [172, 173]. Alvernia et al. reported a case of internal carotid artery pseudoaneurysm owing to skull base mucormycosis [174]. Additionally, Delbrouck and co-authors presented a patient with a carotid artery occlusion due to fulminant rhinocerebral mucormycosis [175].

Diagnosis depends on the demonstration of tissue invasion using biopsy or after surgical debridement. Surgical care is the mainstay of treatment for any form of zygomycosis. In addition, early and aggressive surgical removal of all infected and devitalized tissue is considered the best approach [156, 162]. Amphotericin B is the drug of choice for treatment of mucormycosis and is recommended that therapy should be started as soon as the diagnosis is confirmed. Hyperbaric oxygen therapy can also be given as adjuvant [174].

The mortality rate is around 85 % for patients with the rhinocerebral type of infection, and the overall mortality rate of zygomycosis is about 44 % [156, 176].

Hydatidosis

Hydatidosis is a rare parasitic disease caused by the larval cysts of *Echinococcus granulosis*, a small tape worm currently considered prevalent in Mediterranean countries, the Middle East, Oceania, South Africa, and South America [177]. Liver (60 %) and lungs (30 %) are the common sites of involvement, unlike the skeleton (0.5–2 %) [178]. The skull bones are rarely infected: only 3–4 % of all patients diagnosed as having osseous hydatidosis. About 38 cases were reported in the world literature between 1957 and 2010 [179]. Usually, it does not have any systemic sign unless it becomes ruptured or infected. High index of clinical suspicion is required to diagnose the condition especially in the endemic areas.

Generally, cranial hydatidosis may present with one of the following syndromes including increased intracranial pressure, skull deformity, cranial nerve palsies or focal neurological disturbance [180–184]. Skull base is more rarely infected [185]. CT-scan and MRI are the most important tools for diagnosing the hydatidosis of the skull. Cystic lesion shows density and intensity similar to cerebrospinal fluid on CT-scan and MRI without contrast enhancement. However, if bone lesions become infected by bacteria, cyst wall may be enhanced slightly with contrast medium [186, 187]. The diagnosis may be very difficult if the cranial bones are purely infected without intracranial or extracranial extension. The cyst enlarges and develops irregularly along the path of least resistance, losing its typical spherical shape [184]. If both outer table and inner table are destroyed, intra-cranial and extra-cranial spaces may communicate. Extraosseous hydatid cysts may calcify, while intraosseous hydatid cysts rarely present calcification [179, 188].

Familiarity with imaging findings is important to make a preoperative diagnosis. All patients with suspected hydatid cyst should undergo an abdomino-thoracic CT-scan. Bone and brain tissue evokes minimum or no immunological reaction to hydatidosis, so serologic tests are of little value in diagnosing the condition [189, 190]. Differential diagnosis must be considered with calvarial dermoid/epidermoid cystic tumors, cystic fibrous dysplasia, eosinophylic granuloma, hemangioma and solitary metastases. When intracranial extension occurs, hydatid cyst can mimic abscess formation, arachnoid cysts and other cystic tumors. Oral antihelminthic drug as albendazole/mebendazole has been promising but surgery is the cornerstone of treatment for bone hydatidosis [177].

During operation, every effort should be made to prevent the spillage of the cyst fluid and to remove the cyst completely except in case of basal skull hydatidosis where complete removal of the cyst is not possible and even dangerous [179]. Skull defect is closed by cranioplasty or titanium plate. Then chemotherapy is continued for at least 3 months. Recurrence is the most common complications and need a long follow-up period [186, 191–193]. The treatment of hydatidosis is prophylactic. A good sanitary education and hygiene will reduce the number of people infested in endemic eras [177].

References

1. Tyagi AK, Kirollos RW, Kang NV. Tuberculous osteitis of the skull: a case report and review of the literature. Br J Neurosurg. 1996;10(4):399–401.
2. García-García C, Ibarra V, Azcona-Gutiérrez JM, Oteo JA. Calvarial tuberculosis with parenchymal involvement. Travel Med Infect Dis. 2013;11(5):329–31. doi:10.1016/j.tmaid.2012.11.008.
3. Richardus RA, Jansen JC, Steens SC, Arend SM. Two immigrants with tuberculosis of the ear, nose, and throat region with skull base and cranial nerve involvement. Case Rep Med. 2011;2011:675807. doi:10.1155/2011/675807.
4. Swaminathan S, Padmapriyadarsini C, Narendran G. HIV-associated tuberculosis: clinical update. Clin Infect Dis. 2010;50(10):1377–86. doi:10.1086/652147.

5. Jadhav RN, Palande DA. Calvarial tuberculosis. Neurosurgery. 1999;45(6):1345–9.
6. Strauss DC. Tuberculosis of the flat bones of the vault of skull. Surg Gynaecol Obstet. 1933;57:384–98.
7. Davidson PT, Horowitz I. Skeletal tuberculosis. A review with patient presentations and discussion. Am J Med. 1970;48(1):77–84.
8. Reid E. Mediziniches Correspondenzblatt Bayerischer Erlangen. 1842;33.
9. Mohanty S, Rao CJ, Mukherjee KC. Tuberculosis of the skull. Int Surg. 1981;66(1):81–3.
10. Ramdurg SR, Gupta DK, Suri A, Sharma BS, Mahapatra AK. Calvarial tuberculosis: uncommon manifestation of common disease—a series of 21 cases. Br J Neurosurg. 2010;24(5):572–7. doi:10.3109/02688697.2010.495166.
11. Mukherjee KK, Kaushik R, Nada R, Khosla VK, Khandelwal N, Kak VK. Calvarial tuberculosis. Surg Neurol. 2002;57(3):195–202.
12. Gupta RK, Jena A, Sharma A. Sellar abscess associated with tuberculous osteomyelitis of the skull: MR findings. AJNR Am J Neuroradiol. 1989;10(2):448.
13. LeRoux PD, Griffin GE, Marsh HT, Winn HR. Tuberculosis of the skull—a rare condition: case report and review of the literature. Neurosurgery. 1990;26(5):851–5.
14. Tanioka M, Nakagawa Y, Maruta N, Miyachi Y. Cranial tuberculosis osteitis with symptomless epidural extension. Eur J Dermatol. 2010;20(5):665–6. doi:10.1684/ejd.2010.1046.
15. Chand G, Shafique M, Khan A, Ahmad T. Pott's puffy tumour. J Coll Physicians Surg Pak. 2012;22(3):196–7. doi:02.2012/JCPSP.196197.
16. Tattersall R, Tattersall R. Pott's puffy tumour. Lancet. 2002;359(9311):1060–3.
17. Malhotra R, Dinda AK, Bhan S. Tubercular osteitis of skull. Indian Pediatr. 1993;30(9):1119–23.
18. de Castro CC, de Barros NG, Campos ZM, Cerri GG. CT scans of cranial tuberculosis. Radiol Clin North Am. 1995;33(4):753–69.
19. Akhaddar A, Baallal H, Elouennass M, Elgharbaoui H, Mahi M, Boucetta M. Combined Serratia liquefaciens and Mycobacterium tuberculosis in temporal osteitis with brain extension. Surg Infect (Larchmt). 2011;12(4):329–31. doi:10.1089/sur.2010.100.
20. Sundaram PK, Sayed F. Superior sagittal sinus thrombosis caused by calvarial tuberculosis: case report. Neurosurgery. 2007;60(4):E776.
21. Schuster JD, Rakusan TA, Chonmaitree T, Box QT. Tuberculous osteitis of the skull mimicking histiocytosis X. J Pediatr. 1984;105(2):269–71.
22. Brar T, Mrig S, Passey JC, Agarwal AK, Jain S. Complicated coexisting pyogenic and tuberculous otitis media affecting the temporozygomatic, infratemporal, and parotid areas: report of a rare entity. Ear Nose Throat J. 2013;92(1):E10–2.
23. Sethi A, Sabherwal A, Gulati A, Sareen D. Primary tuberculous petrositis. Acta Otolaryngol. 2005;125(11):1236–9.
24. Mancusi G, Marks B, Czerny C, Thalhammer F, Thurnher D, Riedl M, Dekan G, Knerer B. [Tubercular osteomyelitis of the clivus and the nasopharynx]. HNO. 2005;53(12):1081–4. German.
25. Witcombe JB, Cremin BJ. Tuberculous erosion of the sphenoid bone. Br J Radiol. 1978;51(605):347–50.
26. Kearns DB, Coker NJ, Pitcock JK, Jenkins HA. Tuberculous petrous apicitis. Arch Otolaryngol. 1985;111(6):406–8.
27. Das JC, Singh K, Sharma P, Singla R. Tuberculous osteomyelitis and optic neuritis. Ophthalmic Surg Lasers Imaging. 2003;34(5):409–12.
28. Aggarwal D, Suri A, Mahapatra AK. Orbital tuberculosis with abscess. J Neuroophthalmol. 2002;22(3):208–10.
29. Rajeshwari K, Sharma A. Multifocal skeletal tuberculosis presenting as osteitis skull and atlantoaxial dislocation. Indian Pediatr. 1995;32(11):1214–9.
30. Ikonomopoulos JA, Gorgoulis VG, Zacharatos PV, Manolis EN, Kanavaros P, Rassidakis A, Kittas C. Multiplex polymerase chain reaction for the detection of mycobacterial DNA in cases of tuberculosis and sarcoidosis. Mod Pathol. 1999;12(9):854–62.

31. Gopinath K, Singh S. Multiplex PCR assay for simultaneous detection and differentiation of Mycobacterium tuberculosis, Mycobacterium avium complexes and other Mycobacterial species directly from clinical specimens. J Appl Microbiol. 2009;107(2):425–35. doi:10.1111/j.1365-2672.2009.04218.x.
32. Dharwal M, Gupta DK, Punia VP, Sinha RS. Tuberculous osteomyelitis of skull in a sixty year old female. J Assoc Physicians India. 1995;43(8):575–7.
33. Reddy SS, Penmmaiah DC, Rajesh A, Patil M. Orbital tuberculosis with coexisting fungal (Aspergillus flavus) infection. Surg Neurol Int. 2014;5:32. doi:10.4103/2152-7806.128183.
34. Suchanda B, Alugolu R, Purohit A, Lakshmi V, Sundaram C. A rare concomitant tubercular and Fonsecaea pedrosoi fungal infection of the skull base. J Neurosci Rural Pract. 2012;3(2):189–91. doi:10.4103/0976-3147.98237.
35. Zettel H. [Post-traumatic tuberculosis of the skull]. Monatsschr Unfallheilkd Versicherungsmed. 1961;64:299–307. German.
36. Sundar VI, Shekhawat J, Gupta A, Sinha VD. Post traumatic tubercular osteomyelitis of skull vault. J Neurosci Rural Pract. 2013;4 Suppl 1:S138–41. doi:10.4103/0976-3147.116471.
37. Pandey AS, Surana A. Tuberculous osteomyelitis of the bone flap following craniotomy. Indian J Tuberc. 2011;58(3):129–31.
38. Biniwale SN, Rajshekhar V. Tuberculous osteomyelitis of bone flap following craniotomy for a glioma. Neurol India. 2000;48:91–2.
39. Hayat T, O'Shaughnessy T. Multifocal tuberculous osteomyelitis. Pract Neurol. 2015;15(3):227. doi:10.1136/practneurol-2014-001028.
40. Lynn MM, Kukanesen JR, Khan AW. Troublesome tuberculosis: a case report on multi-focal tuberculous osteomyelitis in an immunocompetent patient. J Clin Med Res. 2012;4(1):73–6. doi:10.4021/jocmr758e.
41. Kurup S, Jose R, Chandy ML. Diagnostic utility of gallium 67 SPECT/CT and role of pentoxifylline-tocopherol in chronic multifocal osteomyelitis. Oral Health Dent Manag. 2014;13(3):821–5.
42. Wedman J, van Weissenbruch R. Chronic recurrent multifocal osteomyelitis. Ann Otol Rhinol Laryngol. 2005;114(1 Pt 1):65–8.
43. Echeverria J, Kaude JV. Multifocal tuberculous osteomyelitis. Pediatr Radiol. 1978;7(4):238–40.
44. Jang YJ, Jung SW, Koo TW, Kim SJ, Park SG. Sinonasal tuberculosis associated with osteomyelitis of the ethmoid bone and cervical lymphadenopathy. J Laryngol Otol. 2001;115(9):736–9.
45. Thandar MA, Fagan JJ, Garb M. Extensive calvarial tuberculosis: rare complication of tuberculous mastoiditis. J Laryngol Otol. 2004;118(1):65–8.
46. Sanjuan-Jimenez R, Morata P, Bermúdez P, Bravo MJ, Colmenero JD. Comparative clinical study of different multiplex real time PCR strategies for the simultaneous differential diagnosis between extrapulmonary tuberculosis and focal complications of brucellosis. PLoS Negl Trop Dis. 2013;7(12):e2593. doi:10.1371/journal.pntd.0002593.
47. Piampiano P, McLeary M, Young LW, Janner D. Brucellosis: unusual presentations in two adolescent boys. Pediatr Radiol. 2000;30(5):355–7.
48. Sohn MH, Lim ST, Jeong YJ, Kim DW, Jeong HJ, Lee CS. Unusual case of occult Brucella osteomyelitis in the skull detected by bone scintigraphy. Nucl Med Mol Imaging. 2010;44(2):161–3. doi:10.1007/s13139-010-0023-2.
49. Tramont EC. Treponema pallidum (syphilis). In: Mandell GL, Bennett JE, Dolin R, editors. Principles and practice of infectious diseases. 5th ed. Philadelphia: Churchill Livingstone; 2000.
50. Mindel A, Tovey SJ, Timmins DJ, Williams P. Primary and secondary syphilis, 20 years' experience. 2. Clinical features. Genitourin Med. 1989;65(1):1–3.
51. Etienne M, Bencteux P, Gueit I, Abboud P, Caron F. Déjà vu in the catacombs: skull syphilitic osteitis. Lancet Infect Dis. 2008;8(7):455. doi:10.1016/S1473-3099(08)70154-3.

52. Coyne K, Browne R, Anagnostopoulos C, Nwokolo N. Syphilitic periostitis in a newly diagnosed HIV-positive man. Int J STD AIDS. 2006;17(6):421–3.
53. Huang I, Leach JL, Fichtenbaum CJ, Narayan RK. Osteomyelitis of the skull in early-acquired syphilis: evaluation by MR imaging and CT. AJNR Am J Neuroradiol. 2007;28 (2):307–8.
54. Samarkos M, Giannopoulou C, Karantoni E, Papastamopoulos V, Baraboutis I, Skoutelis A. Syphilitic periostitis of the skull and ribs in a HIV positive patient. Sex Transm Infect. 2011;87(1):44–5. doi:10.1136/sti.2010.044461.
55. Toby M, Larbalestier N, Kulasegaram R, Teague A, Conway K, White J. Calvarial syphilis in an HIV-positive man. Int J STD AIDS. 2012;23(5):365–6. doi:10.1258/ijsa.2011.011276.
56. Boix V, Merino E, Reus S, Torrus D, Portilla J. Polyostotic osteitis in secondary syphilis in an HIV-infected patient. Sex Transm Dis. 2013;40(8):645–6. doi:10.1097/01.OLQ.0000431351.50346.20.
57. Elopre L, Morell V, Bosshardt C, Geisler WM. A case of syphilitic osteitis in a patient with HIV infection. Int J STD AIDS. 2014;25(10):765–7. doi:10.1177/0956462414522031.
58. Gurland IA, Korn L, Edelman L, Wallach F. An unusual manifestation of acquired syphilis. Clin Infect Dis. 2001;32(4):667–9.
59. Son C, Samples D, Brenner A, Floyd J. Osteolytic calvarial lesions as initial presentation of latent neurosyphilis. J Clin Neurosci. 2015;22(5):909–10. doi:10.1016/j.jocn.2014.11.014.
60. Gómez Martínez MV, Gallardo FG, Cobo Soler J, Babé Romero J, Rios Ferreiros M, Valencia Ortega E. [Osteitis in secondary syphilis]. Rev Esp Med Nucl. 2003;22(6):424–6. Spanish.
61. Waugh MA. Bony symptoms in secondary syphilis. Br J Vener Dis. 1976;52(3):204–5.
62. Thompson RG, Preston RH. Lesions of the skull in secondary syphilis. Am J Syph Gonorrhea Vener Dis. 1952;36(4):332–41.
63. Park KH, Lee MS, Hong IK, Sung JY, Choi SH, Park SO, Shin MJ, Chung HW, Lee SH. Bone involvement in secondary syphilis: a case report and systematic review of the literature. Sex Transm Dis. 2014;41(9):532–7. doi:10.1097/OLQ.0000000000000164.
64. Dismukes WE, Delgado DG, Mallernee SV, Myers TC. Destructive bone disease in early syphilis. JAMA. 1976;236(23):2646–8.
65. el Alaoui Faris M, Birouk N, Slassi I, Jiddane M, Chkili T. [Thrombosis of the upper longitudinal sinus and syphilitic cranial osteitis]. Rev Neurol (Paris). 1992;148(12):783–5. French.
66. Chung KY, Yoon J, Heo JH, Lee MG, Jang JW, Lee JB. Osteitis of the skull in secondary syphilis. J Am Acad Dermatol. 1994;30(5 Pt 1):793–4.
67. Middleton S, Rowntree C, Rudge S. Bone pain as the presenting manifestation of secondary syphilis. Ann Rheum Dis. 1990;49(8):641–2.
68. Kang SH, Park SW, Kwon KY, Hong WJ. A solitary skull lesion of syphilitic osteomyelitis. J Korean Neurosurg Soc. 2010;48(1):85–7. doi:10.3340/jkns.2010.48.1.85.
69. Shore RN, Kiesel HA, Bennett HD. Osteolytic lesions in secondary syphilis. Arch Intern Med. 1977;137(10):1465–7.
70. Trevillyan JM, Yap KS, Hoy J. The great medical imitator: a case of syphilitic osteitis in the setting of HIV infection. Sex Health. 2013;10(3):275–8. doi:10.1071/SH12187.
71. Cohen JI, Bartlett JA, Corey RG. Extra-intestinal manifestations of salmonella infections. Medicine (Baltimore). 1987;66(5):349–88.
72. Arora A, Singh S, Aggarwal A, Aggarwal PK. Salmonella osteomyelitis in an otherwise healthy adult male-successful management with conservative treatment: a case report. J Orthop Surg (Hong Kong). 2003;11(2):217–20.
73. Kamarulzaman A, Briggs RJ, Fabinyi G, Richards MJ. Skull osteomyelitis due to Salmonella species: two case reports and review. Clin Infect Dis. 1996;22(4):638–41.
74. Bhooshan P, Shivaprakasha S, Dinesh KR, Kiran M, Karim P. Chronic subdural empyema and cranial vault osteomyelitis due to Salmonella paratyphi A. Indian J Med Microbiol. 2010;28(1):60–2. doi:10.4103/0255-0857.58733.

75. Meyer F, Sandvoss G, Feldmann H, Töppich G, Dust G. [Osteomyelitis of the skull as a late complication of a Salmonella typhi infection]. Immun Infekt. 1992;20(1):19–20. German.
76. Diwan N, Sharma KB. Isolation of Salmonella typhimurium from cephalhematoma and osteomyelitis. Indian J Med Res. 1978;67:27–9.
77. Schumacher D. [Osteomyelitis of the parietal bone caused by Salmonella typhimurium]. Zentralbl Chir. 1964;89:865–9. German.
78. Aliaga L, Mediavilla JD, López de la Osa A, López-Gómez M, de Cueto M, Miranda C. Nontyphoidal salmonella intracranial infections in HIV-infected patients. Clin Infect Dis. 1997;25(5):1118–20.
79. Thakur K, Singh DV, Goel A. Cranial vault Salmonella osteomyelitis leading to extradural abscess—a case report. Indian J Med Microbiol. 2002;20(4):219–20.
80. Senegor M, Lewis HP. Salmonella osteomyelitis of the skull base. Surg Neurol. 1991;36 (1):37–9.
81. Wu PC, Khin MM, Pang SW. Salmonella osteomyelitis. An important differential diagnosis of granulomatous osteomyelitis. Am J Surg Pathol. 1985;9(7):531–7.
82. Fernández Guerrero ML, Ramos JM, Núñez A, Cuenca M, de Górgolas M. Focal infections due to non-typhi Salmonella in patients with AIDS: report of 10 cases and review. Clin Infect Dis. 1997;25(3):690–7.
83. Belzunegui J, Lopez L, Arrizabalaga J, Gonzalez C, Figueroa M. Salmonella osteomyelitis in a patient with human immunodeficiency virus infection. Clin Rheumatol. 1997;16 (3):319–20.
84. Mastroianni CM, Vullo V, Delia S. Cranial Salmonella abscess with parietal bone osteomyelitis in an HIV-infected patient. AIDS. 1992;6(7):749–50.
85. Mage J, Martin P. [Epidural abscess caused by occipital osteomyelitis; unusual manifestation of a Salmonella paratyphi B infection]. Acta Neurol Psychiatr Belg. 1958;58(10):861–7. French.
86. Suzuki Y, Sugiyama Y, Ishii R, Sato I. Brain abscess caused by Salmonella typhi. Case report. J Neurosurg. 1976;45(6):709–11.
87. Zalagh M, Akhaddar A, Benariba F. Chronic rhinorrhea revealing an actinomycotic rhinolithiasis with ectopic tooth. Int J Oral Maxillofac Surg. 2012;41(3):297–9. doi:10.1016/j.ijom.2011.07.901.
88. Robinson JL, Vaudry WL, Dobrovolsky W. Actinomycosis presenting as osteomyelitis in the pediatric population. Pediatr Infect Dis J. 2005;24(4):365–9.
89. Yenson A, deFries HO, Deeb ZE. Actinomycotic osteomyelitis of the facial bones and mandible. Otolaryngol Head Neck Surg. 1983;91(2):173–6.
90. Roopesh Kumar VR, Madhugiri VS, Gundamaneni SK, Verma SK. Actinomycotic osteomyelitis of the cranial vault presenting with headache: an unusual presentation. BMJ Case Rep. 2014. pii: bcr2013202501. doi:10.1136/bcr-2013-202501.
91. Kolb CM, Ostrander S, Ramsey MJ, Burgos RM, Belnap C. Pathology quiz case 1. Actinomycosis osteomyelitis of the temporal bone. Arch Otolaryngol Head Neck Surg. 2012;138 (2):203–5. doi:10.1001/archoto.2011.1222a.
92. Nomura M, Shin M, Ohta M, Nukui Y, Ohkusu K, Saito N. Atypical osteomyelitis of the skull base and craniovertebral junction caused by Actinomyces infection—case report. Neurol Med Chir (Tokyo). 2011;51(1):64–6.
93. Nugent NF, Murphy M, Kelly J. Scalp abscess—a cautionary tale. J Plast Reconstr Aesthet Surg. 2010;63(8):e619–21. doi:10.1016/j.bjps.2010.02.011.
94. Akhaddar A, Elmostarchid B, Boulahroud O, Elouennass M, Boucetta M. Actinomycotic brain abscess with osteomyelitis arising from frontal sinusitis. Intern Med. 2009;48 (8):619–20.
95. Wadhera R, Gulati SP, Garg A, Ghai A, Kumar S. Frontal sinus actinomycosis presenting as osteomyelitis of frontal bone. Otolaryngol Head Neck Surg. 2008;138(4):544–5. doi:10.1016/j.otohns.2007.12.009.

96. Sundaram C, Purohit AK, Prasad VS, Meena AK, Reddy JJ, Murthy JM. Cranial and intracranial actinomycosis. Clin Neuropathol. 2004;23(4):173–7.
97. Sobol SE, Samadi DS, Wetmore RF. Actinomycosis of the temporal bone: a report of a case. Ear Nose Throat J. 2004;83(5):327–9.
98. Soto-Hernández JL, Morales VA, Lara Giron JC, Balderrama Bañares J. Cranial epidural empyema with osteomyelitis caused by actinomyces, CT, and MRI appearance. Clin Imaging. 1999;23(4):209–14.
99. King AD, Chan YL, Wong KS, Sung JJ, Fung K, Poon WS. Cranial actinomycosis. Singapore Med J. 1998;39(10):465–7.
100. Jewes LA, Laing RJ. Acute actinomycotic osteomyelitis of the skull with subdural empyema. J Infect. 1990;20(3):266–7.
101. Vannier JP, Schaison G, George B, Casin I. Actinomycotic osteomyelitis of the skull and atlas with late dissemination. A case of transient neurosurgical syndrome. Eur J Pediatr. 1986;145(4):316–8.
102. Kirsch WM, Stears JC. Actinomycotic osteomyelitis of the skull and epidural space. Case report. J Neurosurg. 1970;33(3):347–51.
103. Valour F, Sénéchal A, Dupieux C, Karsenty J, Lustig S, Breton P, Gleizal A, Boussel L, Laurent F, Braun E, Chidiac C, Ader F, Ferry T. Actinomycosis: etiology, clinical features, diagnosis, treatment, and management. Infect Drug Resist. 2014;7:183–97. doi:10.2147/IDR.S39601.
104. Akhaddar A, Elouennass M, Baallal H, Boucetta M. Focal intracranial infections due to Actinomyces species in immunocompetent patients: diagnostic and therapeutic challenges. World Neurosurg. 2010;74(2–3):346–50. doi:10.1016/j.wneu.2010.05.029.
105. Bassiri-Jahromi S, Doostkam A. Actinomyces and nocardia infections in chronic granulomatous disease. J Glob Infect Dis. 2011;3(4):348–52. doi:10.4103/0974-777X.91056.
106. Brook I. Actinomycosis: diagnosis and management. South Med J. 2008;101(10):1019–23. doi:10.1097/SMJ.0b013e3181864c1f.
107. Akhaddar A, Gazzaz M, Albouzidi A, Lmimouni B, Elmostarchid B, Boucetta M. Invasive Aspergillus terreus sinusitis with orbitocranial extension: case report. Surg Neurol. 2008;69(5):490–5. doi:10.1016/j.surneu.2007.02.059.
108. Blyth CC, Gomes L, Sorrell TC, da Cruz M, Sud A, Chen SC. Skull-base osteomyelitis: fungal vs. bacterial infection. Clin Microbiol Infect. 2011;17(2):306–11. doi:10.1111/j.1469-0691.2010.03231.x.
109. Chamilos G, Lewis RE, Kontoyiannis DP. Delaying amphotericin B-based frontline therapy significantly increases mortality among patients with hematologic malignancy who have zygomycosis. Clin Infect Dis. 2008;47(4):503–9. doi:10.1086/590004.
110. Stodulski D, Kowalska B, Stankiewicz C. Otogenic skull base osteomyelitis caused by invasive fungal infection. Case report and literature review. Eur Arch Otorhinolaryngol. 2006;263(12):1070–6.
111. Asimakopoulos P, Supriya M, Kealey S, Vernham GA. A case-based discussion on a patient with non-otogenic fungal skull base osteomyelitis: pitfalls in diagnosis. J Laryngol Otol. 2013;127(8):817–21. doi:10.1017/S002221511300145X.
112. Segal BH. Aspergillosis. N Engl J Med. 2009;360(18):1870–84. doi:10.1056/NEJMra0808853.
113. Kountakis SE, Kemper Jr JV, Chang CY, DiMaio DJ, Stiernberg CM. Osteomyelitis of the base of the skull secondary to Aspergillus. Am J Otolaryngol. 1997;18(1):19–22.
114. Gamaletsou MN, Rammaert B, Bueno MA, Moriyama B, Sipsas NV, Kontoyiannis DP, Roilides E, Zeller V, Prinapori R, Taj-Aldeen SJ, Brause B, Lortholary O, Walsh TJ. Aspergillus osteomyelitis: epidemiology, clinical manifestations, management, and outcome. J Infect. 2014;68(5):478–93. doi:10.1016/j.jinf.2013.12.008.
115. Bhatt YM, Pahade N, Nair B. Aspergillus petrous apicitis associated with cerebral and peritubular abscesses in an immunocompetent man. J Laryngol Otol. 2013;127(4):404–7. doi:10.1017/S0022215113000315.

116. van Tol A, van Rijswijk J. Aspergillus mastoiditis, presenting with unexplained progressive otalgia, in an immunocompetent (older) patient. Eur Arch Otorhinolaryngol. 2009;266 (10):1655–7. doi:10.1007/s00405-008-0877-4.
117. Chang PC, Fischbein NJ, Holliday RA. Central skull base osteomyelitis in patients without otitis externa: imaging findings. AJNR Am J Neuroradiol. 2003;24(7):1310–6.
118. Johnson AK, Batra PS. Central skull base osteomyelitis: an emerging clinical entity. Laryngoscope. 2014;124(5):1083–7. doi:10.1002/lary.24440.
119. Seabold JE, Simonson TM, Weber PC, Thompson BH, Harris KG, Rezai K, Madsen MT, Hoffman HT. Cranial osteomyelitis: diagnosis and follow-up with In-111 white blood cell and Tc-99m methylene diphosphonate bone SPECT, CT, and MR imaging. Radiology. 1995;196(3):779–88.
120. Chandra S, Goyal M, Mishra NK, Gaikwad SB. Invasive aspergillosis presenting as a cavernous sinus mass in immuno competent individuals; report of 3 cases. Neuroradiology. 2000;42(2):108–11.
121. Kim DG, Hong SC, Kim HJ, Chi JG, Han MH, Choi KS, Han DH. Cerebral aspergillosis in immunologically competent patients. Surg Neurol. 1993;40(4):326–31.
122. Yuen JC, Puri SK, Feng Z. Scalp necrotizing fasciitis with osteomyelitis of the skull from Aspergillus. J Craniofac Surg. 2002;13(6):762–4.
123. Rodríguez-Hernández MJ, Jiménez-Mejías ME, Montero JM, Regordan C, Ferreras G. Aspergillus fumigatus cranial infection after accidental traumatism. Eur J Clin Microbiol Infect Dis. 2001;20(9):655–6.
124. Srinivasan US. Intracranial aspergilloma in immunocompetent patients successfully treated with radical surgical intervention and antifungal therapy: case series. Ann Acad Med Singapore. 2008;37(9):783–7.
125. Carr MM, Cusimano MD, Muller PJ, Bilbao J. Aspergillosis of the cranial base. Skull Base Surg. 1994;4(3):159–63.
126. Herbrecht R, Denning DW, Patterson TF, Bennett JE, Greene RE, Oestmann JW, Kern WV, Marr KA, Ribaud P, Lortholary O, Sylvester R, Rubin RH, Wingard JR, Stark P, Durand C, Caillot D, Thiel E, Chandrasekar PH, Hodges MR, Schlamm HT, Troke PF, de Pauw B, Invasive Fungal Infections Group of the European Organisation for Research and Treatment of Cancer and the Global Aspergillus Study Group. Voriconazole versus amphotericin B for primary therapy of invasive aspergillosis. N Engl J Med. 2002;347(6):408–15.
127. Walsh TJ, Anaissie EJ, Denning DW, Herbrecht R, Kontoyiannis DP, Marr KA, Morrison VA, Segal BH, Steinbach WJ, Stevens DA, van Burik JA, Wingard JR, Patterson TF, Infectious Diseases Society of America. Treatment of aspergillosis: clinical practice guidelines of the Infectious Diseases Society of America. Clin Infect Dis. 2008;46(3):327–60. doi:10.1086/525258.
128. Parsonage MJ, Stafford ND, Lillie P, Moss PJ, Barlow G, Thaker H. Oral voriconazole for invasive fungal skull base infection. J Laryngol Otol. 2010;124(9):1010–3. doi:10.1017/S0022215109992507.
129. Parize P, Chandesris MO, Lanternier F, Poirée S, Viard JP, Bienvenu B, Mimoun M, Méchai F, Mamzer MF, Herman P, Bougnoux ME, Lecuit M, Lortholary O. Antifungal therapy of Aspergillus invasive otitis externa: efficacy of voriconazole and review. Antimicrob Agents Chemother. 2009;53(3):1048–53. doi:10.1128/AAC.01220-08.
130. Lass-Flörl C. Triazole antifungal agents in invasive fungal infections: a comparative review. Drugs. 2011;71(18):2405–19. doi:10.2165/11596540-000000000-00000.
131. Lodge BA, Ashley ED, Steele MP, Perfect JR. Aspergillus fumigatus empyema, arthritis, and calcaneal osteomyelitis in a lung transplant patient successfully treated with posaconazole. J Clin Microbiol. 2004;42(3):1376–8.
132. Garazzino S, Maiello A, Rosa DEFG, Aprato A, Di Perri G. Post-traumatic osteomyelitis due to Aspergillus flavus successfully treated with voriconazole: a case report. J Chemother. 2008;20(4):524–6.

133. Mouas H, Lutsar I, Dupont B, Fain O, Herbrecht R, Lescure FX, Lortholary O, Voriconazole/ Bone Invasive Aspergillosis Study Group. Voriconazole for invasive bone aspergillosis: a worldwide experience of 20 cases. Clin Infect Dis. 2005;40(8):1141–7.
134. Mohammadpour M, Mamishi S, Oaji M, Pourpak Z, Parvaneh N. Successful treatment of fungal osteomyelitis with voriconazole in a patient with chronic granulomatous disease. Iran J Pediatr. 2010;20(4):487–90.
135. Narozny W, Kuczkowski J, Mikaszewski B. Infectious skull base osteomyelitis—still a life-threatening disease. Otol Neurotol. 2006;27(7):1047–8.
136. Singh A, Al Khabori M, Hyder MJ. Skull base osteomyelitis: diagnostic and therapeutic challenges in atypical presentation. Otolaryngol Head Neck Surg. 2005;133(1):121–5.
137. Baallal H, El Asri AC, Eljebbouri B, Akhaddar A, Gazzaz M, El Mostarchid B, Boucetta M. [Cryptococcal meningitis in a patient with a ventriculoperitoneal shunt and monitoring for pulmonary sarcoidosis]. Neurochirurgie. 2013;59(1):47–9. doi:10.1016/j.neuchi.2012.06.005.French.
138. Rauchway AC, Husain C, Selhorst JB. Neurologic presentations of fungal infections. Neurol Clin. 2010;28(1):293–309. doi:10.1016/j.ncl.2009.09.013.
139. Agadi JB, Madni NA, Nanjappa V, Govindaiah HK. Cryptococcal osteomyelitis of the skull in a patient with transient lymphopenia. Neurol India. 2010;58(2):300–2. doi:10.4103/0028-3886.63798.
140. Corral JE, Lima S, Quezada J, Samayoa B, Arathoon E. Cryptococcal osteomyelitis of the skull. Med Mycol. 2011;49(6):667–71. doi:10.3109/13693786.2011.558124.
141. Amit A, Sudish K, Pople IK. Primary calvarial cryptococcal osteomyelitis in a patient with idiopathic lymphopenia. Acta Neurochir (Wien). 2008;150(7):713–4. doi:10.1007/s00701-008-1608-8.
142. Rerolle JP, Szelag JC, Diaconita M, Paraf F, Aldigier JC, Le Meur Y. Intracranial granuloma and skull osteolysis: complication of a primary cutaneous cryptococcosis in a kidney transplant recipient. Am J Kidney Dis. 2005;46(6):e113–7.
143. Ching N, Lasky J, Lazareff J, Moore TB, Nielsen K. Enlarging parietal mass with lytic skull lesion. Pediatr Infect Dis J. 2004;23(6):589. 595–6.
144. Prendiville S, Bielamowicz SA, Hawrych A, Deeb ZE. Isolated cryptococcal sphenoid sinusitis with septicemia, meningitis, and subsequent skull base osteomyelitis in an immunocompetent patient. Otolaryngol Head Neck Surg. 2000;123(3):277–9.
145. Wood L, Miedzinski L. Skeletal cryptococcosis: case report and review of the literature. Can J Infect Dis. 1996;7(2):125–32.
146. Armonda RA, Fleckenstein JM, Brandvold B, Ondra SL. Cryptococcal skull infection: a case report with review of the literature. Neurosurgery. 1993;32(6):1034–6.
147. Luhr H, Svane S. [Pulmonary pseudotumor caused by Cryptococcus neoformans]. Tidsskr Nor Laegeforen. 1991;111(27):3288–90. Norwegian.
148. Reinig JW, Hungerford GD, Mohrmann ME, Vera CL. Case report 268. Diagnosis: cryptococcal osteomyelitis of the calvaria. Skeletal Radiol. 1984;11(3):221–3.
149. Galloway DC, Schochet Jr SS. Cryptococcal skull granuloma. Case report. J Neurosurg. 1981;54(5):690–2.
150. Woolfitt R, Park HM, Greene M. Localized cryptococcal osteomyelitis. Radiology. 1976;120(2):290.
151. Kong QT, Zhou WQ, Feng J, Sang H, Deng DQ, Wang Z, Li J, Shi QL, Wu B, Liu WD. Isolated skull cryptococcosis in an immunocompetent patient. Mycopathologia. 2012. doi:10.1007/s11046-012-9609-9.
152. Dounis E, Giamarellou H, Peppas T, Sfikakis P. Skull, patella and thigh cryptococcosis after a crashing injury of the temporal bone. J Chemother. 1991;3(2):130–3.
153. Benard G, Gryschek RC, Duarte AJ, Shikanai-Yasuda MA. Cryptococcosis as an opportunistic infection in immunodeficiency secondary to paracoccidioidomycosis. Mycopathologia. 1996;133(2):65–9.

154. Cash JB, Goodman NL. Cryptococcal infection of the temporal bone. Diagn Microbiol Infect Dis. 1983;1(3):257–60.
155. Liu PY. Cryptococcal osteomyelitis: case report and review. Diagn Microbiol Infect Dis. 1998;30(1):33–5.
156. Roden MM, Zaoutis TE, Buchanan WL, Knudsen TA, Sarkisova TA, Schaufele RL. Epidemiology and outcome of zygomycosis: a review of 929 reported cases. Clin Infect Dis. 2005;41:634–53.
157. Islam MN, Cohen DM, Celestina LJ, Ojha J, Claudio R, Bhattacharyya IB. Rhinocerebral zygomycosis: an increasingly frequent challenge: update and favorable outcomes in two cases. Oral Surg Oral Med Oral Pathol Oral Radiol Endod. 2007;104(5):e28–34.
158. Safaya A, Batra K, Capoor M. A case of skull base mucormycosis with osteomyelitis secondary to temporal bone squamous cell carcinoma. Ear Nose Throat J. 2006;85 (12):822–4.
159. Devireddy SK, Kumar RVK, Gali R, Kanubaddy SR, Dasari MR, Akheel M. Mucormycotic skull base osteomyelitis: a case report. J Oral Maxillofac Surg Med Pathol. 2014;26 (3):336–9.
160. Harrill WC, Stewart MG, Lee AG, Cernoch P. Chronic rhinocerebral mucormycosis. Laryngoscope. 1996;106(10):1292–7.
161. Eucker J, Sezer O, Graf B, Possinger K. Mucormycoses. Mycoses. 2001;44(7–8):253–60.
162. Petrikkos G, Skiada A, Lortholary O, Roilides E, Walsh TJ, Kontoyiannis DP. Epidemiology and clinical manifestations of mucormycosis. Clin Infect Dis. 2012;54 Suppl 1:S23–34. doi:10.1093/cid/cir866.
163. Barge RM, Buiting AG, Thompson J, van't Wout JW. [A patient with chronic mucormycosis]. Ned Tijdschr Geneeskd. 1992;136(43):2135–8. Dutch.
164. Kwon-Chung KJ. Taxonomy of fungi causing mucormycosis and entomophthoramycosis (zygomycosis) and nomenclature of the disease: molecular mycologic perspectives. Clin Infect Dis. 2012;54 Suppl 1:S8–15. doi:10.1093/cid/cir864.
165. Bahna MS, Ward PH, Konrad HR. Nasopharyngeal mucormycotic osteitis: a new syndrome characterized by initial presentation of multiple cranial nerve palsies. Otolaryngol Head Neck Surg (1979). 1980;88(2):146–53.
166. Finn DG, Farmer Jr JC. Chronic mucormycosis. Laryngoscope. 1982;92(7 Pt 1):761–6.
167. Ducic Y. Management of osteomyelitis of the anterior skull base and craniovertebral junction. Otolaryngol Head Neck Surg. 2003;128(1):39–42.
168. Effat KG, Karam M, El-Kabani A. Pott's puffy tumour caused by mucormycosis. J Laryngol Otol. 2005;119(8):643–5.
169. Chan LL, Singh S, Jones D, Diaz Jr EM, Ginsberg LE. Imaging of mucormycosis skull base osteomyelitis. AJNR Am J Neuroradiol. 2000;21(5):828–31.
170. Fortún J, Cobo J, Cañal J, Martínez-San Millán J. Post-traumatic cranial mucormycosis in an immunocompetent patient. J Oral Maxillofac Surg. 1995;53(9):1099–102.
171. Buhl MR, Joseph TP, Snelling BE, Buhl L. Temporofacial zygomycosis in a pregnant woman. Infection. 1992;20(4):230–2.
172. Yousem DM, Galetta SL, Gusnard DA, Goldberg HI. MR findings in rhinocerebral mucormycosis. J Comput Assist Tomogr. 1989;13(5):878–82.
173. Terk MR, Underwood DJ, Zee C, Colletti PM. MR imaging in rhinocerebral and intracranial mucormycosis with CT and pathological correlation. Magn Reson Imaging. 1992;10 (1):81–7.
174. Alvernia JE, Patel RN, Cai DZ, Dang N, Anderson DW, Melgar M. A successful combined endovascular and surgical treatment of a cranial base mucormycosis with an associated internal carotid artery pseudoaneurysm. Neurosurgery. 2009;65(4):733–40. doi:10.1227/01.NEU.0000351773.74034.5E.
175. Delbrouck C, Jacobs F, Fernandez Aguilar S, Devroede B, Choufani G, Hassid S. Carotid artery occlusion due to fulminant rhinocerebral mucormycosis. Acta Otorhinolaryngol Belg. 2004;58(2):135–40.

176. Abril V, Ortega E, Segarra P, Pedro F, Sabater V, Herrera A. Rhinocerebral mucormycosis in a patient with AIDS: a complication of diabetic ketoacidosis following pentamidine therapy. Clin Infect Dis. 1996;23(4):845–6.
177. Eckert J, Deplazes P. Biological, epidemiological, and clinical aspects of echinococcosis, a zoonosis of increasing concern. Clin Microbiol Rev. 2004;17(1):107–35.
178. Zlitni M, Ezzaouia K, Lebib H, Karray M, Kooli M, Mestiri M. Hydatid cyst of bone: diagnosis and treatment. World J Surg. 2001;25(1):75–82.
179. Hossain Z. Hydatidosis of the skull. In: Turgut M, editor. Hydatidosis of the central nervous system: diagnosis and treatment. Berlin: Springer; 2014.
180. Aydin Y, Aydin F, Ture U. Intradiploeic and cerebral hydatidosis: a case report and review of literature. Clin Neurol Neurosurg. 1992;94(3):229–33.
181. Siddiqui MA, Rizvi SW, Rizvi SA, Ahmad I, Ullah E. Atypical multifocal hydatid disease of cranial vault: simultaneous orbital and extradural meningeal involvement. Emerg Radiol. 2010;17(5):427–30. doi:10.1007/s10140-010-0885-8.
182. Erman T, Tuna M, Göçer I, Ildan F, Zeren M, Cetinalp E. Intracranial intraosseous hydatid cyst. Case report and review of literature. Neurosurg Focus. 2001;11(1):ECP1.
183. Ennouri S, Ayadi K, Ali HB, Mnif J. Hydatid cyst of the temporal bone: an exceptional location. AJR Am J Roentgenol. 2000;175(3):923–5.
184. Negovetic L, Lupret V, Smiljanic D, Arsenic B. Cranial vault and gigantic intracranial hydatid cyst in a young woman. Neurosurgery. 1990;27(3):480–1.
185. Sureka J, Sarawagi R, Eapen A, Keshava SN, Vedantam R. Skull base hydatid cyst with intracranial extension presenting as vocal cord palsy: a case report. Br J Radiol. 2010;83 (987):e67–9.
186. Limaiem F, Bellil S, Bellil K, Chelly I, Mekni A, Kallel J, Haouet S, Zitouna M, Kchir N. Hydatid cyst of the cranial vault. J Infect Dev Ctries. 2009;3(10):807–10.
187. Hossain MZ, Rahman MM, Badruddoza SM. Cranial hydatid abscess. Trop Doct. 2010;40:255–6.
188. Ciurea AV, Moisa HA, Nica DA. Unusual presentations of hydatidosis of the central nervous system. In: Turgut M, editor. Hydatidosis of the central nervous system: diagnosis and treatment. Berlin: Springer; 2014.
189. Akhaddar A, El-Wartiti A, Mahi M, Boucetta M. Headache due to a large parasitic cyst. Headache. 2011;51(8):1274–5. doi:10.1111/j.1526-4610.2010.01804.x.
190. Arazi M, Erikoglu M, Odev K, Memik R, Ozdemir M. Primary echinococcus infestation of the bone and muscles. Clin Orthop Relat Res. 2005;432:234–41.
191. Benmoussa H, Tamehmacht M, Bellakhdar F. [Hydatidosis of the cranial vault. Two case reports]. Neurochirurgie. 1990;36(3):191–3. French.
192. Kanaka TS, Balasubramaniam V, Meenakshisundaram E, Varadarajan M. Hydatid of the skull. Indian J Surg. 1970;32:200–3.
193. Yazdani N, Basam A, Heidarali M, Kashani SS, Hasibi M, Mokhtari Z. Infratemporal hydatid cyst: a case presenting with blindness. J Laryngol Otol. 2010;124(4):456–9. doi:10.1017/S0022215109991927.

Chapter 15
Special Clinical Situations

Contents

Abbreviations

AIDS	Acquired immune deficiency syndrome
CD4	Cluster of differentiation 4
HAART	Highly active antiretroviral therapy
HIV	Human immunodeficiency virus
POPUT	Pott's puffy tumor

Cranial osteomyelitis, although a relatively uncommon entity, is important, as it may be potentially life threatening if not recognized and adequately treated. Besides the various classic manifestations of skull bone infections, certain unusual presentations merit particular attention. The expression "unusual presentations" of osteomyelitis of the skull, we understand the atypical situations that some clinicians might never actually see in their daily practice. But these appearances can be met and can delay diagnosis and management, so it is important to recognize them. The aim of this chapter is to present and discuss some forms of these unusual presentations including Pott's puffy tumor, infected cephalhematoma, osteomyelitis of the clivus, calvarial sclerosing osteomyelitis, and lastly cranial osteomyelitis in HIV and AIDS.

A. Akhaddar, *Cranial Osteomyelitis*, DOI 10.1007/978-3-319-30268-3_15

Pott's Puffy Tumor

Pott's puffy tumor (POPUT) is an unusual entity characterized by the association of forehead localized swelling with overlying subperiosteal abscess and underlying frontal bone osteomyelitis. Sir Percivall Pott first described this condition in 1760 as a complication of head injury and later of frontal sinusitis [1–4].

POPUT represents a form of cranial osteomyelitis secondary to frontal sinusitis with erosion of the anterior table of the frontal sinus leading to formation of the subperiosteal abscess. When the abscess is at the external table, the clinical picture is the classic forehead swelling mimicking a "unicorn appearance". Posterior table can also be eroded explaining the frequency of intracranial epidural abscess which is less visible, and generally discovered because of neurological symptoms [5]. More serious intracranial complications may occur in up to 80 % of cases including subdural empyema, meningitis, brain abscess or venous sinus thrombosis [6]. Comparatively, intracranial complications have been reported in 0.5–24 % of patients hospitalized with paranasal sinusitis [7–9]. Orbital involvement should also be considered as a regional complication in 29 % of POPUT [5]. Overall, dissemination of the infection may result not only by contiguity but also by hematogenous spread [10].

As all other forms of cranial osteomyelitis, POPUT is considered as rare in the antibiotic therapy era, although, despite the use of broad-spectrum antibiotics, the number of cases reported has increased since 2000 [6, 11–14]. In 2010, 141 cases of POPUT were reported in the world literature by Nisa et al. between 1950 and 2010 [5]. Since then, we collect 49 more cases from MEDLINE between January 2011 and July 2015. The increase in number of reported cases may be explained by improvement in radiological imaging, by increased awareness of this entity and partial (inadequate) antibiotics treatment for chronic sinusitis [5].

POPUT is more common in male (about two-third of patients) and almost always confined to the second decade of life, more rarely in adults and newborns [10]. The prevalence in young males is attributed to the peculiarities of the development of frontal sinuses and by their larger diploic veins, which makes it easier for infections to extend [8, 14] (see Chap. 5). Frontal sinusitis is the main etiology, being acute or chronic it may be associated with other paranasal sinusitis [15]. Other unusual risk factors have been also reported as causes of POPUT such as dental infection, insect bite, acupuncture, hair transplantation, cocaine abuse, intranasal methamphetamine use, infected frontal sinus mucocele and previous craniotomy/cranioplasty [16–24]. Two cases named "Pott's puffy tumor" were previously related to mastoiditis and acute otitis media with temporo-parietal and temporo-zygomatic localization respectively, however these cases do not meet the classic definition [25, 26].

The classic clinical presentation is that of a male adolescent with a history of acute or chronic frontal or pansinusitis with fever and tender frontal swelling (Fig. 15.1). In the beginning, symptoms and signs are insidious and the administration of antibiotic drugs may mask or retard both the neurologic symptoms and intracranial spread of infections. Subperiosteal abscess is usually misdiagnosed as a

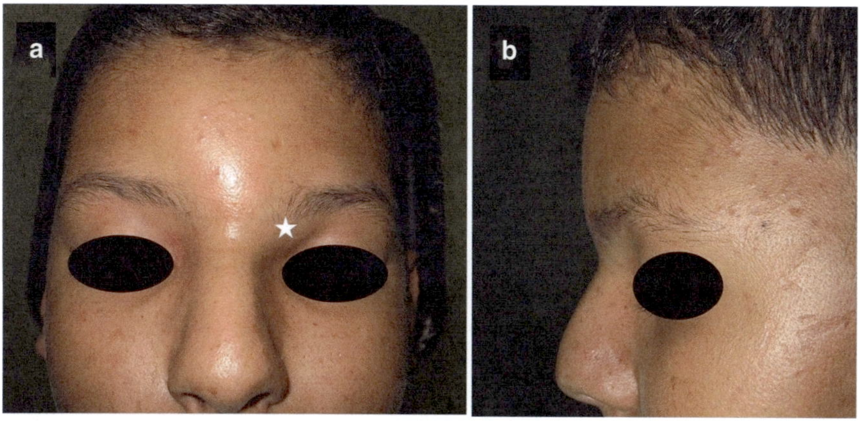

Fig. 15.1 Swelling and edema over the forehead with left superior orbital extension (*star*) (**a** and **b**) (First patient)

primary scalp abscess and sometimes incised and drained [27, 28]. Headache, fever and rhinorrhea are commonly seen [14]. Failure of resolution of symptoms with antibiotics treatment should alert for silent intracranial extension, even in the absence of neurological symptoms and signs because anterior frontal areas of the brain are non-eloquent [14]. When orbital involvement occurs, the most common findings are eyelid and/or periorbital edema (98 %) and proptosis (24 %). Restriction of the extraocular movements (12 %) and diplopia (2.5 %) are more rare [5]. Epidural frontocutaneous fistula may occur and are the expression of periosteal osseous erosion with discharge of purulent secretion via the breached skin of the forehead or orbital area [6, 29–32].

Diagnosis of POPUT is historically made on a clinical basis. Laboratory findings may help in the diagnosis but are unspecific. Inflammatory biomarkers were highly variable in their expression in cranial osteomyelitis. Bone erosions are seen on computed tomography-scan (CT-scan) which is the standard tool (Figs. 15.2, 15.3, and 15.4). CT-scan may also help in diagnosis of paranasal sinusitis and orbital involvement. Magnetic resonance imaging (MRI) is useful in demonstrating intracranial and intraorbital complications, bone marrow edema, leptomeningeal enhancement, extradural and subdural collections, brain abscess and venous sinus thrombosis [33] (Figs. 15.5, and 15.6). Bone scan is very sensitive for detecting cranial bone infection [34] (Fig. 15.7). Ultrasound imaging can be useful in showing subperiosteal abscess associated with erosion of the frontal bone [35, 36].

Differential diagnosis of forehead swelling includes soft tissue infection, benign and malignant tumors, infected hematoma, frontal sinus mucocele and superficial temporal artery pseudoaneurysm [37–40].

Cultures from patients with POPUT often reveal polymicrobial involvement in up to two third of the cases in which culture is positive [4, 5, 11, 28]. However, the most common individual pathogens consisted of microaerophilic streptococci including alpha-hemolytic *streptococcus*, *peptostreptococcus*, staphylococci,

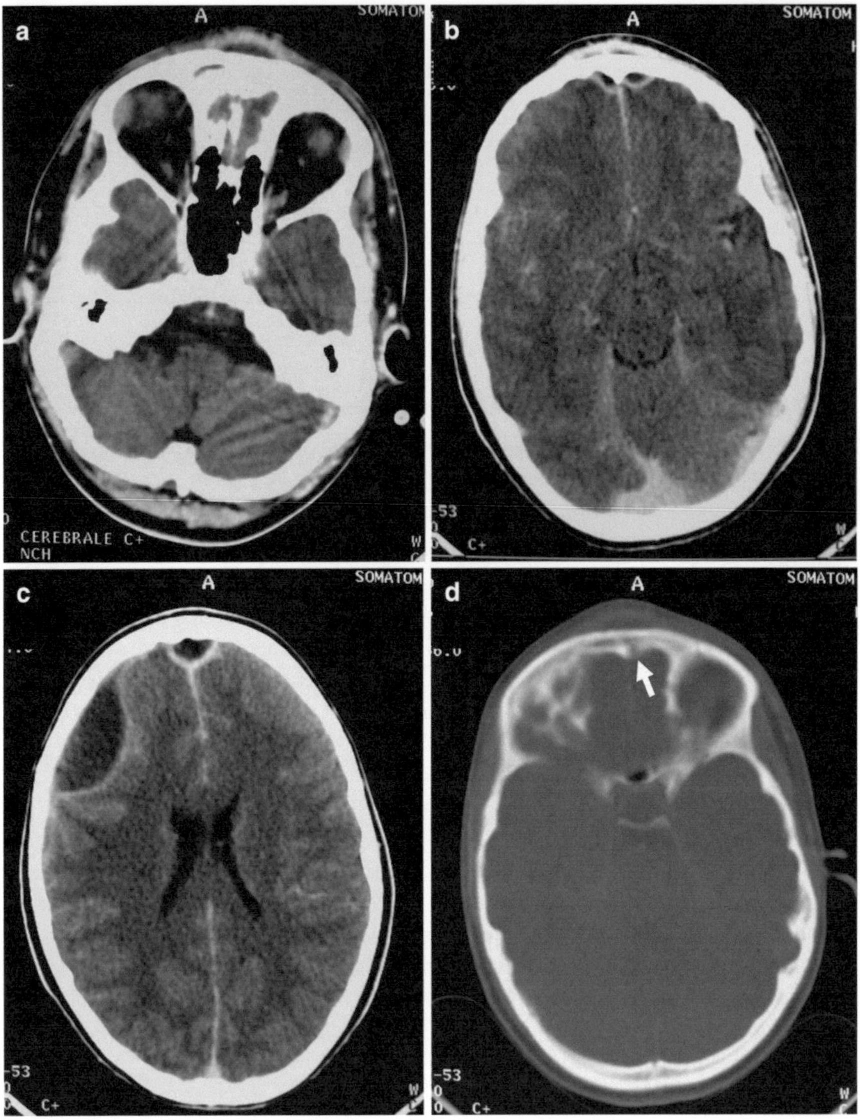

Fig. 15.2 Axial cranial CT-scan after contrast injection showing extracranial frontal subperiosteal abscess (**a** and **b**) and frontal epidural abscesses (**b** and **c**). Axial cranial CT-scan in bone windows demonstrating fronto-basal erosion of the inner table (*arrow*) (**d**) (First patient)

Bacteroides spp., and other anaerobes particularly *Fusobacterium spp.* These microorganisms reflect the bacterial species responsible for sinusitis. Anaerobic bacteria are more frequent in this area, compared to other ear and nose infections, because of the relatively lower oxygen concentration in the frontal sinus caused by compromised ostial patency [41, 42]. Sterile cultures are common, probably

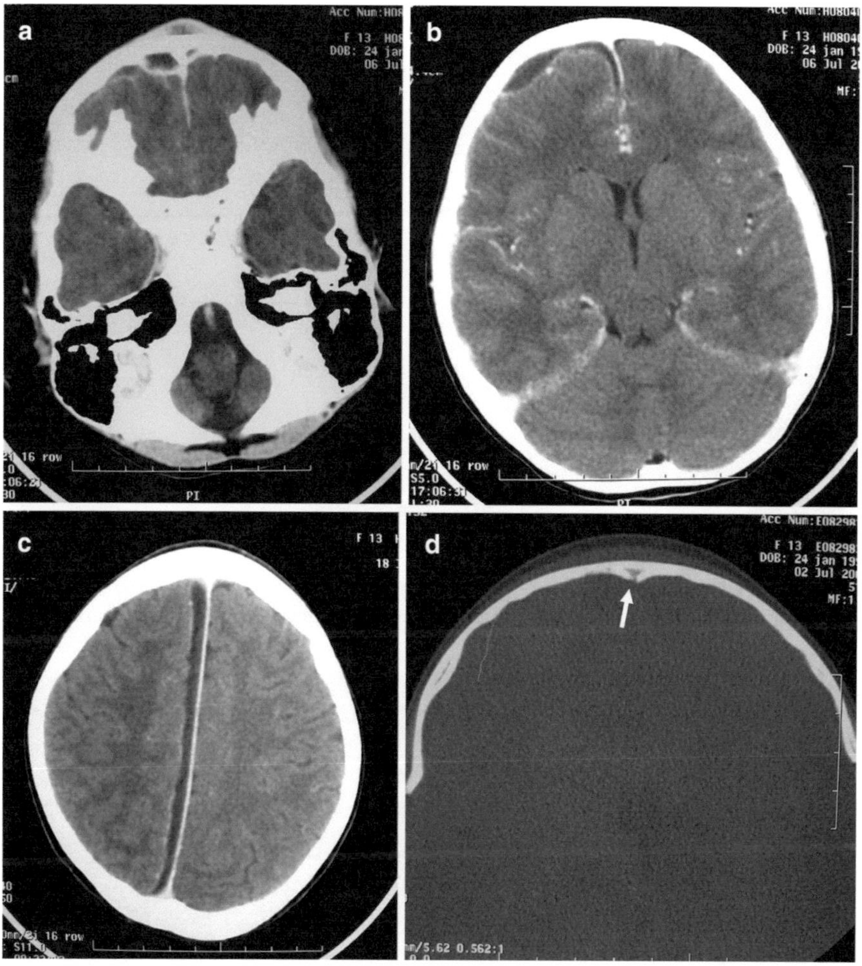

Fig. 15.3 Axial cranial CT-scan after contrast injection showing extracranial frontal subperiosteal abscess (**a**), frontal epidural abscess (**a**), and interhemispheric subdural empyema (**b** and **c**). Axial cranial CT-scan in bone windows demonstrating medial frontal erosion of the inner table (*arrow*) (**d**) (Second patient)

because most patients received antibiotics before surgery. More rarely, numerous other micro-organisms are reported such as *Haemophilus influenza*, *Pasteurella multocida*, mucormycosis and *Candida parapsilosis* [28, 43–45].

Medical management of POPUT typically accompanies surgical treatment. Patients presenting with small subperiosteal collection or epidural abscess without neurological compromise can be treated with antimicrobial drugs associated with close clinical and biological monitoring as well as neuroimaging study to ensure adequate response to treatment. Antimicrobial therapy should include

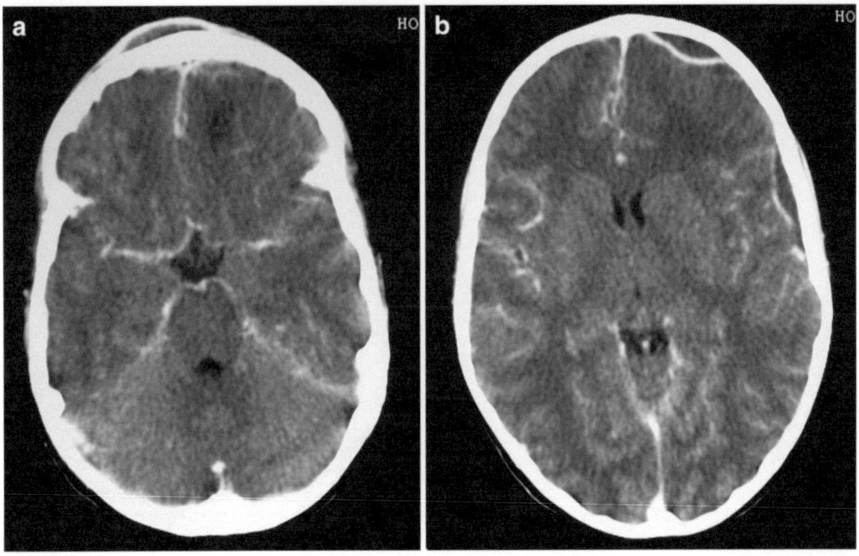

Fig. 15.4 Axial CT-scan of skull after contrast injection revealing extracranial frontal subperiosteal abscess (**a**) and parameningeal extracerebral collections (**b**) (Third patient)

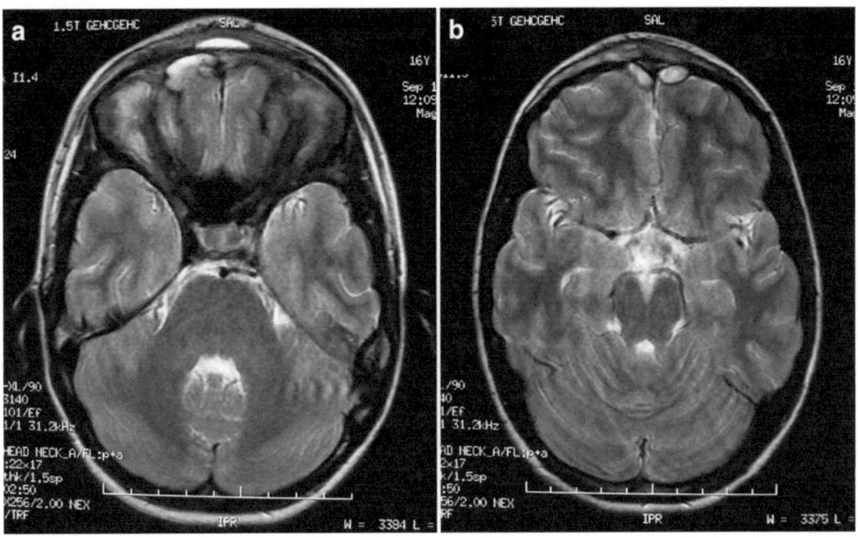

Fig. 15.5 Axial MRI on T2-weighted images showing the frontal extracranial abscess (**a**) and the extradural empyema (**b**) (First patient)

broad-spectrum antibiotics with activity against aerobic and anaerobic cocci and bacilli and adequate central nervous system and abscess penetration [11]. Because of osteomyelitis, the antibiotic should be prolonged for at least 2 months postoperatively.

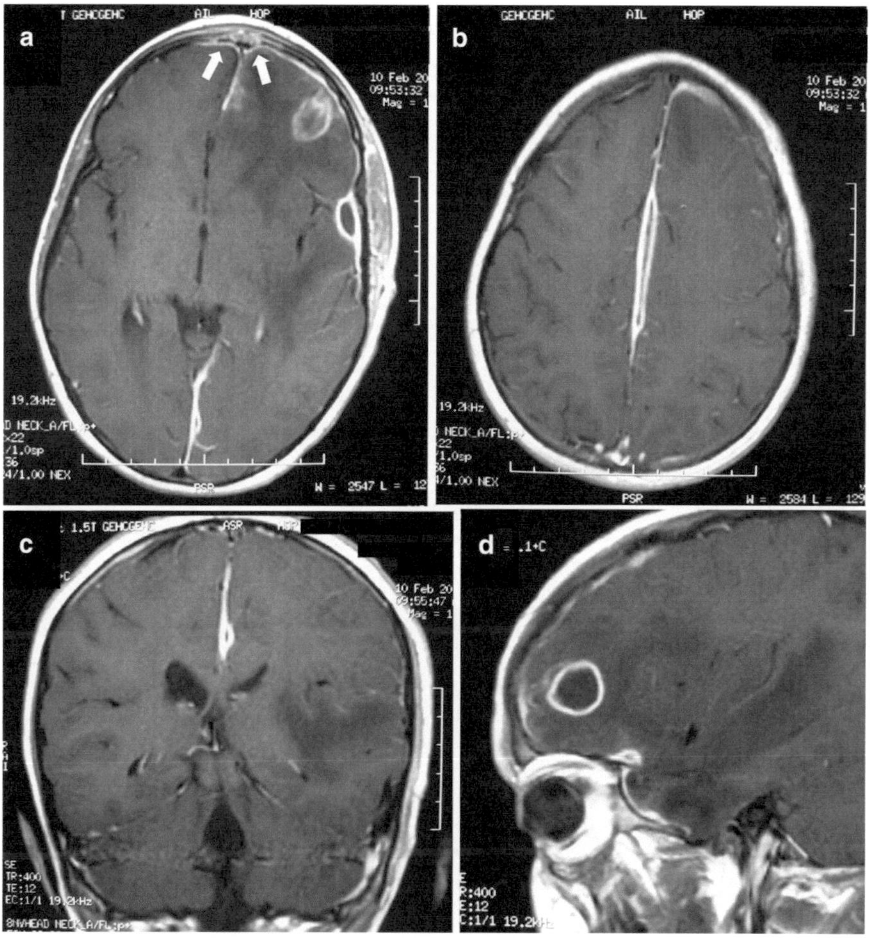

Fig. 15.6 Cranial MRI on T1-weighted images after gadolinium injection. Axial (**a** and **b**), coronal (**c**), and sagittal images (**d**). Frontal bone erosions (*arrows*) are seen with interhemispheric empyema and frontal brain abscess (Third patient)

A multidisciplinary approach (neurosurgical and otorhinolaryngological) is needed to treat frontal sinusitis, osteomyelitis and its intracranial complications. Surgery may be diagnostic (Fig. 15.8), curative and preventive to prevent reseeding of the intracranial area from the infected sinuses. The frontal sinus may be managed via trephination or obliteration and/or exenteration depending on extension of the disease and degree of bony involvement. Endoscopic approach may be effective when there is no intracranial involvement [46–50]. In 2012, a successful experience with balloon sinuplasty in three patients with POPUT was reported by Bozdemir

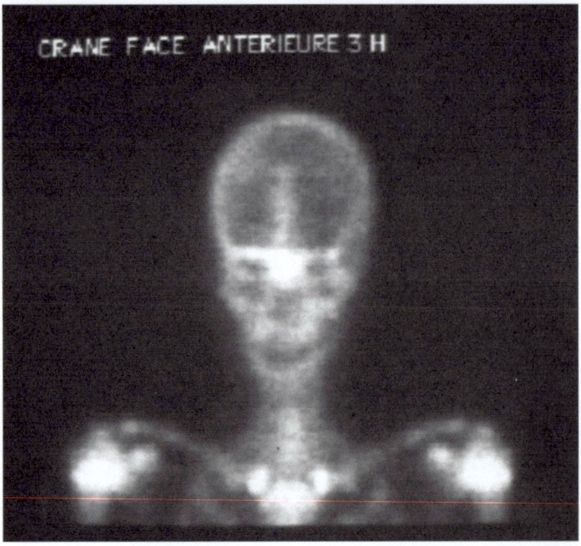

Fig. 15.7 Cranial Technetium-99m methylene diphosphanate bone scan (anterior view) demonstrating an area of increased uptake in the medial basi-frontal bone corresponding to a lytic lesion on CT-scan (First patient)

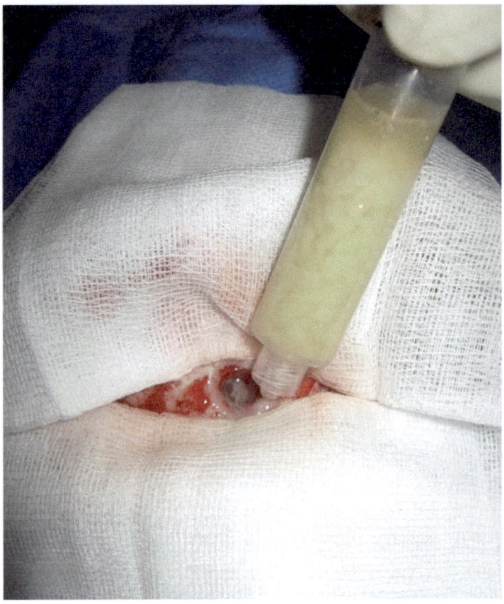

Fig. 15.8 Operative view. A thick yellowish green pus drained from the epidural abscess through a frontal burr hole craniotomy (First patient)

et al. [23]. Craniotomies for draining and debridement can be done with open or minimally invasive approach depending on the exact location of the abscesses. Infected bone with evidence of necrosis must be removed, followed by cranioplasty on a second intervention. Some authors suggest the use of titanium mesh at the time of operation [30]. If accessible, the posterior wall of the frontal sinus should be usually explored during surgery and its canalization might be possible.

Complete clinical recovery is predictable in most patients [6, 50, 51]. The outcome is related to the severity of infection, especially intracranial extension, and to the delay in diagnosis [14, 33]. Nowadays, mortality is considered as low but two deaths (17 %) were recently reported among 12 patients [13, 52]. Long term sequels are rare and may include aphasia, paralysis, enlarged blind spot, seizure, chronic osteomyelitis and facial scar [5, 15, 34, 42, 50, 53].

Infected Cephalhematoma

Cephalhematoma is an effusion of blood under the pericranium (subperiosteal). This hematic collection does not cross suture lines. It is generally due to pressure or injury during labour. Cephalhematomas occur in 1–2 % of spontaneous vaginal deliveries and approximately 4 % of forceps or vacuum-assisted deliveries [54, 55]. Infected cephalhematoma is a relative rare condition. The pathogenesis of infection has been linked to direct extension from needle aspiration, scalp infection or electrodes, and to hematogenous spread in the setting of bacteremia or meningitis [56]. Moreover, complications of infected cephalohematomas include cranial osteomyelitis, epidural abscess, subdural empyema, meningitis, brain abscess, venous sinus thrombosis and death [57–63].

In 1993, Blom and Vreede reviewed the 28 cases of infected cephalohematoma reported between 1818 and 1993 [64]. Through this literature review, 11 cases (39.2 %) had a cranial osteomyelitis. Since then, about a dozen cases were found in PubMed. More recently, Chang et al. reported 28 cases of infected cephalhematoma in newborns over a period of 26 years but they found only one patient (3.5 %) with osteomyelitis. The risk factors include incision or aspiration of the cephalhematoma, placement of scalp electrodes, scalp-vein line insertion, and trauma to the scalp by instruments during vaginal delivery [64, 65]. Osteomyelitis is currently very rare following an infected cephalhematoma but this complication may occur even without a history of scalp trauma [62]. Hematogenous spread of the infection was also suspected by some authors [59, 66, 67].

The mean age of presentation is between 2 and 4 weeks and the most common site of infection was over the parietal bone. Infected cephalhematoma should be suspected when an enlarging erythematous cephalhematoma is noted or in the presence of scalp lesions, sepsis, and meningitis [59, 64]. Misdiagnosis of bone infection as trauma in these mildly ill infants is common. Additionally, because of nonspecific symptoms like irritability, no-localized pain, indolent presentation and isolated fever, the diagnosis of cranial osteomyelitis may be delayed in neonates [63, 66, 68]. CT-scan is the best imaging diagnostic tool to demonstrate osseous erosion and destruction in osteomyelitis. MRI may be used when an intracranial complication was suspected [58]. The systemic approach includes cultures of blood and cerebrospinal fluid (CSF).

Escherichia coli and *Staphylococcus aureus* are the most common etiologic agents associated with infected cephalhematomas [56, 60, 65, 69]. However, when osteomyelitis occurs, *Escherichia coli* is by far the most common pathogens. Less common pathogens include *Staphylococcus aureus*, *Staphylococcus epidermidis*, *Streptococcus pneumoniae*, *Salmonella typhimurium* and *Proteus species* [63, 64, 70, 71].

Management consists of surgical drainage with or without a partial craniectomy in association with 4–6 weeks of intravenous antibiotic therapy covering both *Escherichia coli* and *Staphylococcus aureus* pathogens [56, 58]. Sepsis, meningitis and brain abscess should be considered, as well as the possibility of antibiotic resistance if the clinical condition does not improve with antibiotics.

Although generally a benign condition seen in the newborn infant, cephalhematoma should be closely followed in order to prevent more serious infectious complications and death [64].

Osteomyelitis of the Clivus

The clivus is rarely affected by osteomyelitis. About 18 well-documented cases have been reported in the literature in the last 20 years [72–88]. Nine cases were described in children (50 %). Osteomyelitis of the clivus is often encountered secondary to direct spread of an infectious process involving the sphenoid sinus [77, 78, 86], oropharyngeal area [87, 88], maxillary sinuses and ethmoid cells [85] or adjacent bone of the skull base [73, 76]. Complications are uncommon but may include meningitis, intracranial extension of the disease toward the posterior fossa or the sellar/parasellar areas, and vascular invasion [78, 80, 81, 83, 87, 88]. In addition, clival infection may extend more inferiorly to the craniovertebral junction or even lower in the cervical spine [72, 80, 86].

In an anecdotal publication reported by Prabhu et al., the authors assumed that the fossa navicularis magna can be a potential source of transmission of infection through the skull base from the lymphatic tissue in the pharynx [79]. The fossa navicularis is a notch-like bone defect in the basiocciput that has been considered as an anatomical variant of the clivus.

Clinical presentation may be insidious for a relative long time before occurrence of headache and/or general infectious symptoms. Cranial neuropathies occur as infection progresses, following a pattern which facilitates to define the site of the disease. Lower cranial nerves are more commonly involved in skull base osteomyelitis. However, combined VIth and XIIth cranial nerve palsies suggest the clivus. Some others neurological syndromes may be encountered such as cavernous sinus syndrome and Wallenberg's syndrome [74, 81, 84]. Anyway, brainstem compression remains a serious complication [76]. More acute presentation may also be seen in other diseases interesting ear, neck and throat areas such as retropharyngeal abscess, Lemierre's syndrome or meningitis [85–88].

Diagnosis of clival osteomyelitis requires recognition of characteristic imaging findings such as diffuse clival hypointensity on sagittal T1-weighted MRI due to bone marrow infiltration. Enhanced T1-weighted MRI showed hypertrophic dura mater and sometimes enhancement around the cavernous sinus [87]. Bone CT-scan of the skull demonstrated clival erosion and trabecular thinning, indicating osteomyelitis of the clivus [86]. When CT-scan and MRI are initially reported as normal but there is a high clinical suspicion of skull base osteomyelitis, a SPECT/CT can prove useful [85, 89].

Concerning microbiology, many pathogens have been found including *Staphylococcus aureus*, *Mycobacterium tuberculosis*, *Enterococcus faecium*, *Gemella haemolysans*, *Streptococcus milleri*, *Fusobacterium necrophorum* and *Actinomyces species* [75–78, 80, 81, 83, 85, 87]. Organisms associated with non-otogenic skull base osteomyelitis form part of the normal oral flora and it seems therefore possible that osteomyelitis is the result of first paranasal sinus disease which then spreads continuously to the base of the skull.

Antimicrobial therapy forms the mainstone of management of clival osteomyelitis. Empiric therapy with vancomycin should also be added for adequate methicillin-resistant *Staphylococcus aureus* (MRSA) coverage [78, 86]. As other skull base localization, surgery has a limited role, often diagnosis, being performed primarily to obtain specimens for culture and to exclude malignancy. Though aggressive surgical debridement of affected tissues was once considered first-line therapy, development of many antimicrobials allowed a less radical approach. However, the concrete indications for surgical intervention remain unclear. If suppurative collections are significant, possible craniotomy with abscess drainage would be an option. Endoscopic exploration for biopsy and repair of possible CSF fistula may be achieved [86].

Calvarial Sclerosing Osteomyelitis

Sclerosing osteomyelitis is a rare pathological entity where a chronic osseous process is sustained by slow active infection. The bone reacts to infectious stimulation by the formation of an immature type of new bone outside the normal cortical layer [90]. This disease is well-described in rheumatology and dental literature [91, 92]. In the jaw, sclerosing osteomyelitis is commonly associated with an odontogenic infection resulting from dental caries [93, 94]. Many terms have been used synonymously in the literature such as periostitis ossificans, ossifying periostitis, chronic nonsuppurative osteomyelitis of Garré, Garré's proliferative periostitis, chronic sclerosing inflammation, chronic osteomyelitis with proliferative periostitis, Garré's disease, among others [90, 95]. In 1893, Carl Garré published an article with special forms and complications of acute infective osteomyelitis. Since then, his name has been associated with the disease [96].

The neurocranium is a rare location of sclerosing osteomyelitis (Fig. 15.9). To the best of our knowledge, only two cases were previously published [97, 98]. Klish et al. reported a 15-year-old boy who presented with painful swelling of the head over a period of 2 years without neurological or infectious abnormalities. The imaging findings were no specific. CT-scan demonstrated intradiploic new bone

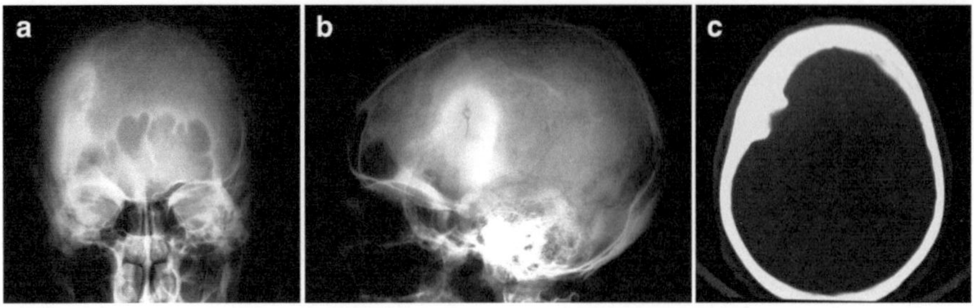

Fig. 15.9 Skull X-rays in antero-posterior (**a**) and lateral view (**b**). Axial CT-scan in bone widows (**c**). Note the thickening of the left frontal skull without respect to the coronal suture. There is no bone erosion

formation and thickening of the left frontoparietal skull. On MRI, the intradiploic lesion was hypointense on T1-weighted images with mixed signal on T2-weighted images. There was a heterogeneous enhancement after gadolinium injection including the adjacent dura. Prior to surgery, the patient was treated with hyperbaric oxygen therapy and antibiotics. The skull lesion was removed but there were no signs of dural infiltration. The craniotomy defect was reconstructed by a titanium implant. Hyperbaric oxygen and antibiotic therapies were continued for 8 weeks and the postoperative course was uneventful without signs of recurrence [97].

The second case report was published by our team in 2009 [98]. A 36-year-old man with a long history of recurrent frontal sinusitis presented with lethargy, meningitis and left hemiparesis. The right frontal scalp appeared swollen, but without inflammatory abnormalities. Plain radiography and CT-scan demonstrated a marked frontal bone thickness without osteolysis. There was also an adjacent subdural empyema with a brain abscess. A rapid craniotomy was performed, but no purulent exudate or abnormal collection was found extracranially. After the bone flap was removed, two purulent collections were drained from the subdural space and the brain parenchyma. Postoperatively, the patient improved dramatically. No microorganisms were growing but antibiotic therapy (ceftriaxone and metronidazole) was administered for 2 months with a good outcome [98].

In both cases, no pathogens growth was obtained in culture and histologic examination revealed numerous thickened bone trabeculae in a dense connective tissue without osteitis or inflammatory infiltration. The trabeculae were often covered by rows of osteoblasts, indicating progressive bone formation. It is clear that the imaging findings are not specific and a wide range of differential diagnosis has to be considered including cavernous angioma, histiocytosis, hyperparathyroidism, Paget's disease, hyperostotic meningioma, osteosarcoma, Ewing sarcoma, bony metastases and fibrous dysplasia among others. As seen in these two cases, complete resection of the diseased bone achieves permanent cure.

In our patient, brain abscess most likely developed slowly and was initially momentarily controlled by antibiotics which were prescribed for recurrent frontal sinusitis. This chronic inflammation may have stimulated calvarial osteoblasts to contain the infection by forming a peudocapsular bone wall [98].

Cranial Osteomyelitis in HIV and AIDS

Acquired immune deficiency syndrome (AIDS) arises from human immunodeficiency virus (HIV) infection. Despite the availability of highly active antiretroviral therapy (HAART) since 1995 and the application of prophylactic antimicrobial regimens, opportunistic infections continue to be a leading cause of morbidity in HIV infected patients [99]. In this population group, skull osteomyelitis is rare and its clinical manifestations vary greatly. Cranial bone infection can occur at any stage, even it may precede the diagnosis of HIV infection [100] and many atypical manifestations may be present. Consequently, a high degree of suspicion is necessary to make an early diagnosis. Spread of infections may be disastrous, not only locally and regionally but possibly even systemically. There is always a chance of a lethal complication. Several pathogens have been described; however the majority of opportunistic cranial bone infections are due to tuberculosis, syphilis, salmonellas and some fungi (see Chap. 14 for more details).

Non-typhoidal salmonella infections are recognized with increasing frequency in HIV-infected individuals [101, 102]. The expected incidence of salmonellosis among patients with AIDS has been 20 to 100-fold more than that among the general population, and 45–78 % of reported patients have presented with bacteremia [103–105]. However, localized salmonella infections have rarely been noted in these patients especially involvement of cranial bones which only two cases were previously reported [106, 107]. Mastroianni et al. reported a 35-year-old HIV-seropositive woman, intravenous drug abuser, with a parietal bone osteomyelitis due to *Salmonella typhimurium*. The cluster of differentiation 4 (CD4) cell count was 9/mm^3. A craniectomy was performed, producing purulent fluid that was drained. The pathogen was isolated from both osseous lesion and stool culture. Medical treatment was conducted by ciprofloxacin with a good outcome [106]. The second case was reported by Aliaga et al., a 35-year-old bisexual man with *Salmonella enteritidis* infection presenting as subdural and epidural cerebral empyema, with concomitant osteomyelitis of the frontal bone. The CD4 cell count was 18/mm^3. The *Salmonella species* was identified in the subcutaneous frontal collection and the same microorganism has grown in stool culture and all blood culture sets. Collections were drained surgically. Therapy with intravenous ciprofloxacin results in rapid improvement. The patient was discharged with trimethoprim-sulfamethoxazole and zidovudine, after that he was cured [107].

Bone involvement is an unusual manifestation of secondary syphilis. In a recent systematic review performed by Park et al. from 1964 to 2013, 37 patients of syphilitic osseous localization were found. Among them, the skull was affected in 21 cases (57 %) [108]. There has recently been an increase in the number of osteitis cases reported, especially in patients with HIV infection. To the best of our knowledge, 11 cases of cranial syphilis were previously reported in HIV infected patients. All of them after the year 2001 [100, 109–117]. Curiously, clinical features and outcome between HIV-uninfected and HIV-infected patients were not different.

Multifocal localization of syphilis was seen in three patients [100, 112, 114]. Gurland et al. reported a case of clinically apparent osteitis of the skull, secondary to acquired syphilis, which was the first manifestation of HIV infection in a 20-year-old bisexual man [100]. The coexistence of HIV infection must be always taken into consideration because about one third of patients with skull syphilis combine HIV disease [108].

Despite the worldwide resurgence of tuberculosis and the increasing number of skull bones tuberculosis (see Chap. 14), only two cases of cranial osteomyelitis due to *Mycobacterium tuberculosis* were previously reported in HIV hosts [118, 119]. Tripathi et al. reported a 40-year-old HIV positive male patient presenting with fever, cough, expectoration and osteolytic, cystic, multiple soft tissue swellings of skull. CD4 lymphocyte count was 11 cells/mm^3. Aspiration from the frontal cystic swelling identified *Mycobacterium tuberculosis*. The patient was put on anti-tubercular treatment and was later discharged but did not come for follow-up treatment [118]. The second case was presented by Mechan et al.; a 33-year-old HIV man has received irregular treatment with highly active antiretroviral therapy in the past. One year later, he complained intense lumbar pain, difficulty walking, hypertrophied cervical lymph nodes, cough and fever. *Mycobacterium tuberculosis* resistant to rifampicin was isolated from the cervical lymph node. Imagery showed several lytic lesions in the skull and thoraco-lumbar vertebrae. There were also renitent swelling in scalp, right forearm and left rib cage. The patient received multidrug resistant tuberculosis treatment for 16 months in addition to HAART with a good outcome [119]. It seems that HIV positivity does not increase the chance of drug resistance but HIV considerably accelerates an infection leading to its development into a disease. It is also appreciated that drug-resistant tuberculosis with HIV infection necessitates particularly rigorous methods to control cross-infection such as confinement of the patient to a negative pressure room and special precautions for nursing [120].

Prognosis of tuberculous cranial osteomyelitis depends on the state of general health, the extent of local lesion, the early establishment of diagnosis and the response to therapy. Overall, this prognosis is usually favorable and mortality due to cranial bone tuberculosis is rare.

Del Val Gomez et al. suggests that many cases of *Mycobacterium tuberculosis* and *M. avium* complex disease remain undiagnosed in HIV-hosts as demonstrated by abnormal Gallium-67 skull uptake in HIV-positive patients with disseminated mycobacterial infection [121].

Nontuberculous mycobacterial infection is a well-known problem for patients with advanced HIV infection. *Mycobacterium avium* complex, *M. kansasii* and *M. xenopi* are the most common pathogens. However, skull bone infection seems to be related only to *M. kansasii* [122]. *Mycobacterium kansasii* is a slow-growing, atypical mycobacterium. It was first isolated about 50 years ago and was initially termed the "yellow bacilli" due to its photochromatogenic properties. The primary route of infection is unknown but may be through inhalation or the digestive tract [123]. Disseminated *M. kansasii* most frequently occurs in immune-compromised patients, especially HIV patients, usually late in the course of AIDS, usually with a

CD4 cell count of less than 50/mL. Osteomyelitis is a rare extrapulmonary manifestation of *M. kansasii*, particularly in HIV patients [124]. To our knowledge, five patients with cranial bone infection caused by *M. kansasii* have been previously reported [125–129]. Intracranial extension was seen in two patients with brain abscess [125, 127]. Multifocal osteolytic infections are common as well as associated systemic lesions. The outcome was fatal for three patients [127–129]. HIV-positive patients with *M. kansasii* have been treated with the same standard antituberculous therapy. However, most patients with disseminated disease died prior to completion of therapy. *M. kansasii* should be considered as a cause of multiple osteolytic lesions of the skull in HIV patients. The clinical course is usually chronic and the time of diagnosis is long. Treatment would be difficult.

Fungal infections are one of the important cause of morbidity and mortality in immunocompromised hosts especially HIV patients. The rate of occurrence of fungal infections has risen over the last decade, as the population of immunocompromised patients has increased. However, cranial osteomyelitis is rarely encountered in HIV patients. Numerous fungi have been described in literature including *Aspergillus species*, *Pneumocystis jiroveci*, Mucormycosis, *Scedosporium apiospermum* and *Pseudallescheria boydii* [130–138]. *Aspergillus spp.* is by far the most frequent fungi in the skull of HIV patients. However, most cases called "skull base osteomyelitis" are in fact lateral otogenic skull base osteomyelitis secondary to necrotizing external otitis or mastoiditis without true bony destruction (see Chap. 1). Considering this latter aspect, a previous literature review found 15 HIV patients with invasive mycoses of temporal bone and lateral skull base: 12 cases with *Aspergillus fumigatus*, 2 patients with *Scedosporium apiospermum* and one patient with *Pseudallescheria boydii* [131]. Mastoidectomy was performed in four patients. According to this review, most of the cases were treated with combination of amphotericin B/itraconazol with a positive response in 8 of 15 patients. However, overall mortality was about 57 %. For many authors, the prognosis seems to depend more on the state of the immunity system than on treatment applied [130, 136, 137, 139].

Concerning mucormycosis, a 33-year-old HIV man presented with progressive right periocular pain, local swelling, rhinorrhea and nasal congestion. His examination revealed right ocular proptosis with periorbital oedema. CD4 lymphocyte count was 20/mm^3. A CT-scan showed involvement of all the sinuses, erosion of the hard palate and sphenoidal osteomyelitis. The patient refused surgery and succumbed to his infection [133]. *Pneumocystis jiroveci* (previously called *P. carinii*) osteomyelitis has been rarely described elsewhere. In HIV-hosts, extrapulmonary *Pneumocystis jiroveci* seems to be less than 1 % of all cases of infection with *Pneumocystis jiroveci*. Among them, only one case was previously reported in the skull. This 51-year-old HIV-positive man had an extrapulmonary *P. jiroveci* infection with multisystemic and multiskeletal involvement particularly osteolytic lesions of the cranial vault bilaterally. The CD4 cell count was 48/mm^3. The patient had a fatal outcome despite appropriate medical therapy [134].

The diagnosis and treatment of fungal infection of the skull is often delayed, as clinical suspicion is often low. For Rothholtz et al., severity of skull base osteomyelitis and the presence of HIV infection significantly affect the duration and charges incurred during hospital stay [140].

An important suspicion of skull base bacterial osteomyelitis should exist in patients with HIV and AIDS due to the significantly worse outcome. The disease presents itself at a much younger age in this patient population, and it is frequently discovered at a more advanced stage of the disease because granulation tissue is often absent from the external auditory canal. Additionally, the multiple species of bacteria (*Pseudomonas aeruginosa*, *Staphylococcus aureus*, *Streptococcus viridans*, *Streptococcus pneumonia and Proteus mirabilis*) that have been cultured from cases in HIV/AIDS patients requires wide early antibiotic coverage while pending culture results [140–142]. Patients with HIV infection are at risk because many take multiple drugs medications and have defects in both cell-mediated and humoral immunity. Hern et al. emphasized that the combination of two antibiotic agents was found to be more effective in treating Pseudomonas infection in HIV patients [143]. Also, association of two anti-Pseudomonas antibiotics may reduce significantly mortality rate [144]. Indeed, *Pseudomonas aeruginosa* infection is frequently fatal and we must think about it in the advanced stages of HIV disease, especially when patients have received co-trimoxazole (trimethoprim/sulfamethoxazole), penicillins or steroids [145].

Although skull infection is unusual in HIV-infected individuals it appears to be an increasing problem. Because fungi, mycobacteria and other specific bacteria are not habitually high on the differential diagnosis of cranial osteomyelitis, it is important to maintain a broad perspective particularly in HIV population. As other co-infectious diseases, cranial osteomyelitis greatly influences the quality of life in respect to physical, mental, social, and economic ground. Early diagnosis and effective management will reduce the morbi-mortality and improve the overall quality of life.

References

1. Flamm ES. Percivall Pott: an 18th century neurosurgeon. J Neurosurg. 1992;76(2):319–26.
2. Pott P. Observations on the nature and consequences of those injuries to which the head is liable from external violence. London: L Hawes, W Clarke, R Collins; 1768.
3. Ravitch MM. Surgery in 1776. Ann Surg. 1977;186(3):291–300.
4. Babu RP, Todor R, Kasoff SS. Pott's puffy tumor: the forgotten entity. Case report. J Neurosurg. 1996;84(1):110–2.
5. Nisa L, Landis BN, Giger R. Orbital involvement in Pott's puffy tumor: a systematic review of published cases. Am J Rhinol Allergy. 2012;26(2):e63–70. doi:10.2500/ajra.2012.26.3746.
6. Salomão JF, Cervante TP, Bellas AR, Boechat MC, Pone SM, Pone MV, de A Pereira B. Neurosurgical implications of Pott's puffy tumor in children and adolescents. Childs Nerv Syst. 2014;30(9):1527–34. doi:10.1007/s00381-014-2480-x.
7. Bradley PJ, Manning KP, Shaw MD. Brain abscess secondary to paranasal sinusitis. J Laryngol Otol. 1984;98(7):719–25.

8. Clayman GL, Adams GL, Paugh DR, Koopmann Jr CF. Intracranial complications of paranasal sinusitis: a combined institutional review. Laryngoscope. 1991;101(3):234–9.
9. Betz CS, Issing W, Matschke J, Kremer A, Uhl E, Leunig A. Complications of acute frontal sinusitis: a retrospective study. Eur Arch Otorhinolaryngol. 2008;265(1):63–72.
10. Cheng S, Vu P. Pott's puffy tumor in a premature neonate: the new youngest case reported in the post-antibiotic era. Orbit. 2009;28(6):412–4. doi:10.3109/01676830903104736.
11. Kombogiorgas D, Seth R, Athwal R, Modha J, Singh J. Suppurative intracranial complications of sinusitis in adolescence. Single institute experience and review of literature. Br J Neurosurg. 2007;21(6):603–9.
12. Suwan PT, Mogal S, Chaudhary S. Pott's puffy tumor: an uncommon clinical entity. Case Rep Pediatr. 2012;2012:386104. doi:10.1155/2012/386104.
13. Ketenci I, Unlü Y, Tucer B, Vural A. The Pott's puffy tumor: a dangerous sign for intracranial complications. Eur Arch Otorhinolaryngol. 2011;268(12):1755–63.
14. Bambakidis NC, Cohen AR. Intracranial complications of frontal sinusitis in children: Pott's puffy tumor revisited. Pediatr Neurosurg. 2001;35(2):82–9.
15. Bannon PD, McCormack RF. Pott's puffy tumor and epidural abscess arising from pansinusitis. J Emerg Med. 2011;41(6):616–22.
16. Elyassi AR, Prenzel R, Closmann JJ. Pott puffy tumor after maxillary tooth extraction. J Oral Maxillofac Surg. 2012;70(3):e190–2. doi:10.1016/j.joms.2011.11.018.
17. Raja V, Low C, Sastry A, Moriarty B. Pott's puffy tumor following an insect bite. J Postgrad Med. 2007;53(2):114–6.
18. Jones JW, Ignelzi RJ, Frank DH, Blacklock JB. Osteomyelitis of the skull following scalp reduction and hair plug transplantation. Ann Plast Surg. 1980;5(6):480–2.
19. Wu CT, Huang JL, Hsia SH, Lee HY, Lin JJ. Pott's puffy tumor after acupuncture therapy. Eur J Pediatr. 2009;168(9):1147–9. doi:10.1007/s00431-008-0892-x.
20. Noskin GA, Kalish SB. Pott's puffy tumor: a complication of intranasal cocaine abuse. Rev Infect Dis. 1991;13(4):606–8.
21. Banooni P, Rickman LS, Ward DM. Pott puffy tumor associated with intranasal methamphetamine. JAMA. 2000;283(10):1293.
22. Sullivan CD, Poetker DM. Anterior table remodeling after treatment for Pott's puffy tumor. Am J Otolaryngol. 2013;34(3):265–7. doi:10.1016/j.amjoto.2012.12.018.
23. Bozdemir K, Kutluhan A, Yalçıner G, Cetin H, Bilgen AS, Tarlak B. Treatment of Pott's Puffy tumor with balloon sinuplasty: report of three cases. Kulak Burun Bogaz Ihtis Derg. 2012;22(6):342–7. doi:10.5606/kbbihtisas.2012.065.
24. Upadhyay S. Recurrent Pott's puffy tumor, a rare clinical entity. Neurol India. 2010;58 (5):815–7. doi:10.4103/0028-3886.72206.
25. Urík M, Machač J, Šlapák I, Hošnová D. Pott's puffy tumor: a rare complication of acute otitis media in child: a case report. Int J Pediatr Otorhinolaryngol. 2015. pii: S0165-5876(15) 00305-5. doi:10.1016/j.ijporl.2015.06.029.
26. Khan MA. Pott's puffy tumor: a rare complication of mastoiditis. Pediatr Neurosurg. 2006;42 (2):125–8.
27. Guillén A, Brell M, Cardona E, Claramunt E, Costa JM. Pott's puffy tumour: still not an eradicated entity. Childs Nerv Syst. 2001;17(6):359–62.
28. Verbon A, Husni RN, Gordon SM, Lavertu P, Keys TF. Pott's puffy tumor due to Haemophilus influenzae: case report and review. Clin Infect Dis. 1996;23(6):1305–7.
29. Goldfarb A, Hocwald E, Gross M, Eliashar R. Frontal sinus cutaneous fistula: a complication of Pott's puffy tumor. Otolaryngol Head Neck Surg. 2004;130(4):490–1.
30. Davidson L, McComb JG. Epidural-cutaneous fistula in association with the Pott puffy tumor in an adolescent. Case report. J Neurosurg. 2006;105(3 Suppl):235–7.
31. Shin JW, Choi IG, Jung SN, Kwon H, Shon WI, Moon SH. Pott puffy tumor appearing with a frontocutaneous fistula. J Craniofac Surg. 2012;23(2):e158–60.

32. Terui H, Numata I, Takata Y, Ogura M, Aiba S. Pott's puffy tumor caused by chronic sinusitis resulting in sinocutaneous fistula. JAMA Dermatol. 2015. doi:10.1001/jamadermatol.2015.0874.
33. Blumfield E, Misra M. Pott's puffy tumor, intracranial, and orbital complications as the initial presentation of sinusitis in healthy adolescents, a case series. Emerg Radiol. 2011;18(3):203–10. doi:10.1007/s10140-010-0934-3.
34. Uren RF, Howman-Giles R. Pott's puffy tumor. Scintigraphic findings. Clin Nucl Med. 1992;17(9):724–7.
35. Vanderveken OM, De Smet K, Dogan-Duyar S, Desimpelaere J, Duval EL, De Praeter M, Van Rompaey D. Pott's puffy tumour in a 5-year old boy: the role of ultrasound and contrast-enhanced CT imaging; surgical case report. B-ENT. 2012;8(2):127–9.
36. Weinberg B, Gupta S, Thomas MJ, Stern H. Pott's puffy tumor: sonographic diagnosis. J Clin Ultrasound. 2005;33(6):305–7.
37. Davis BM, Cofer SA, Aulino JM, Frangoul HA, Boulos FI, Turner KM. Langerhans cell histiocytosis of the frontal sinus mimicking Pott's puffy tumor in a child. Otolaryngol Head Neck Surg. 2007;137(3):515–7.
38. Wong EH, Yang WY, Lowe D. Unilateral non-Hodgkin's lymphoma of the frontal sinus presenting as Pott's puffy tumour. Otolaryngol Pol. 2013;67(4):214–7. doi:10.1016/j.otpol.2012.11.003.
39. Panda NK, Ekambar Eshwara Reddy C. Primary frontal sinus aspergillosis: an uncommon occurrence. Mycoses. 2005;48(4):235–7.
40. Sabatiello M, Vanhooteghem O, Mostinckx S, De La Brassinne M. The Pott's puffy tumor: an unusual complication of frontal sinusitis, methods for its detection. Pediatr Dermatol. 2010;27(4):406–8. doi:10.1111/j.1525-1470.2010.01182.x.
41. Blackman SC, Schleiss MR. Forehead swelling caused by Pott's puffy tumor in a 9-year-old boy with sinusitis. Pediatr Int. 2005;47(6):704–7.
42. Feder Jr HM, Cates KL, Cementina AM. Pott puffy tumor: a serious occult infection. Pediatrics. 1987;79(4):625–9.
43. Skomro R, McClean KL. Frontal osteomyelitis (Pott's puffy tumour) associated with Pasteurella multocida—a case report and review of the literature. Can J Infect Dis. 1998;9(2):115–21.
44. Effat KG, Karam M, El-Kabani A. Pott's puffy tumour caused by mucormycosis. J Laryngol Otol. 2005;119(8):643–5.
45. Patel SA, Chatterjee A, Simonsen K. Recurrent midline frontal mass in a patient with sinusitis. Clin Pediatr (Phila). 2011;50(3):266–8. doi:10.1177/0009922809352680.
46. Jung J, Lee HC, Park IH, Lee HM. Endoscopic endonasal treatment of a Pott's puffy tumor. Clin Exp Otorhinolaryngol. 2012;5(2):112–5. doi:10.3342/ceo.2012.5.2.112.
47. Chandra RK, Kennedy DW, Palmer JN. Endoscopic management of failed frontal sinus obliteration. Am J Rhinol. 2004;18(5):279–84.
48. Deutsch E, Hevron I, Eilon A. Pott's puffy tumor treated by endoscopic frontal sinusotomy. Rhinology. 2000;38(4):177–80.
49. Domville-Lewis C, Friedland PL, Santa Maria PL. Pott's puffy tumour and intracranial complications of frontal sinusitis in pregnancy. J Laryngol Otol. 2013;127 Suppl 1:S35–8. doi:10.1017/S0022215112001673.
50. Parida PK, Surianarayanan G, Ganeshan S, Saxena SK. Pott's puffy tumor in pediatric age group: a retrospective study. Int J Pediatr Otorhinolaryngol. 2012;76(9):1274–7. doi:10.1016/j.ijporl.2012.05.018.
51. Akiyama K, Karaki M, Mori N. Evaluation of adult Pott's puffy tumor: our five cases and 27 literature cases. Laryngoscope. 2012;122(11):2382–8. doi:10.1002/lary.23490.
52. Tsai BY, Lin KL, Lin TY, Chiu CH, Lee WJ, Hsia SH, Wu CT, Wang HS. Pott's puffy tumor in children. Childs Nerv Syst. 2010;26(1):53–60. doi:10.1007/s00381-009-0954-z.
53. Kaabia N, Abdelkafi M, Bellara I, Khalifa M, Bahri F, Letaief A. Pott's puffy tumor. A case report. Med Mal Infect. 2007;37(6):350–3.

54. Broekhuizen FF, Washinton JM, Johnson F. Vacuum extraction versus forceps delivery: indication and complications, 1979 to 1984. Obstet Gynecol. 1987;69(3 Pt 1):338–42.
55. Hankins GDV, Leicht T, Van Hook J, Uckan EM. The role of forceps rotation in maternal and neonatal injury. Am J Obstet Gynecol. 1999;180(1 Pt 1):231–4.
56. Chang HY, Chiu NC, Huang FY, Kao HA, Hsu CH, Hung HY. Infected cephalohematoma of newborns: experience in a medical center in Taiwan. Pediatr Int. 2005;47(3):274–7.
57. Weiss KJ, Edwards MS, Hay LM, Allen CH. Escherichia coli—infected cephalohematoma in an infant. Clin Pediatr (Phila). 2009;48(7):763–6. doi:10.1177/0009922809335669.
58. Chan MS, Wong YC, Lau SP, Lau KY, Ou Y. MRI and CT findings of infected cephalhaematoma complicated by skull vault osteomyelitis, transverse venous sinus thrombosis and cerebellar haemorrhage. Pediatr Radiol. 2002;32(5):376–9.
59. Nakwan N, Nakwan N, Wannaro J, Dissaneevate P, Kritsaneepaiboon S, Chokephaibulkit K. Septicemia, meningitis, and skull osteomyelitis complicating infected cephalhematoma caused by ESBL-producing Escherichia coli. Southeast Asian J Trop Med Public Health. 2011;42(1):148–51.
60. Miedema CJ, Ruige M, Kimpen JL. Primarily infected cephalhematoma and osteomyelitis in a newborn. Eur J Med Res. 1999;4(1):8–10.
61. Van Helleputte C, Dupont V, Barthels S, Aeby A. [Escherichia coli meningitis and parietal osteomyelitis in an infant: a rare complication of cephalohematoma]. Rev Med Brux. 2010;31 (1):57–9. French.
62. Prasad R, Verma N, Mishra OP, Srivastava A. Osteomyelitis of skull with underlying brain abscess. Indian J Pediatr. 2011;78(8):1005–7. doi:10.1007/s12098-011-0369-1.
63. Listinsky JL, Wood BP, Ekholm SE. Parietal osteomyelitis and epidural abscess: a delayed complication of fetal monitoring. Pediatr Radiol. 1986;16(2):150–1.
64. Blom NA, Vreede WB. Infected cephalhematomas associated with osteomyelitis, sepsis and meningitis. Pediatr Infect Dis J. 1993;12(12):1015–7.
65. Wong CS, Cheah FC. Cephalhematoma infected by Escherichia coli presenting as an extensive scalp abscess. J Pediatr Surg. 2012;47(12):2336–40. doi:10.1016/j.jpedsurg.2012.09.029.
66. Levy HL, O'Connor JF, Ingall D. Bacteremia, infected cephalhematoma, and osteomyelitis of the skull in a newborn. Am J Dis Child. 1967;114(6):649–51.
67. Kao HC, Huang YC, Lin TY. Infected cephalohematoma associated with sepsis and skull osteomyelitis: report of one case. Am J Perinatol. 1999;16(9):459–62.
68. Ellis SS, Montgomery JR, Wagner M, Hill RM. Osteomyelitis complicating neonatal cephalhematoma. Am J Dis Child. 1974;127(1):100–2.
69. Vale B, Morais S, Resende C, Taborda A. Neonatal meningitis associated with osteomyelitis and epidural empyema. BMJ Case Rep. 2013. pii: bcr2013009149. doi:10.1136/bcr-2013-009149.
70. Diwan N, Sharma KB. Isolation of Salmonella typhimurium from cephalhematoma and osteomyelitis. Indian J Med Res. 1978;67:27–9.
71. Nightingale LM, Eaton CB, Fruehan AE, Waldman JB, Clark WB, Lepow ML. Cephalhematoma complicated by osteomyelitis presumed due to Gardnerella vaginalis. JAMA. 1986;256(14):1936–7.
72. Azizi SA, Fayad PB, Fulbright R, Giroux ML, Waxman SG. Clivus and cervical spinal osteomyelitis with epidural abscess presenting with multiple cranial neuropathies. Clin Neurol Neurosurg. 1995;97(3):239–44.
73. Hoistad DL, Duvall III AJ. Sinusitis with contiguous abscess involvement of the clivus and petrous apices. Case report. Ann Otol Rhinol Laryngol. 1999;108(5):463–6.
74. Keane JR. Combined VIth and XIIth cranial nerve palsies: a clival syndrome. Neurology. 2000;54(7):1540–1.
75. Rusconi R, Bergamaschi S, Cazzavillan A, Carnelli V. Clivus osteomyelitis secondary to Enterococcus faecium infection in a 6-year-old girl. Int J Pediatr Otorhinolaryngol. 2005;69 (9):1265–8.

76. Mancusi G, Marks B, Czerny C, Thalhammer F, Thurnher D, Riedl M, Dekan G, Knerer B. [Tubercular osteomyelitis of the clivus and the nasopharynx]. HNO. 2005;53(12):1081–4. German.
77. Ng J, Connolly DJ, Rittey CD, Mordekar SR. Skull base osteomyelitis leading to lateral medullary syndrome in a child. Eur J Paediatr Neurol. 2007;11(2):111–4.
78. Laurens MB, Becker RM, Johnson JK, Wolf JS, Kotloff KL. MRSA with progression from otitis media and sphenoid sinusitis to clival osteomyelitis, pachymeningitis and abducens nerve palsy in an immunocompetent 10-year-old patient. Int J Pediatr Otorhinolaryngol. 2008;72(7):945–51. doi:10.1016/j.ijporl.2008.02.025.
79. Prabhu SP, Zinkus T, Cheng AG, Rahbar R. Clival osteomyelitis resulting from spread of infection through the fossa navicularis magna in a child. Pediatr Radiol. 2009;39(9):995–8. doi:10.1007/s00247-009-1283-9.
80. Nomura M, Shin M, Ohta M, Nukui Y, Ohkusu K, Saito N. Atypical osteomyelitis of the skull base and craniovertebral junction caused by Actinomyces infection—case report. Neurol Med Chir (Tokyo). 2011;51(1):64–6.
81. Hayashi T, Uchiumi H, Yanagisawa K, Ogawa Y, Handa H, Tsukamoto N, Nojima Y. Recurrent Gemella haemolysans meningitis in a patient with osteomyelitis of the clivus. Intern Med. 2013;52(18):2145–7.
82. Nabavizadeh SA, Vossough A, Pollock AN. Clival osteomyelitis. Pediatr Emerg Care. 2013;29(9):1030–2.
83. Bhavanam HS, Rajesh A, Uppin MS. Tubercular osteomyelitis of spheno-clival region presenting with lateral rectus palsy. Neurol India. 2014;62(2):198–200. doi:10.4103/0028-3886.132400.
84. Takahashi S, Ito S, Tagashira S, Yasui K, Watanabe Y, Nakashima K. A case of corticosteroid-responsive Lemierre syndrome with clivus osteomyelitis and a mass in the cavernous sinus-suprasellar region. Rinsho Shinkeigaku. 2015;55(5):327–32. doi:10.5692/clinicalneurol.cn-000596.Japanese.
85. Trück J, Thompson A, Dwivedi R, Segal S, Anand G, Kelly DF. Non-otogenic skull base osteomyelitis in children: 2 cases and a review of the literature. Pediatr Infect Dis J. 2015;34(9):1025–7. doi:10.1097/INF.0000000000000782.
86. Tomovic S, Friedel ME, Liu JK, Eloy JA. Community-acquired methicillin-resistant Staphylococcus aureus skull base osteomyelitis with occipital condylar cerebrospinal fluid leak in an immunocompetent patient. Laryngoscope. 2012;122(5):977–81. doi:10.1002/lary.23253.
87. He J, Lam JC, Adlan T. Clival osteomyelitis and hypoglossal nerve palsy-rare complications of Lemierre's syndrome. BMJ Case Rep. 2015. pii: bcr2015209777. doi:10.1136/bcr-2015-209777.
88. Peer Mohamed B, Carr L. Neurological complications in two children with Lemierre syndrome. Dev Med Child Neurol. 2010;52(8):779–81. doi:10.1111/j.1469-8749.2010.03718.x.
89. van der Bruggen W, Bleeker-Rovers CP, Boerman OC, Gotthardt M, Oyen WJ. PET and SPECT in osteomyelitis and prosthetic bone and joint infections: a systematic review. Semin Nucl Med. 2010;40(1):3–15. doi:10.1053/j.semnuclmed.2009.08.005.
90. Baltensperger MM, Gerold KH. Osteomyelitis of the jaws: definition and classification. In: Baltensperger MM, Eyrich GK, editors. Osteomyelitis of the jaws. Berlin: Springer; 2009.
91. Nikomarov D, Zaidman M, Katzman A, Keren Y, Eidelman M. New treatment option for sclerosing osteomyelitis of Garré. J Pediatr Orthop B. 2013;22(6):577–82. doi:10.1097/BPB.0b013e32836330a6.
92. Suma R, Vinay C, Shashikanth MC, Subba Reddy VV. Garre's sclerosing osteomyelitis. J Indian Soc Pedod Prev Dent. 2007;25(Suppl):S30–3.
93. Panders AK, Hadders HN. Chronic sclerosing inflammations of the jaw. Osteomyelitis sicca (Garré), chronic sclerosing osteomyelitis with finemeshed trabecular structure, and very dense sclerosing osteomyelitis. Oral Surg Oral Med Oral Pathol. 1970;30(3):396–412.

94. Belli E, Matteini C, Andreano T. Sclerosing osteomyelitis of Garré periostitis ossificans. J Craniofac Surg. 2002;13(6):765–8.
95. Suei Y, Taguchi A, Tanimoto K. Diagnosis and classification of mandibular osteomyelitis. Oral Surg Oral Med Oral Pathol Oral Radiol Endod. 2005;100(2):207–14.
96. Wood RE, Nortjé CJ, Grotepass F, Schmidt S, Harris AM. Periostitis ossificans versus Garrè's osteomyelitis. Part I. What did Garrè really say? Oral Surg Oral Med Oral Pathol. 1988;65(6):773–7.
97. Klisch J, Spreer J, Bötefür I, Gellrich NC, Adler CP, Zentner J, Schumacher M. Calvarial sclerosing osteomyelitis. Pediatr Neurosurg. 2002;36(3):128–32.
98. Akhaddar A, Albouzidi A, Elouennas M, Elmostarchid B, Boucetta M. Nonsuppurative calvarial thickening: a new form of Garré disease? J Neurosurg. 2009;110(4):808. doi:10.3171/2008.3.17458.
99. Horberg MA, Hurley LB, Klein DB, Follansbee SE, Quesenberry C, Flamm JA, Green GM, Luu T. Surgical outcomes in human immunodeficiency virus-infected patients in the era of highly active antiretroviral therapy. Arch Surg. 2006;141(12):1238–45.
100. Gurland IA, Korn L, Edelman L, Wallach F. An unusual manifestation of acquired syphilis. Clin Infect Dis. 2001;32(4):667–9.
101. Fernández Guerrero ML, Ramos JM, Núñez A, Cuenca M, de Górgolas M. Focal infections due to non-typhi Salmonella in patients with AIDS: report of 10 cases and review. Clin Infect Dis. 1997;25(3):690–7.
102. Belzunegui J, Lopez L, Arrizabalaga J, Gonzalez C, Figueroa M. Salmonella osteomyelitis in a patient with human immunodeficiency virus infection. Clin Rheumatol. 1997;16(3):319–20.
103. Sperber SJ, Schleupner CJ. Salmonellosis during infection with human immunodeficiency virus. Rev Infect Dis. 1987;9(5):925–34.
104. Celum CL, Chaisson RE, Rutherford GW, Barnhart JL, Echenberg DF. Incidence of salmonellosis in patients with AIDS. J Infect Dis. 1987;156(6):998–1002.
105. Gruenewald R, Blum S, Chan J. Relationship between human immunodeficiency virus infection and salmonellosis in 20- to 59-year-old residents of New York City. Clin Infect Dis. 1994;18(3):358–63.
106. Mastroianni CM, Vullo V, Delia S. Cranial Salmonella abscess with parietal bone osteomyelitis in an HIV-infected patient. AIDS. 1992;6(7):749–50.
107. Aliaga L, Mediavilla JD, López de la Osa A, López-Gómez M, de Cueto M, Miranda C. Nontyphoidal salmonella intracranial infections in HIV-infected patients. Clin Infect Dis. 1997;25(5):1118–20.
108. Park KH, Lee MS, Hong IK, Sung JY, Choi SH, Park SO, Shin MJ, Chung HW, Lee SH. Bone involvement in secondary syphilis: a case report and systematic review of the literature. Sex Transm Dis. 2014;41(9):532–7. doi:10.1097/OLQ.0000000000000164.
109. Son C, Samples D, Brenner A, Floyd J. Osteolytic calvarial lesions as initial presentation of latent neurosyphilis. J Clin Neurosci. 2015;22(5):909–10. doi:10.1016/j.jocn.2014.11.014.
110. Elopre L, Morell V, Bosshardt C, Geisler WM. A case of syphilitic osteitis in a patient with HIV infection. Int J STD AIDS. 2014;25(10):765–7. doi:10.1177/0956462414522031.
111. Boix V, Merino E, Reus S, Torrus D, Portilla J. Polyostotic osteitis in secondary syphilis in an HIV-infected patient. Sex Transm Dis. 2013;40(8):645–6. doi:10.1097/01.OLQ.0000431351.50346.20.
112. Trevillyan JM, Yap KS, Hoy J. The great medical imitator: a case of syphilitic osteitis in the setting of HIV infection. Sex Health. 2013;10(3):275–8. doi:10.1071/SH12187.
113. Toby M, Larbalestier N, Kulasegaram R, Teague A, Conway K, White J. Calvarial syphilis in an HIV-positive man. Int J STD AIDS. 2012;23(5):365–6. doi:10.1258/ijsa.2011.011276.
114. Samarkos M, Giannopoulou C, Karantoni E, Papastamopoulos V, Baraboutis I, Skoutelis A. Syphilitic periostitis of the skull and ribs in a HIV positive patient. Sex Transm Infect. 2011;87(1):44–5. doi:10.1136/sti.2010.044461.

115. Etienne M, Bencteux P, Gueit I, Abboud P, Caron F. Déjà vu in the catacombs: skull syphilitic osteitis. Lancet Infect Dis. 2008;8(7):455.
116. Huang I, Leach JL, Fichtenbaum CJ, Narayan RK. Osteomyelitis of the skull in early-acquired syphilis: evaluation by MR imaging and CT. AJNR Am J Neuroradiol. 2007;28 (2):307–8.
117. Gómez Martínez MV, Gallardo FG, Cobo Soler J, Babé Romero J, Rios Ferreiros M, Valencia Ortega E. Osteitis in secondary syphilis. Rev Esp Med Nucl. 2003;22(6):424–6.
118. Tripathi AK, Gupta N, Khanna M, Ahmad R, Tripathi P. Tuberculosis presenting as osteolytic soft tissue swellings of skull in HIV positive patient: a case report. Indian J Tuberc. 2007;54(4):193–5.
119. Mechán V, Salas A, García Y, Llanos F, Cornejo J, Bringas R. [Patient HIV positive with systemic tuberculosis and osteolytic calvarial lesions mimicking multiple Myeloma]. An Fac med. 2010;71(3):207–11. Spanish.
120. Ramdurg SR, Gupta DK, Suri A, Sharma BS, Mahapatra AK. Calvarial tuberculosis: uncommon manifestation of common disease—a series of 21 cases. Br J Neurosurg. 2010;24 (5):572–7. doi:10.3109/02688697.2010.495166.
121. del Val Gomez M, Gallardo FG, Cobo J, Castro-Beiras JM. Abnormal gallium-67 skull uptake: a sign of peripheral marrow activation in HIV-positive patients with disseminated mycobacterioses. J Nucl Med. 1995;36(12):2211–3.
122. Mistry BJ, Kala UK. Palatial erosion caused by Mycobacterium Avium complex in a human immunodeficiency virus infected child. Pediatr Infect Dis J. 2007;26(6):546–8.
123. Witzig RS, Fazal BA, Mera RM, Mushatt DM, Dejace PM, Greer DL, Hyslop Jr NE. Clinical manifestations and implications of coinfection with Mycobacterium kansasii and human immunodeficiency virus type 1. Clin Infect Dis. 1995;21(1):77–85.
124. Yano T, Okuda S, Kato K, Kato K, Kishimoto T. Mycobacterium kansasii osteomyelitis in a patient with AIDS on highly active antiretroviral therapy. Intern Med. 2004;43(11):1084–6.
125. Gordon SM, Blumberg HM. Mycobacterium kansasii brain abscess in a patient with AIDS. Clin Infect Dis. 1992;14(3):789–90.
126. Weinroth SE, Pincetl P, Tuazon CU. Disseminated Mycobacterium kansasii infection presenting as pneumonia and osteomyelitis of the skull in a patient with AIDS. Clin Infect Dis. 1994;18(2):261–2.
127. Flores R, Salvato P, Thompson C, Knight B. Invasive Mycobacterium kansasii brain abscess: a case report. Paper presented at: XI International Conference on AIDS; July 7–12 1996; Vancouver, USA (abstract We, B. 3363).
128. Capdevila O, Zurita A, Domingo E, Corbella X, Alcaide F, Monfort JL, Fernández-Viladrich P. Multiple cranial osteolytic lesions due to Mycobacterium kansasii in a patient with AIDS. Scand J Infect Dis. 1998;30(3):305–6.
129. Mazor Y, Sprecher H, Braun E. Mycobacteria kansassi disseminated disease. Isr Med Assoc J. 2010;12(2):121–2.
130. Wright M, Fikrig S, Haller JO. Aspergillosis in children with acquired immune deficiency. Pediatr Radiol. 1993;23(6):492–4.
131. Stodulski D, Kowalska B, Stankiewicz C. Otogenic skull base osteomyelitis caused by invasive fungal infection. Case report and literature review. Eur Arch Otorhinolaryngol. 2006;263(12):1070–6.
132. Gamaletsou MN, Rammaert B, Bueno MA, Moriyama B, Sipsas NV, Kontoyiannis DP, Roilides E, Zeller V, Prinapori R, Taj-Aldeen SJ, Brause B, Lortholary O, Walsh TJ. Aspergillus osteomyelitis: epidemiology, clinical manifestations, management, and outcome. J Infect. 2014;68(5):478–93. doi:10.1016/j.jinf.2013.12.008.
133. Abril V, Ortega E, Segarra P, Pedro F, Sabater V, Herrera A. Rhinocerebral mucormycosis in a patient with AIDS: a complication of diabetic ketoacidosis following pentamidine therapy. Clin Infect Dis. 1996;23(4):845–6.
134. Panos GZ, Karydis I, Velakoulis SE, Falagas ME. Multi-skeletal Pneumocystis jiroveci (carinii) in an HIV-seropositive patient. Int J STD AIDS. 2007;18(2):134–7.

135. Qiu Y, Zhang J, Liu G, Zhong X, Deng J, He Z, Jing B. Retrospective analysis of 14 cases of disseminated Penicillium marneffei infection with osteolytic lesions. BMC Infect Dis. 2015;15:47. doi:10.1186/s12879-015-0782-6.
136. Slack CL, Watson DW, Abzug MJ, Shaw C, Chan KH. Fungal mastoiditis in immunocompromised children. Arch Otolaryngol Head Neck Surg. 1999;125(1):73–5.
137. Yao M, Messner AH. Fungal malignant otitis externa due to Scedosporium apiospermum. Ann Otol Rhinol Laryngol. 2001;110(4):377–80.
138. Busaba NY, Poulin M. Invasive Pseudallescheria boydii fungal infection of the temporal bone. Otolaryngol Head Neck Surg. 1997;117(6):S91–4.
139. Muñoz A, Martínez-Chamorro E. Necrotizing external otitis caused by Aspergillus fumigatus: computed tomography and high resolution magnetic resonance imaging in an AIDS patient. J Laryngol Otol. 1998;112(1):98–102.
140. Rothholtz VS, Lee AD, Shamloo B, Bazargan M, Pan D, Djalilian HR. Skull base osteomyelitis: the effect of comorbid disease on hospitalization. Laryngoscope. 2008;118 (11):1917–24. doi:10.1097/MLG.0b013e31817fae0d.
141. Ress BD, Luntz M, Telischi FF, Balkany TJ, Whiteman ML. Necrotizing external otitis in patients with AIDS. Laryngoscope. 1997;107(4):456–60.
142. Rubin Grandis J, Branstetter IV BF, Yu VL. The changing face of malignant (necrotising) external otitis: clinical, radiological, and anatomic correlations. Lancet Infect Dis. 2004;4 (1):34–9.
143. Hern JD, Almeyda J, Thomas DM, Main J, Patel KS. Malignant otitis externa in HIV and AIDS. J Laryngol Otol. 1996;110(8):770–5.
144. Mendelson MH, Gurtman A, Szabo S, Neibart E, Meyers BR, Policar M, Cheung TW, Lillienfeld D, Hammer G, Reddy S, et al. Pseudomonas aeruginosa bacteremia in patients with AIDS. Clin Infect Dis. 1994;18(6):886–95.
145. Meynard JL, Barbut F, Guiguet M, Batisse D, Lalande V, Lesage D, Guiard-Schmid JB, Petit JC, Frottier J, Meyohas MC. Pseudomonas aeruginosa infection in human immunodeficiency virus infected patients. J Infect. 1999;38(3):176–81.

Part VI
Prevention of Cranial Osteomyelitis

Chapter 16
Preventive Measures Against Cranial Bone Infection

Contents

Cranial osteomyelitis and its causes remain preventable and treatable although there is no perfect method for the prevention of this infectious disease. Appropriate treatment of conditions and causes that may lead to cranial osteomyelitis in addition to surgical prophylactic measures are the best way to "close the doors" to micro-organisms invasion.

General Considerations

General factors have certainly contributed to the reduction of the incidence of cranial osteomyelitis as in other sites of the skeleton including improved nutrition, good hygiene practices, vaccination, and better availability to medical and dental care. Additionally, good awareness of risk factors (see Chap. 2), their early suspicion and prompt treatment have improved the incidence of this infectious disease. Some comorbidities should also be taken into consideration and actively addressed. These include vulnerability due to metabolic states, unbalanced nutritional states, smoking and tobacco use, specific exposure risks, compromised immune function, malignancy, hemodialysis and extreme old age.

Any infection elsewhere in the body should be diagnosed and treated sufficiently, since it can potentially spreads through the blood to the cranial skeleton inducing an acute hematogenous osteomyelitis.

A. Akhaddar, *Cranial Osteomyelitis*, DOI 10.1007/978-3-319-30268-3_16

Preventing Contiguous Sites of Infections

Paranasal sinusitis, oral/odontogenic infections, otomastoiditis or previous scalp lesions should be suspected and managed promptly. Rhinosinusitis or otomastoiditis symptoms failing to respond to antibiotics or associated with neurological findings (such as seizures, changes in mental status, hemiparesis, or cranial nerve deficits) require prompt attention [1, 2]. Early diagnosis due to more sophisticated imaging modalities and microbiological technologies in addition to adequate antimicrobial treatment has certainly decreased the risk of cranial bones osteomyelitis and intracranial suppurations [3–7].

Special attention should be paid to patients with necrotizing external otitis. The initiating event may be self-inflicted or iatrogenic trauma to the ear canal. Therefore, susceptible patients should be instructed to avoid manipulation of the external auditory canal (i.e., they should not use cotton swabs to remove cerumen). Cleaning of the external auditory canal, including aural irrigation by medical staff, should be carried out with extreme caution to avoid injuring delicate skin in the canal [8]. Eczematous conditions involving the meatus of the canal should be treated topically, because these conditions may result in pruritus that leads to scratching of the irritated skin [9].

In addition, patients with scalp lesion-related superficial bacterial infections should receive close follow-up and, when necessary, antibiotic therapy must be administered [10].

Neurosurgical Prophylactic Procedures

Specifics methods for prevention of postoperative skull osteomyelitis have not been reported. However, several measures are widely used for preventing surgical site infections in neurosurgery as well as patient care and surgical practices from the preoperative preparation to the days following the surgical procedure and even after the patient have left the hospital.

As others surgical site infections, the surgical team remains the most decisive element in preventing post-craniotomy bone infection. Control of the operative theatre with limited traffic, careful patient preparation, adherence to antiseptic principles, minimization of tissue damage, shorter operating times, and meticulous dura and wound closure (to prevent cerebrospinal fluid leak) are crucial [11, 12]. Cushing in the beginning of the twentieth century and prior to the introduction of antibiotics had only 1 % of infection rate in clean neurosurgical procedures. This suggest clearly that technique is extremely important and that surgeons in the pre-antibiotic era would have been particularly meticulous by using just soap and water and simple techniques for sterilizing the operative field, since a bacterial infection had no effective treatment and its consequences were often mortal [13].

A strict pre-operative practice for skin decontamination is important to prevent postoperative wound infections. Often, these varieties of infections can be easily treated, but may extend and result in deeper more severe infection like osteomyelitis of the underlying bone flap. These infections can be considered as incisional infections, acquired at the time of surgery. Their common pathophysiology is suggested by the predominance of saprophyte skin flora microorganisms in a single patient (see Chaps. 3 and 5) [14]. In theory, antibiotic prophylaxis lowers the bacterial inoculum before surgical incision and prevents microbial proliferation during surgery [15].

Prospective studies involving large numbers of patients have demonstrated lower neurosurgical postoperative infection rates when antimicrobial prophylaxis is used [15]. Many studies of clean neurosurgical procedures reported antimicrobial regimens including clindamycin, vancomycin, cefotiam, piperacillin, cloxacillin, oxacillin, cefuroxime, cefotaxime, sulfamethoxazole-trimethoprim, cefazolin, penicillin G, and amoxicillin-clavulanic acid [15–19]. However, no single antimicrobial agent has been demonstrated to have greater efficacy than others [18]. A randomized, open-label, multicenter study of 613 adult patients undergoing elective craniotomy, shunt, or stereotactic procedures found no difference in single doses of cefotaxime and trimethoprim-sulfamethoxazole in postoperative abscess formation, surgical site infections, and shunt infections [19].

Although there is no clear consensus in neurosurgery on the optimal antibiotic regimen for surgical prophylaxis, there is published evidence that the administration of a single dose of cefazolin within 1 h of making the skin incision will reduce the likelihood of postoperative surgical site infection [20, 21]. For patients who are allergic to penicillin, vancomycin is an appropriate alternative treatment choice [21].

Some authors also routinely irrigate copiously with antibiotic-containing saline to prevent intraoperative contamination [22–24]. Although it has become a widely accepted practice, it remains poorly studied, and concrete confirmation supporting or refuting it is deficient.

Recently, intranasal mupirocin administered pre-operatively for decolonization of methicillin-resistant *Staphylococcus aureus* (MRSA) has been proposed in neurosurgical patients to reduce the rate of surgical site infections [25, 26].

Devascularization and devitalization of the craniotomy bone flap have been suggested to contribute to the formation of cranial osteomyelitis because a reduction in the natural resistance to infection in non-vascularized bone. However, there is no statistically significant difference in the incidence of infection in patients managed with free or osteoplastic bone flaps [27]. The surgical drain is left in place for as short a time as possible and never for more than a few days. The draining open system has the danger of contamination and is not recommended.

Some questions have long persisted about the influence of other preventive measures and areas of controversy including shaving the scalp, double gloving (protect against holes in surgical gloves), use of different scalp blades from the skin to the depths surgical field, changing the gloves regularly, use of different variety of surgical drapes (plastic, paper or cloth), and application of incisional antibiotic ointment. However, based on personal conviction, experience or training, some neurosurgeons continue to use some of these methods to prevent the development of infections [28].

Management of cranial bone bleeding is largely based on the use of bone wax and electrocautery. Although effective in stopping bone bleeding, traditional bone wax (composed largely of beeswax) has troublesome adverse effects. The material interferes with bone healing and cause inflammatory reactions. Once applied to the bone, bone wax remains at the surgical site indefinitely. It may become a nidus of surgical site infection and if contaminated, it may cause infection of the soft tissue or osteomyelitis [29–31]. Most surgeons are often unaware of the post-operative complications attributed to the use of bone wax and unfamiliar with the range of alternatives available for bone hemostasis [32]. For Wellisz and co-authors, the possibility of combining topical bone hemostasis materials (such as ostene) with therapeutics (like antibiotics or bone grafts), may in the future enlarge the range of medical tools available to surgeons and reset the role and management of bone bleeding. This measure will be another step toward reducing wound complications and the associated morbidity after bone surgery [31, 33].

Despite the rare occurrence, special attention should be paid not to leave cotton pledgets or other foreign bodies during neurosurgical procedures. Retained foreign bodies may result in chronic, delayed, or recurrent infections [34, 35]. In other side, when the bone flap hits the floor (accidental dropping) during craniotomy, infections can be avoided by autoclaving or soaking the flap in betadine and/or antibiotic solution. Jankowitz et al. highlighted that only a minority of patients needed discarding of the bone and cranioplasty [36].

Adequate postoperative surgical incision care and close surveillance of surgical site is mandatory. Early recognition of superficial infection and prompt treatment are keys to preventing extension to adjacent cranial bones and neurological structures.

In the same way, osteomyelitis and intracranial suppurations have been reported in association with the use of the halo device. This technique should be used with caution and with an awareness of the possible increased risks of pin site infection [37]. Meticulous care of the pin sites of hallo fixation devices is essential to avoid cranial and intracranial infectious complications [38, 39].

Measures Taken Following Scalp Injury

Direct inoculation osteomyelitis can best be prevented with appropriate wound management and consideration of prophylactic antibiotic use at the time of injury.

After a head injury, the entire scalp must be inspected thoroughly and washed to remove debris. The depth of the wound must be checked for skull penetration. Any cerebro-spinal fluid leak should be noted and a skull fracture with dural tear suspected. Because the scalp is highly mobile, a skull fracture may be beyond the limits of the wound. The wound must be thoroughly cleaned with a sterile solution and foreign material and devitalized tissue removed [40]. Generally the wound margins to be apposed will be of equal thickness. Excessive tension on wound closure should be avoided because the scalp tissue would retract leaving a scarred contracted soft tissue envelope inducing an area of denuded cranial bone. Puncture wounds and bites should also be taken into consideration. After that, close surveillance for superficial wound infections is necessary until good healing.

Simple abrasions or small wound can be managed with local anesthesia. Whereas, for extensive scalping injuries it is more reasonable to practice the surgical procedure under general anesthesia in the operating room [41, 42].

From a practical point of view, scalp injuries are adequately managed by using the classic mnemonic acronym **HEDSAT** [41]:

- Hemostasis
- Examination of skull
- Debridement cleaning
- Skin closure without tension
- Antibiotics
- Tetanos prophylaxis.

Nursing Implication

Careful nursing implication in patients with head or face disease or following an injury involves observation, strict awareness to hygiene, appropriate medical drugs administration and dressing, adequate nutrition and hydration. Wound care should constantly be performed with clear procedures considered to avoid contamination. Careful hand washing and proper disposal of dressings and contaminated material are imperative to improve healing and to avoid cranial bone infections [43–45].

Finally, the whole health care team must consider prevention of infection to be a serious problem of such seriousness that it warrants meticulous measures that minimize the risk of cranial infections and deeper extensions.

References

1. Kombogiorgas D, Solanki GA. The Pott puffy tumor revisited: neurosurgical implications of this unforgotten entity. Case report and review of the literature. J Neurosurg. 2006;105 (2 Suppl):143–9.
2. Betz CS, Issing W, Matschke J, Kremer A, Uhl E, Leunig A. Complications of acute frontal sinusitis: a retrospective study. Eur Arch Otorhinolaryngol. 2008;265(1):63–72.
3. Oxford LE, McClay J. Complications of acute sinusitis in children. Otolaryngol Head Neck Surg. 2005;133(1):32–7.
4. Ali A, Kurien M, Mathews SS, Mathew J. Complications of acute infective rhinosinusitis: experience from a developing country. Singapore Med J. 2005;46(10):540–4.

5. Clayman GL, Adams GL, Paugh DR, Koopmann Jr CF. Intracranial complications of paranasal sinusitis: a combined institutional review. Laryngoscope. 1991;101(3):234–9.
6. Salomão JF, Cervante TP, Bellas AR, Boechat MC, Pone SM, Pone MV, de A Pereira B. Neurosurgical implications of Pott's puffy tumor in children and adolescents. Childs Nerv Syst. 2014;30(9):1527–34. doi:10.1007/s00381-014-2480-x.
7. Niv A, Nash M, Slovik Y, Fliss DM, Kaplan D, Leibovitz E, Katz A, Dagan R, Leiberman A. Acute mastoiditis in infancy: the Soroka experience: 1990–2000. Int J Pediatr Otorhinolaryngol. 2004;68(11):1435–9.
8. Rubin J, Yu VL, Kamerer DB, Wagener M. Aural irrigation with water: a potential pathogenic mechanism for inducing malignant external otitis? Ann Otol Rhinol Laryngol. 1990;99(2 pt 1):117–9.
9. Sander R. Otitis externa: a practical guide to treatment and prevention. Am Fam Physician. 2001;63(5):927–36, 941–2.
10. Gallagher PG. Osteomyelitis of the skull after varicella infection. Clin Pediatr (Phila). 1990;29 (1):29.
11. Nabavi A, Knerlich-Lukoschus F, Stark AM. Postoperative intracranial infections. In: Hall WA, Kim PD, editors. Neurosurgical infectious disease. Surgical and nonsurgical management. New York: Thieme Medical Publishers; 2014.
12. Akhaddar A. Infective complications. In: Di Rocco C, Turgut M, Jallo G, Martinez-Lage DJF, editors. Complications of CSF shunting in Hydrocephalus. Switzerland: Springer International Publishing; 2015.
13. Cushing H. Concerning the results of operations for brain tumor. JAMA. 1915;64:189–95.
14. Chiang HY, Steelman VM, Pottinger JM, Schlueter AJ, Diekema DJ, Greenlee JD, Howard III MA, Herwaldt LA. Clinical significance of positive cranial bone flap cultures and associated risk of surgical site infection after craniotomies or craniectomies. J Neurosurg. 2011;114 (6):1746–54.
15. Korinek AM, Golmard JL, Elcheick A, Bismuth R, van Effenterre R, Coriat P, Puybasset L. Risk factors for neurological site infections after craniotomy: a critical reappraisal of antibiotic on 4578 patients. Br J Neurosurg. 2005;19(2):155–62.
16. Bratzler DW, Dellinger EP, Olsen KM, Perl TM, Auwaerter PG, Bolon MK, Fish DN, Napolitano LM, Sawyer RG, Slain D, Steinberg JP, Weinstein RA, American Society of Health-System Pharmacists (ASHP); Infectious Diseases Society of America (IDSA); Surgical Infection Society (SIS); Society for Healthcare Epidemiology of America (SHEA). Clinical practice guidelines for antimicrobial prophylaxis in surgery. Surg Infect (Larchmt). 2013;14 (1):73–156. doi:10.1089/sur.2013.9999.
17. Pons VG, Denlinger SL, Guglielmo BJ, Octavio J, Flaherty J, Derish PA, Wilson CB. Ceftizoxime versus vancomycin and gentamicin in neurosurgical prophylaxis: a randomized, prospective, blinded clinical study. Neurosurgery. 1993;33(3):416–22.
18. Gyssens IC. Preventing postoperative infections: current treatment recommendations. Drugs. 1999;57(2):175–85.
19. Whitby M, Johnson BC, Atkinson RL, Stuart G, Brisbane Neurosurgical Infection Group. The comparative efficacy of intravenous cefotaxime and trimethoprim/sulfamethoxazole in preventing infection after neurosurgery: a prospective, randomized study. Br J Neurosurg. 2000;14(1):13–8.
20. Dempsey R, Rapp RP, Young B, Johnston S, Tibbs P. Prophylactic parenteral antibiotics in clean neurosurgical procedures: a review. J Neurosurg. 1988;69(1):52–7.
21. McClelland SIII, Hall WA. Postoperative central nervous system infection: incidence and associated factors in 2,111 neurosurgery cases. Clin Infect Dis. 2007;45(1):55–9.
22. Alves RV, Godoy R. Topical antibiotics and neurosurgery: have we forgotten to study it? Surg Neurol Int. 2010;1:pii: 22. doi:10.4103/2152-7806.64966.
23. Abdullah KG, Attiah MA, Olsen AS, Richardson A, Lucas TH. Reducing surgical site infections following craniotomy: examination of the use of topical vancomycin. J Neurosurg. 2015;19:1–5.

24. Savitz MH, Malis LI, Savitz S. Topical antibiotics in neurosurgery: a re-evaluation of the Malis technique. Br J Neurosurg. 2000;14(1):69–70.
25. Thompson P, Houston S. Decreasing methicillin-resistant Staphylococcus aureus surgical site infections with chlorhexidine and mupirocin. Am J Infect Control. 2013;41(7):629–33. doi:10.1016/j.ajic.2012.09.003.
26. Kallen AJ, Wilson CT, Larson RJ. Perioperative intranasal mupirocin for the prevention of surgical-site infections: systematic review of the literature and meta-analysis. Infect Control Hosp Epidemiol. 2005;26(12):916–22.
27. Rasmussen S, Ohrström JK, Westergaard L, Kosteljanetz M. Post-operative infections of osteoplastic compared with free bone flaps. Br J Neurosurg. 1990;4(6):493–5.
28. Lal S, McCutcheon IE. Infection after craniotomy. In: Hall WA, McCutcheon IE, editors. Infections in neurosurgery. Park Ridge, IL: The American Association of Neurological Surgeons; 2000.
29. Allison RT. Foreign body reactions and an associated histological artefact due to bone wax. Br J Biomed Sci. 1994;51(1):14–7.
30. Gibbs L, Kakis A, Weinstein P, Conte Jr JE. Bone wax as a risk factor for surgical-site infection following neurospinal surgery. Infect Control Hosp Epidemiol. 2004;25(4):346–8.
31. Wellisz T, An YH, Wen X, Kang Q, Hill CM, Armstrong JK. Infection rates and healing using bone wax and a soluble polymer material. Clin Orthop Relat Res. 2008;466(2):481–6. doi:10.1007/s11999-007-0067-5.
32. Magyar CE, Aghaloo TL, Atti E, Tetradis S. Ostene, a new alkylene oxide copolymer bone hemostatic material, does not inhibit bone healing. Neurosurgery. 2008;63(4 Suppl 2):373–8. doi:10.1227/01.NEU.0000316859.03788.44. discussion 378.
33. Wellisz T, Armstrong JK, Cambridge J, Fisher TC. Ostene, a new water-soluble bone hemostasis agent. J Craniofac Surg. 2006;17(3):420–5. doi:10.1227/01.NEU.0000316859.03788.44.
34. Akhaddar A, Boulahroud O, Naama O, Al-Bouzidi A, Boucetta M. Paraspinal textiloma after posterior lumbar surgery: a wolf in sheep's clothing. World Neurosurg. 2012;77(2):375–80. doi:10.1016/j.wneu.2011.07.017.
35. Akhaddar A, Boucetta M. In reply. World Neurosurg. 2014;82(1–2):e384. doi:10.1016/j.wneu.2012.12.022.
36. Jankowitz BT, Kondziolka DS. When the bone flap hits the floor. Neurosurgery. 2006;59(3):585–90.
37. Niazi T, Quinoñes-Hinojosa A, Schmidt MH. Management of brain abscesses associated with halo fixation. Neurosurg Focus. 2008;24(6):E14. doi:10.3171/FOC/2008/24/6/E14.
38. Garfin SR, Botte MJ, Triggs KJ, Nickel VL. Subdural abscess associated with halo-pin traction. J Bone Joint Surg Am. 1988;70(9):1338–40.
39. Uppal HS, Issa F, Byren I, Johnson D. A case of pancalvarial osteomyelitis: diagnosis and management. J Plast Reconstr Aesthet Surg. 2010;63(2):e159–60. doi:10.1016/j.bjps.2009.05.015.
40. Shehu BB, Mahmud MR, Ismail NJ. Neurosurgical infections. Niger J Surg Res. 2006;8(1–2):1–18.
41. Goodrich JT. Cranioplasty. In: Albright AL, Pollack IF, Adelson PD, editors. Principles and practice of pediatric neurosurgery. New York: Thieme Medical Publishers; 2008.
42. Staffenberg DS, Strauch B. Plastic surgery wound coverage for the neurosurgery patient. In: Goodrich JT, Staffenberg DS, editors. Plastic techniques in neurosurgery. 2nd ed. New York: Thieme Medical Publishers; 2004.
43. Phillips K. Osteomyelitis of the skull. J Neurosurg Nurs. 1982;14(5):280–2.
44. Ameh EA, Wammanda RD, Sabiu L. Complications of scalp vein infusion in infants. Trop Doct. 2005;35(1):46–7.
45. Lane JE, Lane JE, Feltes CH, Johnston KW, Stephens JL, Kent DE. Osteomyelitis of the outer calvarial plate after dermatologic surgery: a case report and review of the literature. Dermatol Surg. 2006;32(9):1182–8.

Index

A. Akhaddar, *Cranial Osteomyelitis*, DOI 10.1007/978-3-319-30268-3

T

U

V

W

Z